Yo

'Detailed, heartfelt account of a movement that inspired thousands of people to wake up and shout about the cruelty that was happening in the heart of England ... This is the book about SHAC. This is the book about *us*.'
—Benjamin Zephaniah, poet and activist

'This is a story of compassion and courage that was crushed by the State. It's a powerful testament to the inspirational campaigns of passionate people who stood for justice and a world without suffering.'
—Peter Tatchell, campaigner for human and animal liberation

'A chilling, honest and true story of individuals who came together to stop an atrocity that every decent person should fight to end. A book to open eyes, hearts, and minds, and a riveting tale of real-life daring-do.'
—Ingrid Newkirk, Founder PETA

'We can all learn something from SHAC and this book is a great place to start that journey. Palestine Action Network wouldn't be doing what we do now without them. Buy it, read it, then be inspired to get out and take action!'
—Richard Barnard, Co-Founder Palestine Action Network

'The raw punk rock spirit of the SHAC campaign leaps from the pages of *Your Neighbour Kills Puppies*. This book is a must-read for all contemporary activists. None of us are powerless, and until every cage is emptied, all of us are needed.'
—Moby, musician

'If you care for animals and people who love them, please read this haunting but crucially important story of SHAC.'
—Jilly Cooper, author

'An excellently written account of one of the most well-planned and hard-hitting campaigns ever waged against animal experimentation, and of the vicious lengths that governments will go to in order to protect the vivisection industry.'
—Ronnie Lee, Co-Founder Animal Liberation Front

'The SHAC campaign rocked the world of animal liberation and inspired a new generation of direct action against state-corporate crimes beyond animal rights. Without SHAC's example there would have been no Smash EDO campaign.'

—Ceri Gibbons, Smash EDO

'Victory for SHAC would create a blueprint for pressure campaigns capable of tearing down any injustice. In the sacrifices of SHAC, contemporary social justice campaigns should find both inspiration and warnings for the future.'

—Dale Vince OBE, Founder Ecotricity

'The SHAC Movement offers vital strategic lessons for those building mass nonviolent civil resistance today. The courage and sacrifice these campaigners showed will inspire you to step up, take action and change the world. This history is a must read.'

—Dan Kidby, Co-Founder Animal Rebellion

'This history of SHAC shows how police action against subversion and domestic extremism widened to encompass crimes against corporate profits, even if those profits are made at the expense of animal welfare or the environment. Non-violent protest has a proud tradition of success in this country which we should all cherish.'

—Baroness Jones of Moulsecoomb, House of Lords

'Thank fuck there are some people out there prepared to take the knocks to defend what is right. With the rise of veganism and increasing awareness of animal rights it can't be long before [SHAC] will be proven right in their defence of the defenceless. In an increasingly insane world the only constants are morality, and defending the rights of animals at all costs is part of that.'

—John Robb, journalist, musician and TV pundit

'This is the story of SHAC; a group of people stirred to action by what they witnessed and inspired to make us all aware of it.'

—David Life, Co-Founder Jivamukti Yoga

'As Harris exposes in [*Your Neighbour Kills Puppies*], when big business directs our policing and our wider legal system, it should terrify us all.'

—Neil Woods, former detective sergeant and spycop

'This is the story of SHAC from the non-state side. Essential reading for any activist. Only time will tell the level of infiltration of this group by the state and corporate spies.'

—Lydia Dagostino, Director of Kellys Solicitors, coordinator of non-state lawyers in the Undercover Policing Inquiry

Your Neighbour Kills Puppies

Inside the Animal Liberation Movement

Tom Harris

Foreword by Chris Packham

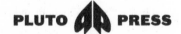
PLUTO PRESS

First published 2024 by Pluto Press
New Wing, Somerset House, Strand, London WC2R 1LA
and Pluto Press, Inc.
1930 Village Center Circle, 3-834, Las Vegas, NV 89134

www.plutobooks.com

British Library Cataloguing in Publication Data
A catalogue record for this book is available from the British Library

ISBN   978 0 7453 4869 8   Paperback
ISBN   978 0 7453 4871 1   PDF
ISBN   978 0 7453 4870 4   EPUB

This book is printed on paper suitable for recycling and made
from fully managed and sustained forest sources. Logging, pulping
and manufacturing processes are expected to conform to the
environmental standards of the country of origin.

Typeset by Stanford DTP Services, Northampton, England

Simultaneously printed in the United Kingdom and United States of
America

Contents

Foreword

Chris Packham

I wish I didn't have to write this Foreword. Not because I'm short of time but because I wish this book, with its horrifying stories of damaged, tortured lives, didn't have to exist. I wish our species could use its conscience to do good, not harm. But wishing is not enough; change needs action, and history tells us that societal reform happens when 25 per cent of the population supports such reform. So, ultimately, this must give us hope.

In 2023, I visited Marcus Decker in Highpoint prison in Suffolk. Terrified for humanity by the science which says fossil fuel extraction must stop now, he and Morgan Trowland scaled the Queen Elizabeth Bridge in east London to hang a banner for Just Stop Oil. Their action stopped traffic for 37 hours. For this, Marcus received a despicably draconian sentence of two years and seven months. A significant chunk of this rational, bright young man's life stolen for peacefully protesting.

Far from being an inalienable right, protest is merely tolerated . . . to a point. When we step off the curb and over the 'lawful' line, the state speaks up to silence our democratic voices. And the consequences can be extreme and violent.

I've always been fuelled by a love for life, all life. I've been fortunate to have spent my life communicating that love while campaigning to make the world a better place for wildlife and the animals we are in closer proximity to. But systemic and institutional exploitation of the planet has exterminated 69 per cent of the world's wildlife since 1970. One-sixth of the UK's monitored species are now in danger of extinction. And, shamefully, despite the monumental scientific shift in our understanding of animal sentience, this hasn't created a paradigm shift in the way we treat non-humans. I know I'm not alone in feeling an enormous weight of guilt for being part of a generation that has failed to get ahead of the curve to deal with these critical and humanity-defining issues.

I grew up in the 1960s under the cloud of a nuclear war. I recall going to bed at night, not knowing if there would be a world to wake up to. Today's youth live with the even greater terror of climate breakdown, orchestrated principally by big oil and animal agriculture. The reckless disdain these industries have for climate science has compelled me to throw my weight behind contemporaries such as Just Stop Oil. Whatever you or I think about their methodologies, their vision and rationale for progress is sound and needs our support.

But it doesn't begin or end with these sorts of existential issues. Animal research is another ugly example of human interaction with nature. It's an archaic branch of science which, by now, should be a dark blemish resigned to history books. With in-vitro and other forms of humane testing, its twenty-first-century relevance to human health is question-able at best. Yet, thousands of wild macaques are stolen from their family groups and bundled into sacks before being transported to sprawling, overcrowded farms. From there, it's a long, miserable journey in cramped, dark cages to the final destination – often a UK laboratory. Fatalities are so normalised that 'deaths in transit' are grimly factored into shipping calculations. These primates share some of our sophisticated mental states, including the capacity to plan, problem-solve, and identify inequity. But despite possessing elements of cognitive function equivalent to young children, these condemned beings are sliced open without pain relief. Have we lost our minds?

Of course, it's not just primates. A sadly diverse assemblage of animal species can be found in research laboratories, from rabbits to cats to horses and deer. But closer to home, as I bed down for the night with my miniature poodles, Sid and Nancy, I'm haunted by the distant howls of dogs in hellholes where, as Tom Harris recounts in the book you are holding, puppies are punched in the face by the 'civilised' species they co-evolved to love and live with. We see the emotions of our canine companions when they are happy, sad, scared, or excited. We smile as we watch them wag in their dreams and marvel as they learn to read us far better, often, than we do them. My dogs quite literally saved my life. And yet, over two thousand beagles are bred in the UK annually for the research industry. It's a painfully short life in small concrete runs or cages, with little stimulation and even less affection. If knowing this doesn't keep us up at night, it should.

We like to view ourselves as a nation of animal lovers. We have comparatively advanced laws aimed at safeguarding domestic animals and wildlife, and we've even begun legally recognising their sentience. Yet, for many animals in laboratories, the level of meaningful protection is pitiful to non-existent. If the Home Office grants a licence, and they usually do, acts of violence towards animals, which would see most of us imprisoned, are legitimised.

From my experience, no one should need to be an activist. But thankfully, some people are simply unable to turn a blind eye to the soulless stare of injustice. Whether it's people like Marcus from JSO trying to slow the climate crisis or Tom and the other brave campaigners of Stop Huntingdon Animal Cruelty who attempted to liberate animals in laboratories. The gentlest, wisest people are often ignored or attacked by those elected to safeguard them. Risking prison, or worse, for trying to shield others from harm, is not a decision anyone takes lightly. These individuals know we cannot allow the narrative to be written by wilful ignorance or vile vested interest.

In *Your Neighbour Kills Puppies*, Tom lays out how the British and American governments responded to the force and influence of the SHAC model. Much of the response was unprecedented, but it did not happen in a vacuum. Just as SHAC were hit with laws to restrict their protests, smears of 'terrorism' or 'extremism', character assassinations, and violent policing, so too are progressive campaigns right now. The tactics developed to end SHAC did not end with SHAC. As leaders fail to keep their side of social contracts to protect civilisation and their inadequate laws laugh in the face of screaming defenceless animals, we must continue to call on our democratic right to shout above the noise. When our leaders respond badly by dialling up the distraction and passing new legislation to attempt to mute us, we must mobilise and follow in SHAC's footsteps.

If we are to win, and we cannot afford not to, we need to learn lessons from the past and draw inspiration from them. This book is essential reading for anyone dreaming of and fighting for a brighter tomorrow.

Ultimately, the world will be destroyed by a lot of good people doing nothing. So, I'll end, before Tom begins, by asking . . . what are you going to do? Please do something.

Chris Packham is a television presenter, writer, photographer, conservationist, animal rights campaigner and filmmaker. As a broadcaster he is a presenter of BBC's BAFTA Award-winning *Springwatch*, *Autumnwatch* and *Winterwatch* series. He also presents notable natural history series such as *Nature's Weirdest Events*, *Inside the Animal Mind* and *Secrets of our Living Planet*.

Preface

In October 2010 I stood alongside my friends in Winchester Crown Court. The hushed chatter from the public gallery above me faded to silence, as time slowed to a crawl and my stomach felt like it might implode. I forced a defiant smile as a British judge sentenced me to four years in prison. One by one he passed similar sentences on my friends. Our crime: coordinating a lawful protest campaign.

The sentence hit me hard, but what hit me harder was standing powerless as those who despised our vision of a more just world dictated a new and distorted narrative to the mainstream media.

Compelled to action by horrifying undercover footage of dogs, non-human primates, rabbits, rats, and countless other species punched, abused, and poisoned, our groundbreaking campaign to close Europe's largest animal testing laboratory (Huntingdon Life Sciences, or HLS) was determined, unapologetic, innovative, and creative.

We were driven by the nightmarish oppression of animals inside laboratories. Our frustration was compounded by the existence of non-animal research models which were consistently ignored through cost-cutting, habit, or indifference.

Tired of pleading for change and ready to force it, the defiant spirit of Stop Huntingdon Animal Cruelty (SHAC) propelled us to victories that have few, if any, comparisons. Our tactics pushed the boundaries of conventional protest and, in doing so, some of the most powerful multinational corporations in the world buckled before us. For fifteen gruelling years, we dominated newspaper headlines, provoked myriad documentaries, featured in novels, and were immortalised in music and pop culture.

Organisations unaffiliated with SHAC, such as the Animal Liberation Front (ALF), waged their own campaigns against HLS. The ALF liberated hundreds of non-human animals from breeders and laboratories, and carried out waves of economic sabotage. These unsolicited actions sometimes accelerated SHAC's momentum, and at other times hindered it. Through it all, the tenacious campaign remained a formidable force in its own right. During its fifteen-year history, SHAC carried out nearly 10,000 protests, far eclipsing the sum of illegal direct actions carried out by others. If at times it seems I have centred the ALF and others, it is because their intentionally attention-grabbing actions frequently impacted the course of the SHAC campaign, as well as the state and media response. With powerful industries being shaken to the core, the British and US governments took a root-and-branch approach to removing the entire campaign from existence.

Amidst hundreds of arrests and prosecutions across the globe, between 2000 and 2020, there were just twelve weeks without an anti-HLS activist in prison; in 2010 over a dozen campaigners languished in jail in the UK alone.

The state intended to send a violent warning and create a climate of fear. By dragging protestors – from teenagers to pensioners – from their beds, locking them in prison for years, and subjecting them to a determined campaign of psychological degradation, they eventually achieved their aim.

The trepidation and trauma which resulted from their scorched-earth approach permeated my research. Tired of their words being twisted or misattributed, most activists would not usually trust a journalist or author with their stories. Many have been so persecuted by their own governments that they are uncertain whether simply discussing decades-old lawful protest activity might somehow invoke an extreme reaction from the authorities. All of the contributors to this text were offered anonymity, and those who chose to speak have read and verified their accounts.

The reason that the state so severely harassed compassionate activists is grounded in the power SHAC wielded at its height. The campaign established a model that had the potential to drive any business out of existence. It was a prototype which threatened to revolutionise the concept of radical protest, and it was an anathema to the entire capitalist system. Even beyond the animal liberation movement, campaigns against the arms trade, logging, fossil fuel industries, and more began effectively emulating the SHAC model. Terrified that the very foundations of global order were at stake, those in power discussed SHAC in fervent tones at the highest levels of Whitehall and Capitol Hill.

Finally, the British and US governments drew a line in the sand; the SHAC campaign could not and would not be allowed to win.

Much like the SHAC campaign itself, crafting this book has been an emotional battlefield. In order to compile a history of SHAC, I spread my research wide. I have conducted over fifty interviews, hired private investigators, lodged dozens of Freedom of Information requests (FOIs), spoken with former spies and the heads of secretive police units, collated and studied scores of magazines and newsletters, trawled newspaper archives, poured over parliamentary records, and watched hours of video footage. Using modern technology, I have retrieved once-redacted data from documents revealing secret meetings between government officials and the pharmaceutical industry. I also reached out to politicians and pharmaceutical executives from the other side of the fence in hopes of securing their stories. Most chose to remain silent.

I offer my gratitude to everyone who played a part in this campaign, and to all those who helped me to preserve a history which has proven more intense, inspiring, and intriguing than any of us could have appreciated. It is a tale of idealistic hope, governmental conspiracy, high action, and heartbreak. Amidst sadness and joy, there is innocence and there is pain, but at its heart is the reason we fought so hard. It was not our voice we wanted heard, but that of the non-human animals who lay scared, tortured, and dying on their cage floors; they never knew the love we held for them or the desperation we had to free them.

I hope this book may act as a seed, for even scorched earth can give birth to new life. Let it serve as inspiration to anyone who questions their own potential to achieve change. This story may not have the happiest of endings, but between 1999 and 2014 a committed group of determined campaigners brought one of the largest industries in the world to its knees and compelled some of the planet's most powerful governments to resort to measures not seen before or since.

Special thanks must go to Nicola Harris, Chas Newkey-Burden, David Castle, James Gorman, Jamie McGhee, and Rolanda Bellairs for their tireless help in editing, funding, and publishing this work. Without the retention of materials and knowledge by Heather Nicholson, Aaron Zellhoefer, Gamal, Sue Hughes, Lee Culley, Lynn Sawyer, Gerrah Selby, Dawn Hurst, and everyone I interviewed, this project would not have been possible. I offer my sincere apologies to anyone whose testimony I missed. There were many people from across the world whom I hoped to interview but could not track down. Their identities and stories sadly remain untold.

For those fighting for justice, be prepared for your own success. Changing the world will never be easy.

PART I

The Genesis: 1996–99

I want, just as much as the Animal Liberation Front, to stop using animals, but it's just a question of when.[1]

– Colin Blakemore, animal researcher

1
Consort Beagles: 1996–97

Every revolution begins with a single act of defiance.

A hooded figure stood atop the roof of Consort Bio Services, protective over the liberated beagle trembling in the crate beside him.

He looked out over the sea of protestors – a surging tide of fury and compassion – and debated how to get the dog into their hands and away from harm. Scanning the formidable rows of police and razor wire, he had no idea that his action would ignite a global rebellion – a rebellion which convinced the *Financial Times* that 'A tiny group of activists is succeeding where Karl Marx, the Baader-Meinhof gang, and the Red Brigades failed.'[2]

* * *

Five months earlier, in December 1996, twenty-eight-year-old animal liberation activist Gregg Avery launched a campaign against the animal research industry. A quiet young man from a middle-class family in Buxton, Gregg singled out Consort Bio Services in Ross-on-Wye near Hereford, which bred and supplied beagle puppies to vivisection laboratories. The UK was a major centre in the international trade of laboratory animals, shipping beagle puppies to researchers all over the world.[3] Gregg had no firm ideas of how he and his friends would close the facility, but they needed to show Consort they meant business:

At first, we protested outside and issued leaflets and so on, and the staff going in laughed at us. But we were very professional; we were there every day from 6:30 am to 6:30 pm. After a while, the staff stopped laughing.[4]

Throughout the early 1990s, animal rights activists waged intense campaigns against the live export of farmed animals from the UK to Europe. The three major ferry operators,[5] and several airlines,[6] buckled to pressure and refused to accept animal transporters on their vessels, forcing the industry to use smaller firms operating out of quaint seaside towns or small airports. Breeders crammed huge, articulated lorries full of desperate, terrified animals and subjected them to torturous twenty-four-hour journeys, without food or drink, to far distant slaughterhouses. Seeing the trucks roll past was too much for Little England, which prided itself on being a 'nation of animal lovers'. Protestors took to the streets in their thousands; the majority middle-class women who had never protested anything before in their lives.[7]

On several occasions, the police warned or arrested live export drivers for putting protestors in danger.[8] The aggression reached a head on 1 February 1995, when a lorry crushed thirty-one-year-old Jill Phipps to death outside Coventry Airport.[9]

In 1996, BSE ('mad cow disease') consumed the British livestock industry, and the EU banned the import of British meat.[10] This temporarily ended live exports from the UK and hundreds of freshly radicalised activists needed a new campaign.

With this surge of energy behind them, a core of Consort campaigners began developing tactics to force the company to its knees. Working tirelessly, often with little food or sleep, they devoted themselves to their cause. Heather Nicholson co-founded the campaign with Gregg. A warm, gentle, and infectiously passionate campaigner, Heather never once doubted that they would succeed:

I remember being interviewed by a local journalist and he said, 'I agree with you, this is an awful place and should close, but you'll never do it.'

I looked him in the eye and said, 'Oh yes we will', and I meant it.

One worker used to come out and taunt us with a beagle in his arms. I remember looking at him and thinking, 'You'll be out of a job soon.' I had never felt so determined in all my life; after years of feeling sad and helpless for the animals, I finally felt we were going to win for them.

Alongside relentless protests, Heather and Gregg devoted hours to researching the ins and outs of the multi-million-pound company, down to every cog in its machine. Heather quickly learned the fate destined for the beagle trapped in the Consort employee's arms:

We followed vans of beagles to see which laboratories they were sending them to. They were sneaking out at three o'clock in the morning to avoid us. It wasn't easy, and many of us tried and failed; we kept losing them. One day I followed them all the way. I nearly lost them twice and it was a three-hour drive, but I did it. I watched them go up the drive to AgrEvo, an agrochemical company.

As soon as I got home, I sat down and cried, and cried, and cried. I hated myself because I let them go up there. I knew where they were going and knew what hell they were going to go through. But what could I do? I hated myself for not rescuing them, but it would have been impossible.

AgrEvo used the dogs to test the toxicity of a weedkiller called iodosulfuron-methyl-sodium. They laced the dogs' food with varying doses of weedkiller and observed as they suffered symptoms including persistent coughing, bloody faeces, watering eyes, blood discharged from the nose, and an inability to walk. Researchers removed the bone marrow from the puppies before killing them and dissecting their organs.[11]

The Consort campaign revealed these disturbing discoveries in their newsletter and on high-street outreach stalls, and their ranks continued to swell. The daily protests developed into all-night vigils, but to be truly effective, the campaigners wanted to make it personal. For Heather, Consort wasn't a faceless business entity, behind which its employees could hide. Those employees were individuals with names and addresses:

> We found out where some workers lived and took the protests to their doorsteps. It was wrong these people could send beagle puppies to live in a barren cage and be tortured to death, and those same people could just go home to their cosy house and forget about what they'd done.
>
> We'd stand outside their homes with banners and megaphones, causing them huge embarrassment. A lot of the local community thought Consort was a boarding kennel, they didn't have a clue. Consort operated secretively, so we made it our mission to drag them into the spotlight and make everybody aware of what they really were. No one wanted a place like that in their town. They became a pariah.

As well as making it personal, the Consort campaign also began secondary targeting against the breeder's customers. If they could dissuade enough companies from buying the dogs then the entire business would become unviable. Any company identified as a Consort customer was subjected to protests of their own.

As the activists increased their pressure, the wider animal liberation movement was experiencing a momentous resurgence. While on remand in prison – charged with leading his own militant campaign against the fur and animal research industries – veteran animal liberation activist Barry Horne began a hunger strike for laboratory animals. It was the first of a series that would eventually cost his life. Refusing to allow incarceration to silence him, he called on the government to 'give a commitment to end its support for the vivisection industry, both financial and moral, within a period of five years'.[12]

The hunger strike lit a fire under the animal liberation movement, and a flurry of direct action swept the country. One of these actions occurred during a protest at Consort in January 1997. It was the largest protest the farm had ever seen, and they hired a new security team to keep protestors at bay. Overconfident in their abilities, security goaded demonstrators at the main entrance; oblivious to the small group of activists sneaking around the back. In broad daylight – and in a matter of minutes – the activists carried ten beagle puppies across the fields to freedom.[13]

As security realised their mistake, the police were scrambled. A helicopter roared across the sky as riot vans scoured the area. The activists and dogs they hunted hid safely under their noses, in the garden shed of a supportive neighbour. However, one of the dogs didn't make it to the immediate safety of the shed. Walking around the side of the farm, a Consort campaigner saw another activist hurtling towards them with an army of police officers and security guards on their heels:

They sprinted towards me, thrust a six-month-old puppy into my hands, and kept running. The police hadn't noticed and continued to pursue the other activist. I instinctively turned and ran as fast as I could. One security guard had noticed and started to follow me, but he deliberately slowed to let me escape. I could see and hear police closing in, so I hid against a wall in an embankment beside the road. Police vans were parked above me, and I could hear them discussing tactics. The police dogs were making so much noise. I prayed the puppy wouldn't bark and give us away. The helicopter hovered overhead, but I was so close to the police above me that it must have thought I was one of them.

I stayed hidden there, protecting and comforting that puppy for over an hour. Eventually one of the cops muttered something, and one by one they left. As the helicopter and the last few police vans peeled away, I took a deep breath and left my hiding place.

I ran through the night, not knowing where I was going, but desperate to get that dog as far away from Consort as possible. As I crossed a road, a car pulled up beside me. My heart sank fearing the police had found me, but it was one of my friends searching for me. The puppy was safe.

Heather and her fellow campaigners were delighted:

It was amazing. The Consort Campaign itself always remained lawful, but we never criticised direct action like that. We did things our way, but it was never our place to tell people how best to help the animals; it was life and death for those beagles. We just wanted them out of there, and I would be the first to cheer when that happened.

As the campaign celebrated the brazen liberation, a significant political shift appeared to be on the horizon for Britain. In 1996, Tony Blair, as leader of the opposition, had signed up to the Plan 2000 pledge to end vivisection.[14] With the 1997 election looming, he produced a pamphlet entitled *New Labour: New Life for Animals*, in which he promised a Royal Commission into the efficacy and ethics of animal testing. Behind the scenes, Tony Blair's representatives met with supporters of hunger-striker Barry Horne giving him confidence that a new future for non-human animals could be on the horizon. Based on their promises, he called off his hunger strike after thirty-five days.

* * *

Since 1979, 24 April has been observed as World Day for Animals in Laboratories, with protests and actions held across the globe.[15] In 1997, World Day was the perfect date to get all eyes on the Consort campaign.

When the big day arrived, the police were prepared. Expecting a sizeable turnout, they stretched rolls of barbed wire around the perimeter. This created a second barrier beyond the razor-capped wall which had already been erected. It was a formidable defence, aimed at deterring any further incursions.

The police's show of force surprised American activist Josh Trenter, who was visiting England:

The premises were completely surrounded by police officers wearing riot gear. Helicopters hovered in the air, probably the largest security presence I had encountered at a demonstration. The police's demeanour was threatening and hostile as we arrived. Dogs could be clearly heard barking within the facility, which incensed the crowd, and there was a definite sense of urgency.

I remember that the protestors and police started clashing almost immediately as we tried to approach Consort, but the police presence was overwhelming and Consort seemed surrounded.

For Gamal, a young activist fresh from environmental protest camps at Manchester Airport, a few hundred armour-clad police officers, rolls of barbed wire, and a fortified wall weren't going stop him:

We were in a field running beside the razor wire. I spotted a friend jump up and grab a low-hanging branch that went over the razor wire. I ran over and followed him.

Once inside, we got to the back of a large stable block, my friend grabbed the gutter with two hands, put his feet up against the wall, and was up on the roof in a matter of seconds. After a couple of failed attempts, I followed him onto the roof.

I ran across and slid down the other side of the building into a courtyard. There was a pen with half a dozen dogs inside, and a small room with a big pile of dog carriers. Next to the pen was a high-pressure hose.

One of the dogs was in the corner of the pen looking terrified. As the others ran out to explore the courtyard, I scooped her up and put her in a carrier. I threw the hose to my friend on the roof, and we hoisted the dog up and away.

We moved to the front of the building as a police helicopter looped around in the sky above us. We expected to see everyone inside the razor wire, but we were in for a surprise. No one else had breached the perimeter, and no one knew we were on the roof. We had no choice. I started shouting, 'Come on!' and waving.

The crowd responded and rushed forward. This act of defiance would inspire a generation of activists and revolutionise a movement. But in that moment, no one was thinking about the future; this was animal liberation in action, and a life was at stake.

Austrian physicist Martin Balluch was in the crowd and ready to act:

It was when all the people in the crowd saw the dog and the two men surrounded by police and razor wire, that protestors showed their true strength of feeling. They tried with all their means to get into the place and to free the men and the dog ... Some protestors broke through the razor wire by dragging a bathtub to the fence, tearing the fence down and putting this tub over it. Within minutes, hundreds of protestors entered the inner area, surrounding the building with the two men and the dog on top.[16]

The crowd piled through the fences. Desperate to do all he could to help the dog, Josh attempted to stall the police:

I surged forward with the crowd and made a semicircle at the base of the wall with our arms linked to keep the police at bay. Once the beagle was on the ground, everyone took off their sweatshirts, and bundled them in their arms to look like they were holding dogs. We ran in different directions trying to obscure from the police who was holding the beagle. The group I was with was surrounded by police who attacked the crowd. I saw the police knock the beagle out of someone's arms. She dropped to the ground, only to be snatched up again by demonstrators who fought their way through the police lines and ran.

As a keen hunt saboteur – used to running for hours across the countryside – Martin seized the moment, and the dog. He sprinted for several miles before things took a turn for the worse:

A police car spotted me and set a dog loose on me. It bit me and was clinging to me till police caught up.

Thirteen protestors piled together on top of me to protect the beagle underneath their bodies. More and more police officers moved in to beat the thirteen away and take the dog. They arrested all of us under suspicion of theft.

On the drive to the police station, I had the beagle dog on my lap while I was handcuffed, which made it impossible to comfort the poor soul in the way she would have needed. The dog was a young female, and pregnant. They drove me to the police station, where they took the dog away by force.[17]

Behind Martin, the protest raged on. The daring rescue attempt empowered the remaining campaigners and infuriated the police. With his friend vanishing into the crowd, police arrested Gamal and loaded him into a minibus with several other activists. The remaining protestors rounded on the vehicle to prevent it leaving, but the police responded with unprecedented force.

Writing for the *Independent*, Michael Ricks reported this as the first-ever use of CS gas during a protest in mainland Britain:

Eyewitnesses claim officers fired the spray without warning above the heads of a crowd trying to stop a van carrying people who had been arrested. One middle-aged woman who suffers from severe arthritis and cancer claims a police officer hit her in the chest with a riot shield and then sprayed the liquid into her throat from a few inches in front of her face. She was among eight people treated by paramedics at the scene ...

Mr Barrett claims his fingers were broken after he was hit by a police baton and that he and his fiancée were sprayed with CS spray. He said: 'I was not doing anything. I was standing by a gate and then the police charged out. I had my hands on the gate and suddenly a policeman whacked me across the knuckles with a baton ... then I felt this tingling and it was as if my eyes were on fire. I had not said anything, and I certainly wasn't threatening anybody.'[18]

As the dust began to settle, Consort and the police appeared unconcerned by negative publicity. Rather than sparing the pregnant beagle and giving her freedom, the police decided to return her to the farm. A Consort employee arrived at the police station, and under police escort dragged the dog back to meet her fate – and that of her unborn pups. The action caused outrage. Later that evening, the farm's owner and three employees received home visits and their property was vandalised.[19]

Home visits were a tactic employed by individuals acting under the banner of groups such as the Animal Liberation Front (ALF). Unlike a home demonstration, home visits were acts of illegal direct action and involved criminal damage to the house or vehicles of the target. By operating outside of the law, the ALF differentiated themselves from lawful protests groups such as the Consort campaign. Outlining the ethos of the ALF, one anonymous activist explained:

The ALF are nobody, and somebody. The ALF is just a person who decides to go and do an action off their own back, something for animals. They're not sent by anybody, they're not an organisation. If you go and do a direct action for an animal, you are the ALF.

In May 1997, the ALF broke into Consort and carried twenty-five beagles to freedom. The beagles were never to be seen again. At least, not by the police or Consort. As it turns out, some rescued dogs were hiding in plain sight. While not involved in the raid, regular Consort protestor Barney Sheldon adopted two:

Consort claimed that such dogs would never be able to live in a home because they had been bred for experimentation, but Murphy and Ted lived good, fulfilled lives.

Initially they feared everything, even just feeling the grass seemed traumatic for them. But they grew confident quickly. I recall when my partner said it was time to try going off-lead. We stood at the top of a grassy bank and I reluctantly let Murphy go. He ran so fast, his mouth in the widest grin I've ever seen on a dog, and his ears were flying like he was about to take off. I watched him run the entire circle of the vast mound and straight back to us. It was such a happy moment; it proved that every second we spent campaigning for these beautiful animals was worth it; their freedom meant everything to them.

During the same month as the Consort liberation, New Labour were elected to power. With the fanfare of their promises for laboratory animals, the movement waited with bated breath for the Royal Commission into animal experiments.

Four months later, no political progress had materialised. Even the director of pro-vivisection lobby group the Research Defence Society (RDS) noted the government's failure to deliver an increase in funding to non-animal research models was a damning indication of 'how much importance it attached to alternatives.'[20]

With New Labour backtracking, the Consort protestors continued their campaign with dogged determination until Consort Bio Services could take no more. In July 1997, they announced their closure.

Liz Stewart from Dorset Animal Rescue convinced the owner of the farm, Charles Gentry, to sell her fifty Consort beagles for £15,000:[21]

The BUAV and Last Chance for Animals put up a lot of the money, but I had to take out a bank loan too. I couldn't bear the thought of them dying in a laboratory. Consort was closing, and Gentry was retiring, so I knew the money wouldn't be used to breed more dogs.

When I collected them, I noticed at the back of the farm a bank of cages, which contained many more dogs. I asked Gentry if I could take those too, but he told me they were going to a cosmetics laboratory in Spain. He hated the idea of selling them to the people who had forced him out of business, and he wanted to make a point of not letting us have them. Eventually though, I convinced him that he would feel better taking our money, and he reluctantly agreed to sell me the other 126 dogs.

The market value of a laboratory beagle was £300, and I had no idea where I could find £40,000. We put out an appeal, and individuals and groups around the country raising thousands almost overnight. Paul and Linda McCartney contributed £8,000, but we were still a little short, so I sold the story to the *Sunday Mirror*, who paid the final £6,000.

Charles Gentry allowed three campaigners to enter Consort to remove the beagles. As they were loaded onto vans, a *Sunday Mirror* reporter took a look around:

We walked down the now empty rows of tiny dog runs, stinking of faeces and fear. It was here the pups spent their early weeks, without love or affection, before being sent off to the vivisection labs.

Stella, one of the few beagles to have a name, walked out slowly on the lead of Liz Stewart. Stella had fifty pups at Consort. All had been snatched from her at an early age. Liz and Stella stopped at the entrance to Consort and laid a bouquet of purple flowers at the roadside.

Several hours later, the rescued dogs were almost unrecognisable as they played together on the grass at an animal centre. The fear and the haunted look in their eyes were gone. They had experienced love for the first time and they were looking forward to the start of the rest of their lives.[22]

For the campaign founders the closure of Consort was just the beginning. Gregg Avery recalls:

There were no big parties ... but it gave us an inkling of what we could achieve.[23]

2
The Battle of Hill Grove: 1997–99

The numbers of protestors will dwindle and fade away.[24]
– Thames Valley Police

With excitement and passion coursing through the movement, Gamal recalls the speed with which the Consort activists
turned on their new target:

It was late on a Friday when Consort announced that they
would close. The owner deliberately waited until the night
before a large protest, knowing that we'd invested a lot of
time and money into the event. However, his last attempt
to frustrate us backfired on the entire vivisection industry
as overnight we transferred the protest to a new target: Hill
Grove. In 1997, most people didn't have mobiles, or even
email, so we organised everything over landlines and word
of mouth.

Diverting hundreds of people from one target to another
in a matter of hours was a remarkable feat, and I'm not sure
it had been done before.

Hill Grove Family Farm was the UK's last commercial
breeder of kittens for vivisection laboratories. It had long been
regarded with horror by the animal liberation movement.
Speaking to a local newspaper, a former employee of the farm
in Minster Lovell, near Witney in Oxfordshire, made it clear
why:

Chris Brown [the farm's owner] is not an animal lover. He didn't seem to care about his cats at all.

A lot of cats were born deformed, and their mothers would eat them. I found several cats dead for no apparent reason.

They used to go mad when he came in; climbing the walls of their cages. Cats were frequently ill and suffered from diarrhoea a lot. We used to report such illnesses to Farmer Brown, and the next day the cats … just disappeared.

I never saw a vet, and I saw no [government] inspectors.[25]

Tragically for the cats, Farmer Brown's facility was just the start of their wretched lives; they were all destined to be blinded, poisoned, cut open, and killed inside laboratories. Farmer Brown offered little reassurance when he asked the *Daily Mail*, 'How do you know they feel pain? … I've seen kittens with electrodes in their heads running about and playing with each other.'[26]

Activist Cynthia O'Neill had spearheaded a local campaign against the farm for six years. She was later joined by Natasha Dallemagne, a young activist with a quick smile and sharp wit. Following their success at Consort, Natasha asked Gregg and Heather to throw their weight behind the Hillgrove campaign.

Though not to the scale of what had come before – or what was to follow – the protest which launched the Hillgrove campaign was lively, loud, and set the tone for a movement on the march. Undeterred by the last-minute venue change, hundreds of activists converged on the conveniently central location of Witney. As half the protestors besieged the farm, the rest marched through the town's streets, highlighting the realities of Brown's farm to his neighbours.

Following the mass mobilisation, the Hillgrove campaign ensured that daily demonstrations, home demos, and all-night vigils became part of the new normal. Using their newsletter, they launched an unequivocal defence of focusing on Hill Grove's employees:

> It must be understood that without [the staff's] compliance, Hill Grove could not function, and these people cannot hide behind the idea that they didn't know where the cats were going.[27]

To our critics we would argue; ask the cats if it's personal.[28]

Hill Grove Farm fell under the jurisdiction of a different police force to Consort, and Thames Valley were clear from the outset that they were not fans of the campaign's tactics. With senior officers dismissing lawful home demos as 'not nice',[29] a police constable assaulted and shoved a twenty-three-year-old protestor outside a Hill Grove employee's house. The homeowner's friend then mowed him down. Eyewitness Craig Stevens witnessed the incident:

> The car reversed over him. When it happened, everything stopped. He looked in a bad way. When the paramedics arrived, they strapped him for fear of spinal injuries. He was unconscious and badly injured round the head.[30]

Despite the severity of the incident, and witnesses claiming it was a deliberate attack, police failed to arrest the driver of the car, or the officer who shoved the protestor behind it. The injured activist made a full recovery and was eventually discharged from hospital, but tensions between protestors and police ran high.

Every fortnight, protestors hosted all-night vigils outside Farmer Brown's house. The vigils were peaceful but made the farmer uncomfortable, and often police outnumbered protestors six to one. On at least one occasion, armed police appeared in a show of force.[31] With protestors making relentless noise outside his house, the police helicopter thundering in the sky above, police lights flashing, and the occasional firework bursting, the protests began to have an impact. Hill Grove Farm decided to fight back.

Multiple activists suddenly and mysteriously became severely ill after standing on the grass verge beside Hill Grove during a protest. Police forensic officers were called in to investigate. They concluded that someone had sprayed the verge with high doses of an organophosphate called dimethoate, a derivation of nerve agents developed during the Second World War.[32] The agents are suspected to be responsible for 'Gulf War Syndrome' which caused chronic fatigue, long-term sickness, diarrhoea, and arthritis in British and North American soldiers returning from the first Gulf War.[33] Amongst those affected by the Hill Grove poisoning was Linda Abrey:

> On the way home I felt very unwell with a sore throat and a tightness in my chest. My husband, Brian, was actually sitting on the verge where there were some yellow marks and when he stood up, he found a hole burnt in his jeans.[34]

Other protestors reported difficulty in breathing, mouth ulcers, diarrhoea, and vomiting. Once again, the police took no further action and accepted at face value Farmer Brown's rebuttal:

> I don't know anything about it. It is a mystery to me. I think there are many of us getting fed up with these people. Some want to take action, but I dare not.[35]

Regardless of whether Farmer Brown dared to act himself, the poisoning attack was not an isolated incident. Hill Grove employee Brian Butler spat on a female protestor and tried to smash her car window; he was convicted and fined.[36] In retaliation, ALF activists broke several windows of his home. The situation escalated fast. Campaign co-founder Cynthia O'Neill had her house windows smashed, and someone attempted to break down her door with a hammer before her son chased them away.[37] Brian Butler was arrested, but later released without charge. The tit-for-tat altercations reached a head when Cynthia reported that someone connected to the farm had stolen her cat.[38] In a separate incident, the son of an Oxford University vivisector 'karate kicked' an activist's car window, smashing the glass just inches from her face.[39]

There was a clear disparity between the massive police effort spent investigating every crime against Hill Grove Family Farm and the minimal resources expended investigating crimes against animal liberation protestors. This did nothing to ease the ever-widening fissure, as policing costs soared towards £500,000.[40] Following an aggressive police response to yet another large-scale protest, Gregg Avery declared:

> The police went intending to teach everyone a lesson, but this kind of treatment makes people see the injustice of it all and far from making them reluctant to come next time, they will come back with twice as many supporters.[41]

Indeed, the numbers on large national protests continued to rise. However, heavy-handed policing also drove more and more activists underground, leading to an increase in direct action. In a clear correlation, every time the police attempted to suppress people's legal right to protest, there was a notable increase in illegal home visits, during which employees saw their cars vandalised and covered with paint stripper. On one such occasion, ALF activists broke the windows at the house of notorious vivisector Professor Colin Blakemore, who had purchased kittens from Hill Grove and stitched their eyelids shut during experiments for the condition 'lazy eye'. He bemoaned to the media he wanted animal testing to end 'just as much as the ALF',[42] though he continued to profit from animal research for at least two more decades.

The Hillgrove campaign refused to publicly condemn or analyse the tactics of others – regardless of how controversial they were. While they did not call for, or encourage, illegal protest actions, they welcomed everyone's contribution towards their aim of closing Hill Grove Farm. Regardless of their personal viewpoints, their newsletter reported all actions, from Rev James Thompson blessing protestors, to Farmer Brown's Range Rover being set on fire.

The inclusive nature of the campaign regularly saw those dubbed the 'granarchists' of the movement marching side by side with teenagers in balaclavas. When ninety-four-year-old Marion Tyrrell handed a 11,000-signature petition calling for the closure of the farm to the District Council, a journalist asked how she felt about more militant activists. She replied, 'I just wish I could join them.'[43]

There was one form of direct action which campaigners like Marion could take part in. Prior to March 1997, there were no anti-harassment laws in the UK. Protest movements often encouraged nuisance phone calls, unwanted mail-order subscriptions and the like, with minimal fear of arrest or reprisal. When the popular Teletubbies dolls sold out one Christmas, free ads appeared offering them at discount prices, listing Farmer Brown's number. Even the passing of the Protection from Harassment Act in 1997 gave no suggestion that it would deter protests of this sort.

Day by day, and week by week, the campaign grew and evolved. The efficacy of home protests was unmistakable – more and more staff decided that such a low-paid job was not worth the hassle and jumped ship in search of better pay, and less drama. Activists took the secondary targeting strategies they'd implemented at Consort and refined them. Farmer Brown found himself banned from his local shop, his B&B adverts blocked from everywhere he tried to place them, and his final side-hustle scuppered as the Caravan Club withdrew his campsite licence.

Desperate to stop the protests, Farmer Brown used the new Protection from Harassment Act and paid around £5,000 to secure a High Court Injunction, effectively buying a ban on protests near his business. It even criminalised activists from advertising protests, in a move which civil rights group Liberty described as an abuse of the law.[44] It was the second such injunction granted in the UK, and the lawyer who secured it admitted to the *Oxford Mail* that its implementation would mean the police having to suppress the right to protest. He later complained that 'The police are trying to keep the peace and allow a peaceful protest. You can't blame them for that. But to do it, they are turning a blind eye to the injunction.'[45]

The police denied they were 'turning a blind eye' to anything. To prove it, they arrested Cynthia O'Neill simply for using a loud hailer outside the farm. She was determined to resist the draconian order:

What the 'powers that be' cannot grasp is that it isn't a game, it is serious, and the nightmare of animals in laboratories is something we all have to live with twenty-four hours a day, every day. So, if they think anyone is going to be put off by this harassment law, they can think again, and this charge will be fought all the way.[46]

As World Day for Animals in Laboratories approached, the police began visiting key activists, including Natasha Dellemagne and Lynn Sawyer, and served them with the injunction. If they breached it, they'd be summonsed to court.

* * *

In January 1997, before the Hillgrove campaign had started, a group of activists inspired by Barry Horne's first hunger strike attempted to liberate fourteen cats from Hill Grove Farm. Amongst them was Tony Gatter:

> During a small protest, a group of us went around the back and got into one of the cat units. We grabbed a dozen cats and got out of there as fast as we could, but the police were waiting. They gave chase as we spread out across fields; there was a helicopter circling the sky above us and they followed us through rivers, woods, wherever we went. We couldn't get away and were cornered one by one. When arrested, we were allowed to keep hold of the cats on our laps as they drove us to the station. We hoped it was a sign that they may allow us to rehome them – we didn't care what happened to us, we just wanted to prevent those cats from ending up in the hell of a laboratory.
>
> When we got to the police station, we begged them to let us keep the cats, but they just laughed and returned them to Hill Grove. The cats were supposed to be 'pathogen free' and having been exposed to the outside world were now of no value to the industry – they didn't care, and took them anyway.
>
> It completely broke my heart, knowing those cats who were in my hands were returned to a place like that.

Now, with World Day 1998 just weeks away, and injunctions being handed out left, right, and centre, all eyes were on the high-profile court case. Of the activists who had been arrested, three were brought before the court: Nicola Maddocks, Kevin Hickey, and Brian Shiel. Following accusations of police officers attempting to 'stitch up' the activists,[47] all three were acquitted of burglary,[48] but not before Farmer Brown had given evidence. Brown openly told the court about mother cats eating their offspring, kittens breaking each other's necks, and others being bitten through the head. Describing him as 'a heavy, suspicious-eyed man with a faintly aggressive smile', the *Independent* observed:

Questioned about his business, by journalists or by lawyers, he tends to answer unhelpfully and, often, inconsistently. He clearly distrusts the outside world – and the outside world distrusts him.[49]

For Farmer Brown, everything he described in court was just another day at the office, but for the supporters of the Hillgrove campaign it was like tinder to a flame. In the preceding year, their mailing list had soared from a few hundred to 4,000, and as their biggest protest approached, not even the organisers could predict how many people would heed their call.

The police braced themselves for something big during the World Day demonstration. They had seen what happened to Consort's temporary fencing the year before and decided to go bigger and better; raising twelve-foot-high walls of metal around the farm. At strategic points, police officers with cameras perched in cages above the fortification, and officers attached a police radio mast to Farmer Brown's chimney to ensure coverage didn't drop out at the rural location.[50] Police established a new unit labelled 'Operation Stile' to find a 'permanent solution' to the protests. The officer in charge of Stile expressed his fears when he stated, 'If the farm closes, the demonstrators will go somewhere else, strengthening their resolve that these kinds of demonstrations work.'[51] He was adamant: the farm could not close, the protestors could not win, and one way or another they had to be removed.

As nearly 2,000 activists converged on Oxfordshire, police stormed coaches and minibuses, filming everyone on board. They snatched masks from the faces of those who tried to avoid being photographed and confiscated any item deemed 'suspicious'. Many of the protestors spent over an hour navigating through police blockades, only to find themselves confronted by the new fence around the farm.[52] The crowd grew larger and more irate. As anger grew, protestors identified undercover police officers and agent provocateurs, whose uniformed colleagues grabbed and ushered them back through police lines.

Predictably, the crowd attempted to storm the barricades to get to the cats, but over 500 riot police blocked the way. Officers wielded shields, batons, and horses to violently and effectively keep the cats in, and the protestors out. The *Sunday Express* reported:

> Violence replaced peaceful protest as a hard core of 300 activists used homemade battering rams to demolish a 12-foot metal fence …
>
> A 63-year-old man was knocked unconscious after he was hit by a police riot shield.
>
> A 32-year-old woman had a heart attack and six others sustained minor injuries.[53]

The media missed the irony of reporting on violent protests when activists were the only ones injured; not a single police officer was hurt.[54] Barney Sheldon witnessed the aftermath of one incident:

I was walking back to our minibus and saw Zab Phipps standing at the side of the road, clutching his hand to his body. I asked if he was okay; said he was, and an ambulance was on its way. It wasn't till later I learned that the end of his finger had been cut off.

Zab had already lost far more than a part of his finger. Just a few years before, the driver of a live export lorry had killed his sister Jill Phipps as she peacefully protested. That attack compelled him to join the movement. Now, at Hill Grove, a police officer threw a stone that struck him on the hand, and he required emergency amputation to save what was left of his digit. Eager to report on the protestors' perceived aggression, the press failed to acknowledge that stones were flying in both directions.

As activists used a five-bar gate to prise open the metal barrier, two sections of the wall swung open, and a horde of mounted police in armour rode out, charging down anyone who didn't leap out of their way. On the other side of the farm, protestors used a telegraph pole to lever open another gap in the fence, but a rain of blows from shields and truncheons drove the protestors back. In another location, activists tunnelled under the fence, but police officers rebuffed them, following orders to 'prevent the alleged aim of the protesters, the liberation of the cats'.[55]

Described by activists and journalists alike as reminiscent of a medieval siege,[56] the battle waged on, but it had become clear to those protesting that their voices would not be heard.

As their desperation rose, so too did their anger. Protestor Anne Edwards, declared to reporters:

> This is the largest event we have had here – they breed these cats for torture. People must realise the pain they suffer.
>
> This barbaric farm will be shut by public pressure, by peaceful means or any we can muster.[57]

A cry went up. Activists had found a weakness. While the breeding centre was impregnable, the wall around Brown's house was unguarded, and large rocks littered the freshly ploughed fields. Over the next two hours, protestors bombarded the house with anything they could get their hands on. Holes appeared in the roof, and the holes grew until there was more air than tiles. Eighty panes of glass were smashed,[58] leaving curtains torn and billowing out of empty frames. For the protestors who unleashed their fury, it seemed too good to be true. The police simply let them do it. One eyewitness observed with suspicion that 'the mounted police sat on their horses in a line for some time, just watching and doing nothing'.[59] Farmer Brown's wife Katherine echoed the sentiment, complaining that she 'wondered what the police were doing'.[60]

Eventually, the police gave one last push, and the battle of Hill Grove was over. The metal wall remained mostly intact. The cattery was untouched, and the cats remained locked inside. Farmer Brown's house, however, resembled something from a war zone.

As the dust settled, protestors began to question the unguarded house, the plain clothes agent provocateurs, the phalanx of police evidence gatherers with video cameras, and the photographing of every single protestor as they had arrived. For many it seemed that Operation Stile had laid and baited their trap, and more than a few activists had fallen into it. In the weeks that followed, Thames Valley Police carried out scores of early morning raids. Kicking down activists' doors while they slept and dragging them from their beds, the police arrested dozens of people. Most found themselves facing the courts – and in many cases prison – for their part in the disorder.

If the police aimed to stop the campaign by shock and awe, they failed. The Hillgrove campaign stuck to its message, and while its organisers hadn't carried out or facilitated the criminal damage, they maintained their refusal to criticise those who did. When questioned by the press, Heather acknowledged:

> I wouldn't encourage anyone to break the law, but I fully understand the pain and anger people are feeling. They've written to their MPs, they've petitioned the Home Office, they've been laughed at by Brown's workers ... and they've had to listen to Brown saying on TV that he's an animal-lover. At the end of the day, I've no sympathy if someone's roof gets broken.[61]

The police grew increasingly frustrated at the protestors' determination and power. Officers detained forty-nine activists at roadblocks on their way to the next national protest. They arrested and questioned them over hypothetical future offences which had neither been planned nor threatened.

If the police were getting more serious, so too were the Hillgrove campaign. In 1998, most grassroots campaigning groups didn't use computers. Gamal fundraised for an Apple Mac computer, and together with Gregg and Heather, put together the first newsletter with a full-colour cover. It featured two of four kittens rescued in an impromptu grab-and-run during a protest at the farm. From that point on, they designed all the campaign's literature on a computer and printed it in colour. This professional approach made the Hillgrove campaign stand out and appeal to a far wider audience. Outside the office, campaigners continued to search for new and inventive ways to close the cat farm as well.

Having cauterised Farmer Brown's income from his guest house and campsite, they selected a new secondary target which marked the start of a truly national campaign. Par Air was an Essex-based company which shipped animals between laboratories and breeders, including Hill Grove. Campaigners in Essex were quick to take notice, and regular protests began.

Back at the farm itself, an activist parked her car outside the front gates as the workers were about to leave, and D-locked her head to the steering wheel to trap the employees inside. She, along with two accomplices who deflated the car tyres, was promptly arrested and removed.

Others outside of the animal liberation movement were also trying to save the Hill Grove cats. Former farm employee Allie Moore confessed to the *Oxford Mail* that she had rescued her favourite cat 'Buddy' from the farm and had lost her job as a result. She suggested that over the years, employees had covertly removed and rehomed 'hundreds' of cats.[62]

It wasn't just cats being removed from the farm; in May 1998 the Hillgrove campaign acquired a bundle of breeding records. They passed the documents on to the *Daily Mirror*, which reported the tragic story of young kittens being sold to laboratories:

Many were born deformed and were destroyed. Others are listed as 'eaten', 'disappeared' or 'squashed'. One in ten cats die or are killed by their mother before they can be reared and sold.

A 90g kitten was sent to [a] university … when he was five weeks old … they were blinded in one eye, anaesthetised and put in a head frame while their brain was injected with dye. They were then destroyed and the brain dissected.

Maureen Hutchinson, veterinary adviser for the Cat Action Trust, said: 'It is not normal for kittens to be eaten by their mother. This is stress related. Life as a breeding cat in such sterile conditions could make a cat quite psychotic.'[63]

When pushed on the fate of the kittens he sold, Brown responded brusquely, 'When you buy a car, no-one asks where you're going to drive it.'[64]

With the campaign benefiting from Farmer Brown's adverse publicity, Thames Valley Police and Operation Stile were keen to ensure their presence was not forgotten. After arresting thirty-nine protestors – including a ten-year-old boy – during a protest in May 1998, they took drastic action to prevent the next protest march.

Home Secretary Jack Straw had a second home in Brown's village and attended the same church. Mr Straw approved an exclusion zone which stretched for a 5-mile radius around the farm. This kept protestors – and disruption – away from his own house too.

The *Independent* observed battle lines being drawn:

The animal rights community is resolved that, whatever it takes, Christopher Brown's cat-breeding establishment must be closed. The Government is resolved that, whatever it takes, he must be allowed to keep it open.[65]

By pushing a large protest away from the small towns of Minster Lovell and Witney, Jack Straw unintentionally ensured much wider disruption. The march was moved to Oxford, and the unexpected protest brought the entire city to a standstill. A jubilant Heather Nicholson told the gathered media:

> It has been a good day. It just shows you, when the police try to stop us going to Witney, the anger comes out somewhere else. It can't be stopped. They would have been better off letting us march.[66]

Following the protest, a local newspaper reported that 95 per cent of their readership supported the closure of Hill Grove. A 200,000-signature petition calling for the farm's demise was handed to the Home Office. In Parliament, over a hundred MPs signed an Early Day Motion calling for a ban on the breeding of cats for vivisection,[67] and the local council pressured the police to justify spending over £1 million on protecting a single business from protests.[68] Realising their mistake – both in terms of publicity for the campaign, and the disruption caused to a major city – Thames Valley Police allowed protests to return to the farm.

Across the country secondary targeting was in full swing. Activists frequently protested outside Par Air in Essex, and other groups had mobilised too. Regular demonstrations occured across the UK, against customers including Pfizer, Merial, and the Universities of Bristol, Oxford, Cardiff, and Glasgow. The campaign newsletter declared:

> The campaign aims to widen the net until all who deal with Hill Grove Farm fall fully under the spotlight, until the lesson is learnt that if you deal with Hill Grove Farm, you will be targeted. Dealing with a place that sells kittens from days old is an ugly business, and those who do will be exposed.[69]

These secondary targets were subjected to a diverse range of tactics including road blockades, run-ins, pickets, and vigils, in what would become a blueprint for the future of the movement. Finding himself outflanked, Farmer Brown admitted to the *Independent*:

Financially it's been a disaster, devastating. We're existing, not living. And you can only withstand so much. I just wish I could see a future.[70]

Oxford city centre hosted further protest marches, and campaigners climbed to the top of the city's famous Carfax Tower, padlocked the doors, and draped an enormous banner down the side. To spread their message further, the campaign purchased adverts in *The Big Issue*. The Hillgrove campaign phone lines had to be manned twenty-four hours a day to cope with the influx of support.

By the start of 1999, the campaign mailing list totalled 8,000. A second petition, backed by the cast of the musical *Cats*, was handed in at the Home Office, containing a further 150,000 signatures.[71] Farmer Brown was beginning to crack.

He suggested to a newspaper that he would consider closing his farm if he received £200,000 in compensation – twice the retail value of the cats he held in captivity.[72] Despite policing costs spiralling towards £3 million, the government and police were resolute that the campaign could not succeed, and ignored the offer. After Consort, they feared the closure of Hill Grove could cause an entire chain of dominoes to fall.

The campaign itself simply could not afford £200,000, and lambasted the offer as 'emotional blackmail'.[73]

The Hillgrove campaign remained eager to exploit the cracks, and extended their list of secondary protest targets. That list now included Home Secretary Jack Straw, and other

Home Office staff who defended the farm.[74] With Brown wavering, the police doubled down. During a protest near the farm, a police horse rode down a young mother named Debbie Hillier, breaking her leg and damaging her kidneys. When she attempted to speak to the media from hospital, the police barred her from making phone calls and sealed off her ward to everyone except her husband.[75]

With the police and government desperate to keep the farm open, and Farmer Brown on the ropes, frustration mounted on all sides. As police investigated who had chopped down Hill Grove's telegraph poles, they were alerted to allegations of a far more serious incident. Farmer Brown's wife Katherine, whose parents founded Hill Grove, claimed she had been assaulted while out walking. In a statement to the police, she claimed she had been shackled to a fence with a bag over her head. The police found no evidence, and no arrests were made. A local officer privately told campaigners that he believed it had been staged.

Having endured a campaign which had seen over 350 activists arrested and twenty-one people sent to prison,[76] Farmer Brown reached his tipping point.

On 9 August 1999, the campaign received the phone call they had been waiting for. An RSPCA volunteer revealed they were on standby to accept 800 cats. The only facility in the country with that kind of capacity was Hill Grove.

In the middle-of-the-night, the RSPCA collected the Hill Grove cats in a convoy of sixteen vans and took them away for rehoming. The entire movement watched in delight as national television news broadcast footage of the vehicles leaving the facility, and images of the cats adorned the morning's front pages.[77]

And just like that, it was over. Hill Grove Family Farm was closed.

Inspired by the success at Hill Grove, activists launched similar grassroots campaigns against vivisection breeders Shamrock Monkey Farm and Newchurch Guinea Pig Farm. Shamrock closed in a few short months, and the organisers switched their attention to Regal Rabbits, who shut after just twelve days. Newchurch campaigners faced a far tougher fight; it would take six gruelling years of protest and direct action before they could claim success.

With the blueprint being replicated against new targets across the UK, Heather, Gregg, and Natasha set their sights on a bigger prize. Their victory newsletter carried a very clear message:

We know for a fact that similar places to Hill Grove are shaking in their shoes, wondering if they are next. You will find out soon enough where that place is. We hope you want to be part of a third victory however long it takes. The animals don't have a single day to lose. They are dying now.[78]

PART II

The Battleground: 1989–99

The ferocity of the battle, its unexpected twists and turns, and the devastation of the company's finances were all underestimated at the outset.[1]

– Christopher Cliffe, HLS executive

3

Where Blood Runs Cold: 1989–97

I've seen hell, and it's called Huntingdon Life Sciences.
> – Michele Rokke, undercover investigator

Petrified beagles cowered in terror at the back of their cages as Sarah Kite reached in to grab them. Their pleading eyes implored her to show mercy, their legs pushed out in front of them in hopeless resistance. The dogs shook with fear as one by one she lifted them out and carried them towards her co-worker, Andrew Mash. He seized them roughly and clamped their small bodies between his legs, cranking their heads backwards to force a long gavage tube down their throats. Mash administered three and a half syringes of an experimental plaque remover directly into their stomachs before the dogs were returned to their barren cages.

Leaving Room 20 at Huntingdon Research Centre (HRC) in Cambridgeshire, UK, Sarah wiped a tear from her eye and tried to steady her trembling hands. During her coffee break, she snuck into another room, where dogs had been shaved and their skin deliberately cut. Sarah's colleagues had smeared a trial psoriasis cream into the wounds and covered them in surgical plasters. When she crept into the room, most of the cages were empty; the dogs had been taken away and killed.

It was the final straw. On 16 September 1989, seven years before the start of the Consort campaign, she walked out of the gates of HRC for the last time. Staff turnover at HRC was high, but unlike those who had walked out before, Sarah was not seeking less traumatic employment. She had been carrying out another job all along, as an undercover investigator for the British Union for the Abolition of Vivisection (BUAV).

Sarah spent two months compiling a dossier of evidence. Based on diaries and photographs she had collated over eight months inside the laboratory, she handed her report to *Today* newspaper, who splashed it across their frontpage. Animal research companies were, and remain, amongst the most secretive and impenetrable facilities in the UK. The newspaper revealed an exclusive glimpse behind locked doors and razor wire fences to a readership who had seen little like it before.

Suddenly, HRC's sinister slogan, 'Your secrets are our secrets', became painfully disingenuous. Their secrets were out.

Today journalists visited the home of HRC director David Anslow. Anslow threw a dustpan and brush at them as he attempted to incite his docile labrador to attack.[2] The following day, the newspaper ran a second multi-page spread on the horrors uncovered inside the HRC 'torture labs'.[3]

More and more media joined the fray, with television, newspaper, and radio interviews revealing the gruesome details to a mass audience. HRC remained conspicuously silent.

On 26 November 1990, less than a week after the story broke, over 150 people gathered outside the laboratory to call for its closure. Sarah joined the protest:

> The company had been exposed for what it was, and now everyone knew of the suffering that it was responsible for. I had fulfilled my promise to the animals, yet it was with great sadness that I thought of all those animals that were still imprisoned in their cages, being pumped with noxious substances, unaware of the outcry that their suffering had caused.[4]

Following the protest, the BUAV organised a public meeting packed with over 100 concerned members of the public in Huntingdon town centre. Several attendees united in agreement to close HRC and formed Huntingdon Animal Concern (HAC).

HAC's first protest marked the end of an experiment exposed by Sarah. Protestors gathered outside the laboratory, each wearing a beagle mask and holding a number: one for every dog used in the test. Inside the laboratory, the animals were taken from their cages and, in the words of HRC, 'sacrificed'. For an entire year, the beagles had been force-fed varying doses of dimethoate, the same toxin which would later poison protestors outside Hill Grove Cat Farm.

The demonstration received widespread publicity and prompted HAC to organise a funeral service outside HRC for a second group of dogs condemned to death. As well as these attention-grabbing stunts, campaigners hosted regular demonstrations, greeting employees on their way to or from work. Protestors tied purple ribbons to the fences and left crosses in memory of the animals killed.

HRC was in a rural location, with no public transport connection. For staff members without cars, Duncan's Coaches supplied private buses to pick up HRC employees from local estates. It was a vital service, as the low-paid jobs at HRC meant that for many, cars were an unaffordable luxury. Lee Culley from HAC decided to strike:

If HRC's staff couldn't get to work, they couldn't kill animals. We waited by the Duncan's bus stop on a nearby estate, and as the bus pulled up, I dived underneath and chained myself to it. My friend got on the bus, posing as an HRC employee, and alerted the driver. No one had mobile phones back then, so my friend offered to go to the nearest shop to call the police. The driver waited patiently beside me, with a coach load of HRC employees becoming increasingly frustrated at not being able to get to work. The driver got suspicious when my friend failed to return after two hours, but a police patrol car happened by. I unchained myself as the cop spoke to the coach driver and ran through a bush to get away.

As local campaigners used civil disobedience to pressure HRC and Duncan's, others chose a far more direct approach. On 28 October 1990, seven years before his first hunger strike, Barry Horne sat in a van less than a mile from HRC. His heart must have sunk when a police car pulled in behind him, though they were unaware of his plot; they were on the lookout for youths who had been throwing fireworks. Barry assured them he had seen nothing.

The police were preparing to leave when they spotted a stolen car, containing four men in overalls, parked nearby. As the men leapt from the vehicle and made for the fields, the police discovered 10 gallons of petrol and a pile of incendiary devices – intended to destroy Duncan's fleet of coaches as they lay unguarded overnight.[5] The police made chase, apprehending and arresting Barry Horne and Gary Allen. Both were sentenced to three years in prison for attempted arson.

Above-ground and underground activism continued for many years, but as the decade wore on, the intensity and momentum slowed. By 1997 – seven years after Sarah Kite's investigation – actions had become sporadic. Thanks to a young journalist named Zoe Broughton, that was all about to change.

Following in Sarah Kite's footsteps, Zoe carried her favourite beagle puppy down the same narrow corridor, trying to suppress her grief. The only notable difference since Sarah had walked through this building was that the Huntingdon

Research Centre had rebranded as Huntingdon Life Sciences (HLS).

The preceding weekend had been torturous for Zoe, and this final walk was the culmination of one of the hardest decisions of her life. For fifty-seven days, she had been aware of the bulky battery equipment strapped to her body, constantly waiting for one of her colleagues to notice it and ask questions she didn't have answers to. But as she slowly lowered the dog into one of the 'Death Row' cages, it was the last thing on her mind.

The conflict she wrestled with was a lose–lose situation. She could attempt to smuggle her favourite dog to freedom, perhaps saving their life, or she could place them in the cage, finish her job, and potentially save thousands more.[6]

Zoe turned her back on the dog and left the room. At the end of her shift, she walked out of the gate for the final time and wrote the last entry into her journal, later printed in the *Guardian* under the title 'Where blood runs cold':

> I wanted to say goodbye and pet the dogs, but I've found it so hard loving those about to be put down that I kept my distance at the end. I don't think anybody suspects me. I have followed the whole process with my puppies, from the settling-in weeks, through experiments to the post-mortem. As I was leaving, they told me my chores for the next morning – nobody knew I would not be there, but in the editing suite, assembling the evidence of their cruelty.[7]

* * *

In March 1997, before Hill Grove, and with the Consort campaign in full swing, most British television sets had just four channels, the internet was in its infancy, and Netflix hadn't yet posted out their first rental DVD. As a result, at 9 o'clock on a Wednesday evening, millions of families gathered eagerly in their living rooms to watch a new series: *Countryside Undercover* on Channel 4.

As the premiere episode, 'It's a Dog's Life', aired, Europe's largest animal testing laboratory faced the stark realisation that their former animal technician Zoe was an investigative journalist.

The footage shocked the nation. Zoe showed workers punching eight-week-old beagle puppies in the face, shaking dogs, and throwing them against the wall. She had evidence that staff were falsifying scientific data and poisoning dogs, all caught on camera in a document of institutional violence and abuse.[8]

There was outrage. A local resident claimed neighbours accosted the employee filmed punching a puppy, stating, 'About ten people gave him what he'd done to the dog.'[9]

After reviewing over twenty hours of unaired footage, interviewing former and serving staff members, and scrutinising the company's own records, Home Office minister George Howarth conceded there had been 'shortcomings relating to the care, treatment, and handling of animals'.[10]

For the first time in British history, two animal technicians were arrested and prosecuted, and HLS had their licence to experiment on animals temporarily revoked. The staff members, Robert Waters and Andrew Mash, pleaded guilty to 'cruelly terrifying' animals, were fined £250, and ordered to do sixty hours of community service.[11]

Despite hours of damning footage, mass public outrage, and a government investigation resulting in unprecedented sanctions, HLS' Chief Executive Christopher Cliffe struggled to comprehend what his staff had done wrong. He complained to a local paper, 'I don't understand why they pleaded guilty.'[12]

Unlike Christopher Cliffe, HLS' customers could see the growing storm, and hurried to cancel contracts with the laboratory. Revenue plummeted by 30 per cent over the following year, driving HLS to the brink of bankruptcy. In a fruitless charm offensive, the company spent over £1 million on advisers' fees, marketing, and management changes.[13]

Unknown to HLS, as Zoe Broughton gathered evidence in their UK lab, over in the USA, animal rights group PETA had been running a simultaneous investigation inside HLS' New Jersey laboratory. As investigator Michele Rokke recalls, two HLS' facilities being investigated at the same time was entirely serendipitous:

I had a list of a dozen CROs [Contract Research Organisations]. I put out applications at some of the places and while driving around the area, I passed a sign that said Huntingdon Life Sciences. I thought, 'That sure sounds like a biomedical research facility.' I went in and applied for a job.

I was asked if I understood that no animals leave the lab alive, and then I was given a tour of the facility. I remember seeing a beagle being held down on a cart in the hallway. His tail was wagging, but it abruptly stopped when the workers did something to him – I couldn't see what.

Incredibly, I got the job. I ended up working at HLS as an entry-level technician in the cardiovascular unit for about nine months. That was a unit that did experimental surgeries on the animals. I mostly cleaned the cages and held animals for dosing and saw them get sick, and suffer, and die.

Going undercover in the mid-1990s was a risky affair. As with Zoe, the video camera's battery pack was bulky and hard to conceal in a close-proximity environment. Even the camera she used for still photography put her in danger; when the roll of film finished, the camera made a loud whirring sound, forcing her to dive into an empty room or make enough noise to cover the sound. Nonetheless, by writing detailed notes, taking photos, and filming as much as she dared, Michele amassed a catalogue of evidence – evidence which proved beyond a shadow of a doubt that the behaviour Zoe Broughton exposed in the Cambridgeshire laboratory was endemic:

I've watched chickens ripped apart after weeks of suffering in factory farms, pregnant mares strapped to hard rubber urine bags to produce Premarin, miserable 'purebred' dogs locked in tiny cages in filthy puppy mills, and countless animals being hit, kicked, stabbed, and choked. But nothing prepared me for what I saw at Huntingdon Life Sciences.

In addition to cleaning their cages, I held the animals down for dosing with all sorts of toxic substances. I scrubbed blood from the floor after unnecessary surgeries were performed by inept, poorly trained employees. When chemicals were pumped into the animals – into their noses, mouths, skin, veins, stomachs, and lungs – I recorded the effects and worried about their misery while others shrugged and walked away.

When I saw Zoe Broughton's report, 'It's a Dog's Life', I shook my head in amazement at the mirror image of what we've both seen. Falsified records, dosing errors, blatant animal cruelty, and a lack of regard for animal welfare. The careless attitude of HLS technicians as they handle animals and perform tests that are of no use to human beings is truly and thoroughly sickening.

One day, after Zoe's exposé broke, I was pushed up against the wall and felt up by a male technician who made a joke of saying, 'For all we know you could be taping things.'

He pinned me against the wall and groped me all over as if feeling for a recording device. Luckily, I wasn't wearing the equipment that day. The supervisors at that time didn't say, 'Don't ever, ever, ever do any of these things,' they said essentially, 'Don't get caught doing these things.'[14]

When PETA went public and released a nine-minute excerpt of Michele's video footage, the United States Department of Agriculture (USDA) slapped HLS with a $50,000 fine.[15] However, the laboratory took legal action against PETA. HLS failed to get the $10 million in damages they sought, but were awarded a strict gagging order.[16]

The order meant only the nine minutes of footage already released could be used by PETA, or anyone else. However, alongside Michele's diary, the horrors revealed in those nine minutes were enough to spark widespread condemnation. Her diary documented a catalogue of abuse:

The terrible insensitivity and disconnectedness of the workers, the administration, and the 'scientists' is what always gets me. Animals are victims of inept techniques, cruel treatment, and tests that are designed to garner a desired result. I remember one technician violently shaking a very, very sick dehydrated beagle. That dog had been one of many who had had a series of tubes surgically implanted to deliver the test substance. The dogs were so sick from whatever was being put into them, you could hear them dry heaving and retching from way down the hall. The tech took hold of two handfuls of that dog's skin and slammed him through the air to unkink the tubing sewn in under his skin, so that it would deliver the test substance into his otherwise healthy body. It was so violent and unnecessary that another technician, who was not any nicer to the animals, couldn't help but say the tech's name and give him a dirty look. And that was all she did. She was a peer to him. It didn't stop him. He didn't act ashamed. He wasn't reprimanded. He wasn't disciplined. That's just the way the animals were treated. The animals were just in the way of people getting their work done so they could go home. It is like the animals weren't allowed to have any sentience – they weren't allowed to be living, breathing, perceptive beings – they were a test tube who annoyed the technicians because they did react to pain and make messes, and they did get sick and resist having painful, awful things done to them.

The disregard for life and science was so commonplace that HLS staff devised a 'Platinum Club' for technicians who made a fatal mistake, such as misusing a nasal gastric tube. The tube is meant to be fed through the animal's nose and into the stomach, so a test substance can be administered. However, technicians often accidentally inserted the tube into the windpipe and delivered the substance into the lung. When a 'lung shot' happened, the animal dropped dead, and the technician joined the Platinum Club.

As she filmed a litany of horrors, including a young monkey being slit open without anaesthesia from the groin to the throat as their hand clenched against the unimaginable pain, Michele came to a horrifying conclusion:

Contract research organisations [CROs] exist for one single purpose; to get their customers' products approved for sale on the market. It's irrelevant whether the product is safe; the customer has invested a small fortune in it, and are paying the CRO to tick whatever boxes are needed to satisfy the regulators. They will use any number of tricks to ensure that happens; if they don't, then they will lose that client forever.

A career vivisector told me data from animal research is easily manipulated, and that the industry relies on that susceptibility to meet goals and metrics.

No one knows how any substance will affect a human until a human uses it, no matter how many other animals have suffered and died to get it to market. The animals in those laboratories do not differ from the dog or cat one has at home. They are lovely, sentient beings who feel pain and terror at the hands of sadistic and narcissistic entry-level employees.

While PETA were prohibited from campaigning against HLS, actress Kim Basinger resolved to help. Michele Rokke had revealed the intended fate of thirty-six beagles due to be mutilated on behalf of the Japanese pharmaceutical company Yamanouchi. HLS planned to saw into each dog's leg before wrapping a steel wire around the bone and pulling until it snapped in half.[17] They had dosed the dogs with a trial osteoporosis drug, intending to see whether the drug affected bone healing.

Days before the experiment was due to commence, Kim wrote to Yamanouchi, pleading:

I beg you to cancel this cruel experiment immediately. I will personally adopt each and every one of the animals now held in small barren metal cages in your contract laboratory.[18]

Amidst an international barrage of outrage and horror, Yamanouchi suspended the tests and held an inquiry to determine a more humane testing method. Two weeks later, the pharmaceutical giant agreed to hand the beagles over to Kim, who headed straight to HLS' New Jersey laboratory to collect them.

As she held a press conference on their front lawn, HLS released a statement declaring that the dogs belonged to them, not Yamanouchi, and they would not be handing them over. Kim Basinger declared she would do 'anything it takes' to secure their freedom.[19]

Under increasing pressure, HLS grudgingly caved and handed the dogs over to rescue centres. The director of one of those shelters told the press, 'We want them to have a good life, to be a family member, to be loved.'[20]

4

Huntingdon Death Sciences:
1997–99

In 1997, an organised international assault almost succeeded in the company's destruction.[21]

– Christopher Cliffe, HLS executive

In the dead of night, Gamal patrolled HLS' perimeter. He stopped for a moment and shook the fence, setting off the motion sensor alarms within the security hut, before resuming his patrol. A moment later, he shook the fence again. A security officer sauntered towards Gamal, slinging insults at the young activist through the razor wire. Gamal muttered back, 'I'll be coming in later', as he stalked back the way he had come.

It was the first night of Camp Rena. In response to Zoe Broughton's *Countryside Undercover* documentary, Huntingdon Animal Concern (HAC) established a small settlement in front of HLS' flagship laboratory in Cambridgeshire. Launching a new group, Huntingdon Death Sciences (HDSC), they intended to maintain a constant presence outside the laboratory, and Gamal was determined that his warning would not be empty. He scouted the small camp for a piece of carpet, or thick fabric, which he could throw over the razor wire fence to protect himself from the lacerating spikes:

I had absolutely no plan. I just wanted to get onto the roof and occupy it for as long as I was able. I wanted to let HLS know that we were on their doorstep, and that we were coming for the animals.

I found some heavy material to drape over the top and was up and over the fence in seconds. The first building I came to had a metal rail beside it, which I could stand on to reach the roof.

I got onto the huge metal chimneys and stayed there for about an hour until the police arrived. I tried to climb higher, but two cops grabbed my legs, pulling me down. I refused to leave, so they called the fire brigade, who tied me to a stretcher and carried me down. A few days later the fire brigade came to the camp and apologised. They promised they would never intervene again.

Manchester activist Max Watson became a regular at Camp Rena. Inspired by Gamal, Max concocted a plan. During Barry Horne's second hunger strike, the national Animal Rights Coalition (ARC) hosted a meeting at Camp Rena. With hundreds of fresh faces showing up, Max seized the moment to call attention to the campaign and the plight of his close friend Barry:

My mate and I hid in a ditch while a protest kicked off at the front. We waited for our moment, took the chance, and ran for it, climbing up the narrow gap I'd found in the fencing, and squeezed between the razor wire.

I jumped down and ran for the nearest building. I got up onto the first low roof and looked over my shoulder. My friend was right behind me, but another friend – Brendan – had spotted us and decided to join in.

The rooftops were all joined and seemed to go on forever, higher and higher. Eventually we got as high as we could get and saw the protest by the gate. We shouted down and could see a whole new dynamic to the demonstration.

We intended to stay for as long as we could, to raise as much publicity as possible. In solidarity with Barry, we refused to eat for as long as we were up there.

We persuaded the police to give us two blankets, which they brought up in a cherry picker while they worked out what to do. As it got colder, we all lay on one of the blankets and huddled together with the other one on top of us. It was lovely and warm during the day, but at night it was horrifically cold. We sunbathed and slept during the day, and just huddled and suffered at night. We found a bit of rubber, which we used to mark a draughts board on the roof and used moss and stones as playing pieces, which helped pass the time.

After a couple of days, Brendan wanted to get down; he had joined us on the spur of the moment without knowing we intended to stay up there indefinitely and hadn't prepared for it mentally. We convinced the police to swap him for a much-needed bottle of water.

After three freezing nights, no food, and little water, we were told there had been national media coverage, so we agreed to come down. As soon as I got in the police car, I came over really ill due to dehydration, hunger, and exhaustion.

Max, Brendan Mee, and Nicholas Newbury were taken to court over their action, which the prosecution insisted 'went beyond the right to protest'.[22] They claimed that by moving about to keep warm, the three men had caused damage, including rusting, melting plastic around heat ducts, and decades of natural weathering. The magistrates called the trial to a halt and dismissed all charges.

No charges were brought against an HLS employee who drove their car into activists, resulting in a protestor being hospitalised. A Cambridgeshire Police superintendent casually labelled the incident 'accidental'; in the same breath, he lambasted an impromptu, but thoroughly peaceful, sit-down protest to support Max and his friends as 'unlawful'.[23] Police arrested several of the sit-down protestors while the driver continued their journey home unchallenged.

Greta, a Camp Rena stalwart, witnessed the daily changes at HLS:

HLS were under siege, and as the siege mentality set in, the effects of a 24/7 presence became clear. Slowly and surely, and at ever-increasing cost, they blocked themselves in. Each day saw a fresh roll of razor wire around the perimeter, fences added within, and more security guards put on patrol. Staff spotted inside hurried through the shadows with their heads hung low.

The night brought no respite to those under siege. As the staff left the animals to suffer, the activists moved under the cover of darkness – huge holes appeared in the fences, razor wire was squashed down, and alarm wires cut.

HLS applied to the High Court to evict the camp. Bailiffs were ordered to clear the site – but campers were ready to resist. Veteran campaigner John Curtin told the press, 'We won't be going easily. We look forward to the eviction.'[24] And he meant it.

Several activists had cut their teeth at protest camps against the expansion of Manchester Airport, where they dug tunnels and built defences to prevent the construction of a second runway. HDSC also liaised with campaigners from the

Newbury bypass occupations and environmental direct action group Earth First!

According to John, the police remained wilfully ignorant of their plans:

> When we prepared for the eviction, we weren't subtle. We built defences and dug tunnels. When the police asked, we told them we were digging a toilet. They would laugh and go back to what they were doing. They knew exactly what we were up to, and they didn't care. We had a huge safe delivered on the back of a truck, and we told them it was for our valuables. They didn't believe us for a second, but they let us unload it, anyway.
>
> One of our tunnels was taking a while to get ready, and we needed more time. Luckily, we found a problem with the way HLS had applied for the eviction and a magistrate delayed the eviction for nearly a month. It gave us all the time we needed to get ourselves prepared.

They erected structures for the camp's defenders to lock on to, both above and below ground. The pièce de résistance was the industrial safe, which they buried in the ground and encased in concrete. From the outside, only the steel door was visible, acting as a fortified hatch into the ground. Beneath the surface, they had removed one side of the safe, which led to a hidden passage, ten-foot long. In places, the tunnel was almost tall enough to crouch in. Should it become necessary, a person could just about fit into the safe itself – if they curled into a tight enough ball. For Greta, who volunteered to barricade herself inside, it was a reassuring backup if the tunnel collapsed.

In the early hours of 30 September 1997, two veteran activists, Pat and Sue, finished their stint on lookout duty and drifted off into a much-needed sleep. Unfortunately for the campers, the replacement shift also struggled to stay awake. Sue Hughes can't remember what woke her, but as she opened her eyes, a formidable sight greeted her:

> An army of police officers in riot gear marched towards us. There were 130 officers involved in the eviction, and it looked as though they were all marching up the road at once. Pat and I jumped out of our car where we had been sleeping and ran towards the camp screaming and shouting.
>
> We didn't have time to run to the entrance of the camp; we just threw ourselves through the bushes, telling everyone that the moment had finally come.

The campers scrambled to their stations. They chained themselves to metal bars embedded into the ground, padlocked themselves up trees, and attached themselves to one another.[25] Perhaps counterintuitively, as Greta climbed into the safe, she felt protected by the steel and earth walls around her:

> As the bailiffs, cherry-pickers, tunnellers, and riot police made their way down Woolley Road, the war cries of protestors greeted them. It was the last thing I saw or heard as the safe door closed.
>
> My thoughts weren't focused on my own plight, but that of the animals across the way, and everything they were going through. My isolation and deprivation gave me no insight into what they must suffer, and that was the very thought that chilled me to the bone and filled me with a burning fury.[26]

Two other activists locked themselves to concrete tubes and lay across the entrance to the safe. From within her tunnel Greta made daily reports to local broadcaster Anglia News via telephone, and was interviewed by *Cambridge News*:

> The only detail I can release is that it is extremely unsafe. There is a high risk that I might be killed. It's a dangerous place to mess with. I'm hoping they will leave me here to peacefully make my protest.
>
> If I have to risk death, then that is what I will do.[27]

HLS had no intention of leaving her there. They employed professional cavers, bailiffs, and a team of specialists. Oxygen was pumped into the tunnel, as police and bailiffs struggled to work out how to free her from 'an incredibly dangerous situation'.[28] Over the course of three long days, they dug cautiously around the safe and attempted to pick or cut through the locking mechanism. In fact, the lock didn't function. Instead, the safe was secured from the inside by a deadbolt which Greta could open at any point if she wished. The bailiffs spent three days – and over £200,000 – on a complex, delicate, and risky digging operation. Finally, they reached Greta:

> As I emerged, the first thing to hit me was the destruction of the land the camp had been on; the area had been obliterated. The second was a question from the press asking what I thought about the announcement, a few hours prior, that the Home Office had granted HLS a new certificate to continue animal experiments. I was numb, but not surprised.[29]

As police dragged Greta from her tunnel, HLS' temporary licence suspension had been lifted, and they were free to resume testing commercial products on animals for the first time since Zoe Broughton's investigstion. The protestors strengthened their resolve; if HLS wouldn't stop, then neither would they.

While the police had been arresting Greta and eight other campaigners,[30] Pat and Sue snuck around to a patch of land behind HLS and taped off a new campsite.

At a cost of more than £250,000, HLS had successfully moved the protest camp from their front gates to their back fence.[31] The landowner of the new site was unknown, and HLS had no grounds to request the camp's eviction. Both sides hurried to determine the owner in a bid to buy the land. HLS narrowly won the race and purchased the land. Having caused HLS this extra expense, the protestors moved on willingly.

HLS sought an injunction to end the daily protests. However, HLS' Chief Executive, Christopher Cliffe, had no idea exactly who to name on it:

It is very difficult to pin responsibility on anyone. What is clear is that these demonstrations and activities are organised to a greater or lesser degree.[32]

The proposed order would have stopped all protests by groups including the British Union for the Abolition of Vivisection (BUAV), including publishing factual articles about the laboratory. Justice Eady, the High Court judge hearing the case, removed the BUAV from the order and noted his concerns over how the Act was being interpreted. *The Big Issue* described it as 'a blow to firms which expected to restrict the powers of legitimate protest groups'.[33] However, orders against HDSC activists John Curtin and Max Watson were granted.

Campaigners set up a third encampment, 'Camp for Justice', on land donated by a local supporter. Protestors marched from the camp along the busy A1 dual carriageway to HLS, staging a sit-down protest which caused diversions and tail-backs lasting several hours.[34]

While HLS' management threatened to sue *Channel 4 News* if they covered protests against them,[35] their security guards took a more hands-on approach. During one incident in June 1998, they grabbed a young protestor and threw her into the road. She was rushed to hospital for treatment.[36] The security guard was subsequently arrested and cautioned.

* * *

In 1995, HLS had begun a bold expansion strategy. Borrowing £19 million from NatWest Bank, they purchased facilities in Occold in the UK, and New Jersey in North America.[37] The exodus of customers following Michele Rokke and Zoe Broughton's exposés devastated HLS' finances, and should have curtailed HLS' plans for growth.[38]

However, Christopher Cliffe pushed forward regardless. In 1997, he purchased a new laboratory in Wilmslow, Cheshire, from one of HLS' competitors. He borrowed an extra £1 million from NatWest to make a down payment on the £5 million facility.[39] To pay the balance, he agreed a two-year payment plan, deferred for a year.[40]

Max and his local group now had an HLS facility right on their doorstep. Branding themselves Huntingdon Action Group (HAG), activists from Manchester and Liverpool subjected the Wilmslow site to the full gamut of protest tactics. With regular run-ins, marches of over a thousand people, and another protest camp, HLS' bright new opportunity was just as besieged as their flagship in Cambridgeshire.

At one protest, police sprayed campaigners at point-blank range with CS gas.[41] Several activists were arrested and banned from protesting at all HLS sites. In response, HAG activists launched demonstrations against NatWest, demanding that they recall their loan. Kate Jones was a regular:

For our first NatWest protest, we went into the Manchester branch. We photocopied bank notes splatted with red paint and joined the queue. We told the cashiers, 'We want to bank this blood money,' and then we sat on the counters. A giant rabbit came in, with someone on a megaphone, and a protest started outside. The bank was evacuated and closed for the day.

When we did the same in St Helens, black shutters suddenly dropped down in front of the counters. Within seconds we could hear sirens coming down the street. Armed police charged in and bundled us to the floor. The giant rabbit and the person with the megaphone were arrested for breach of the peace. They were held overnight and released the next day. It didn't put us off though!

The internet was not as big back then, and there was no social media, so being on the high street was vital. The public were horrified that their bank continued to finance HLS after the Channel 4 documentary. People would march into the bank, close their accounts, come out, and snap their bank cards up in front of us. It was amazing; it made us emotional and motivated us so much.

Alongside the NatWest campaign, HAC activist Rob White helped devise a new strategy:

We drew inspiration from the campaign against mining company Rio Tinto, which had caused the deaths of over 10,000 civilians in Papua New Guinea. They had begun protesting the company's shareholders, and it was proving very effective.

We obtained HLS' shareholder lists from Companies House, which revealed their corporate shareholders, as well as the small but significant individual holdings.

As a bonus scheme, HLS awarded all their employees shares. Their home addresses were listed in the paperwork, and home demonstrations surged as a result. The shareholder list also named companies such as Co-operative Insurance Services (CIS). As part of the Co-op brand – which included banks and grocery stores – CIS provided a plethora of high-street protest targets.[42] Despite a rigorous ethical policy, they proved reluctant to concede to a pressure campaign which included regular demonstrations, rooftop occupations, and publicity stunts.[43]

As the financial campaign escalated, HLS' second-largest shareholder, Robert Fleming Holdings, divested from the laboratory. HLS' share price plummeted by 50 per cent overnight.[44] With losses spiralling out of control, thirty employees at the Wilmslow facility were handed redundancy notices.[45] A month later, HLS made the closure of the laboratory public just a year after it had been purchased, before HLS had made a single repayment on it. HLS were now saddled with an empty laboratory which they owed nearly £4 million on, as well as loan repayments – and interest – from the £1 million down payment. The building lay abandoned for over a year before HLS sold it at a loss to a property developer.[46] In total, the Wilmslow fiasco lost HLS over £3 million.[47]

HLS also intended to build an in-house dog breeding facility at their Occold site.[48] Ipswich Animal Rights (IAR) raised fierce opposition and the local council vetoed the plans.[49] The government, who had only just returned HLS' licence, overruled the council decision. IAR continued their protests until building work was postponed, and later scrapped.[50]

More bad news faced HLS when ALF activists snuck into Duncan's Coaches' yard. They commandeered double-decker buses and drove them into the coaches used to transport HLS staff, causing £15,000 of damage. The action convinced Duncan's, and every other coach company in the region, to refuse their services to the beleaguered laboratory.[51]

In 1998, HLS moved their Annual General Meeting (AGM) to Boston, USA, to avoid protests. Activists discovered that a single share allowed them access to HLS' financial documents within the facility itself. At mere pennies per share, they bought 200 and opened a 'share shop' outside HLS' Occold laboratory. Armed with their shares, two campaigners flew to the USA to make their case in person, while the rest attempted to walk into HLS. Breaching their own articles of association, HLS only allowed five inside – the others were arrested for breaching the peace.[52]

HLS' real shareholders had endured enough. They demanded an Emergency General Meeting (EGM) in London. With a £250,000 golden handshake, they gave Christopher Cliffe his marching orders and brought in a new team to revive HLS.[53]

Accountant Andrew Baker had been working for HLS' competitors and service providers since the 1970s. In 1997, as financial disaster rocked HLS, Andrew Baker formed an investment group called Focused Healthcare Partners (FHP) which invested in up-and-coming companies connected to the vivisection industry.[54]

While HLS was no start-up, a successful recovery had the potential to make someone very wealthy. Andrew Baker saw an unmissable opportunity. FHP orchestrated an investment package, creating 177 million new HLS shares for FHP's customers, immediately netting HLS over £20 million. Anticipating a sharp rise in the company's share price, FHP bought 11 million of the new shares themselves. HLS' existing shareholders eagerly approved the investment, and allowed Andrew Baker to effectively buy himself his position as HLS' new CEO.[55]

Andrew Baker brought with him Brian Cass, another former accountant who had been the corporate vice president for HLS' rival Covance.[56] Cass became the new managing director, and the face of the company.

* * *

In 1999, the National Institute of Clinical Excellence (NICE) decided not to approve a new Glaxo Wellcome flu drug for NHS prescription. Glaxo's chief executive, Jean-Pierre Garnier, warned Tony Blair that it could 'not be taken for granted that the UK would remain an attractive location for pharmaceutical research and development (R&D)'.[57] Fearful of losing British research jobs – and the financial benefits his government reaped from them – Tony Blair set up the Pharmaceutical Industry Competitiveness Task Force (PICTF), comprising pharmaceutical executives and government ministers. PICTF met regularly and reported to the prime minister on the steps needed to appease the pharmaceutical industry.[58] As protests against HLS intensified, these meetings took on increasing significance.

While Tony Blair succumbed to corporate blackmail, Huntingdon Animal Concern founder Joan Court received a note through her letterbox. The note was signed by the Animal Liberation Front and reported an action they had taken against HLS' beagle suppliers, Harlan Interfauna.

To avoid razor wire and a ten-foot alarmed fence, the ALF constructed a scaffold frame to bridge the fortifications. The plan worked perfectly, and they liberated seventy-one beagles. One activist dubbed it a 'textbook' ALF raid:

A few of us got onto the roof and straight away we could hear the pups yapping. It gave us a big kick. As soon as we heard them, there was no way we would leave empty-handed. Time for the trusty old crowbar. We used it to make a little hole, and then we ripped big bits of the roof off with our bare hands.

I looked through the hole and saw two of the most beautiful big eyes looking back up at me, probably wondering why some nutter in a balaclava and a grin was shining a torch at her. As I jumped down into her pen, she went crazy, jumping up at me and squealing with excitement.

There was no time for fussing her, that would come later. She went straight into the sack my partner was holding and was lifted through the roof into the safe hands of another friend. She went along the chain of people, over the fence and into the field ... There were four pens with roughly fifteen pups in each, aged four to six months old, and one pen with older dogs in it – about eighteen months old. Whereas the puppies had all been jumping up yapping and pissing themselves through excitement, these older dogs were cowering in the corners, pissing themselves through fear.

It was gutting, absolutely heart-breaking, to see an animal so scared. They were terrified of human beings. Within an hour we had bagged up and passed out down the chain seventy-one beagles, and what was once a packed, noisy puppy unit was now eerily silent, and best of all, empty.

Now was the hardest part of all; a ten-minute run ferrying the dogs to the vehicles. We hoisted a sack over each shoulder and legged it. After two minutes everyone was knackered but running on adrenalin. All the time running back and forth across the fields I kept expecting to hear an alarm going off, or the guard to come out, or the police to turn up, but luck was on our side and nothing happened.[59]

As ALF activists waited beside the road with the liberated beagles, a fleet of cars pulled up. One by one they loaded the dogs into the vehicles. The cars sped off in different directions to freedom.

At another Harlan facility, BUAV investigator Jane East-wood witnessed dogs eating new-born pups, tearing off each other's ears, biting to the bone, and being forced to eat their own faeces. Any slight deformity resulted in a dog being declared a 'non-conforming product' and killed. Technicians killed roughly 300 dogs per year simply because breeding out-paced demand.[60] Several dogs were sent to HLS to be used in genital mutilation experiments for Viagra. As she went public with her evidence, Jane admitted:

> If I had known before how horrific it would be, I don't think I could have done it. I don't think the memories will ever leave me.[61]

Following the BUAV exposés and the ALF raid, Home Sec-retary Jack Straw launched an investigation of his own, before declaring that he was going to ban puppy farms which sup-plied animal research establishments. This move would save about 6,300 dogs per year. A statement from the Home Office clarified that he wasn't just going to end the trade in labora-tory beagles – he aimed to stop experiments on them entirely:

> If laboratories cannot legally obtain dogs within the UK, then the experiments will cease.[62]

For campaigners who hoped their expectations in the New Labour government were finally being realised, relief was short-lived. The Home Secretary abruptly U-turned on his promise, declaring that animal researchers were 'decent people doing legitimate jobs'.[63]

The seventy-one beagle puppies rescued by the ALF lived out their natural lives as beloved companion animals, knowing safety and security. For HLS, a very different fate was in store.

PART III

The Beginning: 1999–2001

To animal rights sympathisers, SHAC – the most successful group of its kind in the world – has become a beacon of hope, an organisation that is seen to get results.[1]

– Guardian

5
The Birth of SHAC: 1999–2000

This was the beginning of a campaign that essentially says, 'I am going to grab hold of your air hose and squeeze it until you die.'[2]

– Richard Michaelson, HLS' director

I peered out from behind a dumpster. The coast was clear. I zipped a camouflaged chem-suit over my school uniform and rolled a two-hole balaclava over my face.

I was sixteen years old and preparing to carry out my first-ever action in the name of animal liberation. I didn't know any other activists, but I had seen newspaper articles and magazines. I had no idea how to rescue animals from a laboratory, but there was something I could do to help.

Striding towards my local NatWest, I began pasting anti-vivisection posters to their windows.

Unconcerned by my ludicrous outfit, two older ladies ambled over to see what I was up to. When I told them, they tutted and shook their heads. I prepared to defend my actions but instead, they shouted furiously into the bank, directing their disgust at animal testing towards everyone working inside. As I headed back to school, their impromptu protest echoed down the road behind me.

It was a tiny, almost insignificant, action by a teenager in a small town, but similar actions – and far more besides – were taking place daily across the country. Something exciting was happening, and I was part of it.

* * *

As I took my first small steps into the animal liberation movement, HLS were floundering. Their share price had plummeted
from £1.13[3] to just 17p,[4] and their debt to NatWest ballooned
to £24.5 million.[5] For Andrew Baker and Brian Cass, the two
accountants running HLS, dreams of a golden future were
fading fast.

The founders of the Hillgrove campaign, Heather, Gregg,
and Natasha, had taken a brief pause. They needed to pay off
debts and recoup the losses from running a campaign which
printed and distributed over half a million free leaflets, hired
coaches, and posted newsletters to up to 10,000 people at a
time. Then there were the stickers, fact sheets, megaphones,
petrol, phone bills, and myriad other costs of running a full-
time campaign.

But now they were back, and ready for the biggest fight of
their lives. They'd launched what would become the largest
grassroots animal rights campaign the world had ever seen.

HDSC had been inventive, passionate, and dedicated – but it
was missing the surgical focus many felt was required to finish
the job. The Hill Grove veterans joined with HDSC, and in
November 1999 launched a new campaign: Stop Huntingdon
Animal Cruelty (SHAC). In a public statement, they outlined
their intentions:

> HLS has been exposed by three undercover investigations.
> Each investigation told the same story; routine, vicious
> abuse of the animals, and routine breaches of the Animals
> (Scientific Procedures) Act 1986.
>
> Surprise, surprise, after each investigation the animals are
> still suffering violence and torture at the hands of HLS staff.

Nothing changes for laboratory animals until we step in and force a change by closing these places down.

Together we can end the nightmare of the animals imprisoned at HLS. They live their lives in fear, not knowing they have any friends.

But we are here for them, we will fight for them with all our strength, and we will win.[6]

SHAC's reach and relentless targeting hit NatWest with a surge of pressure. Local animal rights groups across the country mobilised and united for the cause, replicating the stunts HAG devised in Liverpool and Manchester. They subjected branches of NatWest all over the UK to protests, occupations, and varying levels of civil disobedience and direct action.

Like the campaigns which preceded it, SHAC toed a delicate line between publicising ALF actions taken against HLS and encouraging them. Buoyed by their repeated success, the nascent SHAC campaign exuded a naive hubris and occasionally strayed across that line. The second *SHAC Newsletter* reported:

The week before Christmas in London, over eighty NatWest cash machines were 'disabled' in one night. It would appear that people have been getting hold of supermarket loyalty cards, such as the Tesco Clubcard, covering them with superglue and pushing them into the slot on the cash machines, rendering the machine out of action. It is thought the activists covered their faces with a hat and scarf to avoid being filmed on the hidden cameras which some cash machines contain.[7]

They didn't know it, but that issue of the newsletter would later prove to be a step too far for SHAC's founders. In the meantime, Gregg, Natasha, and Heather focused on how to take on, and take out, a multinational company. They needed to render HLS uninvestable to prevent another bank taking over the NatWest loan.

Gregg infiltrated the City of London, Britain's financial heartland:

HLS is in the middle of nowhere; we could go there and shout at people, but they just don't care. We decided most of the damage could be done from hundreds of miles away if we did our homework.

Reuters provided a service called Citywatch, which offered information on shareholders. I posed as a potential customer – the service cost £200 a month – and asked what information they could give me. I said I might be interested in investing in Huntingdon Life Sciences and asked for an example of the information they could provide. I was emailed a list of the main HLS shareholders, and we got a big shock. Not only were we shown who the nominees were – big investment bankers like Phillips and Drew – but also the beneficiaries, the people they were investing for, usually big pension funds. They included the Labour Party pension fund, and those of Camden Council, Hammersmith and Fulham Council, Rolls-Royce, and Rover.[8]

It turned out the Labour Party had bought 55,000 shares after the 1997 documentary about HLS aired. Gregg Avery bitterly commented to journalists, 'No wonder their license wasn't revoked.'[9] Shadow Home Secretary Ann Widdecombe echoed the sentiment, declaring that Labour's talk on non-human animal welfare reforms was nothing more than 'hollow rhetoric':

This is hypocrisy of the worst kind. In opposition, Labour talked tough on outlawing vivisection. Now we discover that Labour are alleged to have used money from their superannuation fund to buy shares in a condemned vivisection laboratory.[10]

The mainstream press felt the same way, and after a few embarrassing headlines, Labour sold their shares. With protests, phone blockades, and letter-writing campaigns introduced across the country, other shareholders followed suit. Rover, Hammersmith Council, and others dumped their shares in HLS almost immediately.

SHAC's first major scalp was Philips and Drew Fund Management, one of the world's largest fund managers. Just two months after SHAC formed, Phillips and Drew ditched their entire portfolio of HLS stock for 1p per share, costing themselves millions.[11]

The sudden and dramatic dispersal of corporate shareholders spurred on the campaign. Activists watched HLS' market value plummet from a height of £330 million in 1990, to just £23 million in 2000.[12]

With companies flocking to divest in HLS, the campaign switched its focus to private shareholders. They sent every shareholder a letter explaining the cruelty the repeated undercover exposés had revealed. It urged them to sell their shares within two weeks, before the launch of a 'campaign tour'. Despite Cambridgeshire Police acknowledging the letters and proposed tour were entirely lawful, they arrested the letter's writer for 1,700 counts of blackmail. After seven hours in a police cell, he was released without charge.

Over 250 investors contacted the campaign to inform them that collectively they had sold nearly a million shares, wiping a further 40 per cent from HLS' share price. The laboratory called on the government to keep shareholder details secret, and wrote to their remaining investors, begging them not to sell.

Encouraged by a media response they described as 'hysterical', the campaign tour went ahead. The first shareholder subjected to a twenty-four-hour protest home demonstration was retired businessman David Braybrook, who owned 22,000 shares. While unquestionably irritated by the demonstration outside his home, he appeared more concerned about the journalists and camera crews, who easily outnumbered the activists. As reporter after reporter knocked on his door, he finally snapped, 'I'm more pissed off with all the media than with the protesters.'[13]

Thanks to the international news coverage, by the end of the protest HLS' share price had plummeted to just 1.5p. David Braybrook's holding was worth £300 less than it had been at the start of the day.[14]

The tactic drew the attention of other campaign groups. Tony Juniper, director of Friends of the Earth, observed:

The City is an important bastion, a source of enormous power that campaigners and activists have not been able to influence very much. But it's just sitting there. Most people have a stake in the City through their pension or insurance funds. But it's not the City's money, it's ours. This sort of protest turns faceless people into individuals.[15]

Pushed for his opinion by the *Guardian* newspaper, Green Party peer Sir Jonathon Porritt added:

The City has argued for years that all they are doing is investing other people's money, that they are just middlemen. That whole illusion is eroding fast. People don't like their names in lights. I suspect that the sort of protests against Huntingdon, the personalising of the protest, will become much more common. The animal rights campaigners are drawing on a huge hinterland of support.[16]

Driven by Gregg's remarkable understanding of the financial world, SHAC seemed unstoppable. As Steve Boggan from the *Guardian* later observed:

To talk to the man at the centre of the process is sometimes uncomfortable. But to do so is to wander through the mind of the protester of the future.[17]

The *Independent* newspaper went further, exploring the possibilities of SHAC's fresh approach:

The situation at Huntingdon is very unpleasant, and not just for the animals. But the surprising thing is that it is not familiar forms of intimidation which are crippling Huntingdon. Rather, it is a new strategy employed by the activists – which focuses on company finances – that may yet close it.

Huntingdon is the largest company to be targeted by animal rights activists so far. It is also the first to be listed on the London Stock Exchange – and it is this that has opened up a new world of possibilities to the Stop Huntingdon Animal Cruelty campaign. SHAC, which distances itself from the most extreme behaviour of its supporters, is now waging a concerted financial offensive, not just against Huntingdon but the financial institutions necessary to its survival.[18]

The situation was indeed unpleasant for HLS – but for some of the animals due to be experimented on, it became demonstrably less so. During night-time raids the ALF liberated 400 rats and 64 guinea pigs from two of HLS' animal suppliers in Essex and Sussex. An activist involved in the action against one of the facilities recalls how they carried out the operation:

> Harlan's Firgrove Farm looked a lot like a chicken farm, with long rows of low wooden buildings. We skirted around the side to avoid any security on the front doors. Halfway along the side of the unit was a small wooden door, which we popped open, and stepped inside.
>
> Suddenly, alarms started wailing across the whole site. It should have been terrifying, but one of my friends appeared behind me and informed us all that there was no staff on-site, and that we were miles from anywhere. We had all the time we needed.
>
> When I stepped into the shed, I immediately presumed we were in the wrong place, as I had been expecting to see pens full of guinea pigs, Instead, there were rows and rows of shelving. Each shelf was packed with plastic boxes, and it quickly became apparent that these boxes each contained several guinea pigs.
>
> We each grabbed a box and calmly walked back to our vehicles, before driving off into the night, without seeing a single member of staff or any sign of the police. The sixty-four guinea pigs were all placed in loving homes, where they got to live out their natural lives in comfort, rather than being tortured to death in some bizarre experiment. Firgrove closed a few years later.

* * *

By March 2000, HLS were in serious financial trouble. Desperate to raise an additional £75 million,[19] they called an Emergency General Meeting (EGM) in New York.[20]

SHAC sent four campaigners to the USA, where they met with a group of American activists-come-shareholders in order to disrupt the EGM. Heather was one of the four:

I stepped into the building, and the security all had guns. I was terrified. In the UK you might get beaten or arrested, but you weren't likely to get shot. The guy presenting the EGM knew exactly who we were, and started by saying, 'Okay, I hope we'll all be civilised now.'

We asked a lot of awkward questions and clarified that even in the USA they could not escape SHAC. It was worth it for that. I wish I had said more, but … they had guns.

While we were out there, we did a load of other protests too, including one at the Bank of New York, a major HLS shareholder. I walked into the building, dressed in a suit, hoping to find somebody important. I entered a room with a security guard and some staff, who were chatting about SHAC. One of them turned and said, 'Can I help you?' So I replied, 'Sure, I'm SHAC.' They were completely panic-stricken, but I only wanted to give them an information pack.

Unfortunately for HLS, their articles of association still allowed shareholders to access their Huntingdon and Occold offices. Despite risking civil action from campaigners, HLS and the police began escorting known activists off their premises. In response, protestors blocked the gates at Huntingdon while demanding access and trapping workers in the car park. Other activists with megaphones scaled trees overlooking the fence. One campaigner climbed between the two rolls of razor wire which surrounded the complex, forcing the police to cut through it to remove her.

HLS had installed the extra razor wire in the run-up to the first major SHAC protest at HLS in December 1999. Despite HLS spending thousands of pounds installing new fences, cameras, and the spiked barricades, police issued a Section 14 order at the last minute, essentially banning any protest outside the laboratory. SHAC re-routed the demonstration to Huntingdon town centre. Hundreds of protestors filled the town, forcing the local NatWest to shut, holding a sit-down protest on the ring road, and protesting at the homes of HLS employees.

Following this and the shambolic EGM, police were keen to take the bite out of the next national protest, especially as World Day for Animals in Laboratories had a history of civil disobedience. Unlike at Consort or Hill Grove, SHAC now had a website to publicise their actions. Nobody could predict what impact that would have on the turnout or nature of the protest.

In what many saw as a deliberate attempt to disrupt the organisation of World Day, police arrested Gregg Avery during a routine picket outside HLS. They accused him of shouting at an HLS executive, 'We've got your car number. We missed you last night. The police don't want to protect scum like you.' Charged with breaching the Public Order Act, he was sentenced to four months in prison.[21] It was a blow for the campaign, but activists had a point to prove: SHAC was never about one person or personality.

With Gregg unavailable – and perhaps hoping that without him things may be a little less coordinated – the police allowed the campaign to host World Day outside HLS. Gamal was one of those who stepped forward to organise:

We asked the campaign to put out a message to everyone that it would be a day to remember the dead, and that people should wear black clothes and skull masks. We thought this theatrical element would make everyone look the same and keep people's identities hidden.

What we intended was to get as many people inside the laboratory as possible. The police laid down two simple rules: don't go into HLS and don't block the main road. We accepted the challenge.

Richard England Snr, a paramedic whose family were all passionate animal rights campaigners, made portable frames from the stakes used for estate agent signs. Campaign posters were attached to both sides, leaving a narrow void between them which was just wide enough to securely – but discretely – hide sets of bolt cutters.

Getting inside HLS would be no mean feat, as the laboratory had gone all-out to secure itself. Besides their already extensive protections, two soaring parallel fences topped with razor wire now surrounded the site. Behind them stood a freshly dug water-filled moat. Nonetheless, protestors like Gamal were eager to try:

We planned to march along one side of HLS and, once we were around the top corner, rip the signs open and cut the fence. We'd devised a simple signal using fireworks. Once the fireworks went off, we were to start chopping.

What we hadn't anticipated was other people bringing fireworks. We'd only just started walking along the perimeter when fireworks went off. Too soon! I ran up to the end of the fence along the back edge and started cutting, as did at least five other groups. With each group cutting several holes in the space of minutes, the next job was to herd people inside. This worked well, and we soon had a few hundred people inside the HLS perimeter.

Lynn Sawyer, a midwife and long-time activist, was one of those who got inside. Taking advantage of the confusion, she – along with Tony Gatter – made it a little further than most:

First stop was the cattle unit where cows were being milked. We ran down the main thoroughfare trying doors, observing the numerous riot vans speeding towards our colleagues on the far side.

It wasn't long before we found a ladder and accessed the roof of a lab, to the horror of the emerging HLS employees and security guards.

The police were busy elsewhere. The helicopter was circling around the breach in the fence. Its job became more difficult when protestors on the ground marched onto the A1 carriageway.

After some time on the roof, we were joined by Inspector Dougal. He and three of his men grabbed us. They physically dragged us off the roof and into the waiting police van, despite the danger they put us all in by forcing us over various pipes and fixtures on the roof and down the ladder.

With protestors trapped between rolls of razor wire, it hadn't taken long for the police to usher the bulk of them back out the way they'd come. In their frustration, activists spilled out of the laboratory and onto the busy A1 which ran beside it. For hours, protestors marched along the road – now devoid of cars – barricading it with branches, road signs, and anything else they could find.

Blocking a major road garnered far more media attention than the activists who had stormed the fences. It gave Lynn and Gamal an idea. Over the next few months, the pair hatched a plan. Gamal recalls:

We practiced repeatedly for some months, so when we eventually did the action, it was fairly straightforward. Two activists brought cars that they drove side by side along the dual carriageway beside HLS. As they slowed down and stopped, we ran out and put up the tripods.

Gamal scaled one of the 7m structures, constructed from three scaffold poles, with a large protest banner stretched between the two. Lynn climbed the second tripod, aware that the drivers in the now congested road would be furious:

Almost immediately, a man approached my tripod and said, 'You are coming down from there.'

He grabbed one of the legs of my tripod, and pulled it out, causing me to plummet 24 feet to the tarmac. My assailant swiftly mounted his motorbike and rode away. Half of my cheek was hanging off and blood was splashed across me and all over the road. My leg felt like jelly and I knew it was badly smashed, but there was no actual pain. I tried to move my leg, but couldn't.

Gamal sat by me, stopping anyone from moving me, and without doubt saved my life. He got the registration number of the motorbike and phoned it through to his partner. Someone gave me a handkerchief, and I held it to my face until the police arrived and put a bandage on. Gamal was handcuffed and arrested for Obstruction of the Highway. They remanded him to prison, while I was taken to Hinchingbrooke Hospital in Huntingdon.

It took a team of orthopaedic and plastic surgeons five hours to repair my leg and face. I lost a litre of blood. I remember being surrounded by doctors, seeing my mother crying, and blood everywhere. I refused a plasma expander made of bovine collagen and went back to sleep.

Two days later, the police showed up at my bedside. I gave a statement against my assailant while attached to a morphine drip. As I drifted in and out of consciousness, the police failed to tell me they were interviewing me under caution with a view to prosecuting me.

Two months later, in late September, I attended Huntingdon magistrates to plead guilty to Obstructing the Highway. I had to attend court in a wheelchair, and for the first time in eight weeks I put the story into the public realm. I received a conditional discharge.

Because of my injury, I am permanently disabled; my left leg is shorter than my right by about an inch, meaning I have a permanent limp and regular discomfort.

It took just weeks to bring Lynn before the courts. But it would be over a year before the man who attacked her, off-duty police officer PC Manton, faced the legal system:

David Manton told the court that he was testing to see how heavy the leg of the tripod was so that he could move it. When I fell, he claimed his 'nerve just went', and he fled. He went to a relative's party. When he came back to his home he was arrested by his colleagues, his house was raided, and he was taken to Cambridge police station and interviewed.

The witnesses who had seen Manton attack me were the reason the case ended up in court. A squadron leader, a teacher, an accountant, and a senior nurse all testified that he had attacked me and was very angry. It was not enough, though. In less than an hour, with the police sitting around us in the public gallery whooping for joy, he was acquitted.

A year later, I bumped into one witness. She told me that from the moment she had come forward she had received death threats and police harassment. Her car was pulled over at least three times a week by police, and when she reported it she was told that her safety could not be guaranteed if she was a witness.

While searching PC Manton's house in August 2000, the police also raided several addresses related to SHAC. The search warrant showed that they were looking for anything to do with tripods. They found no such items, but the police did storm the offices of the printing company which produced the *SHAC Newsletter* and leaflets, seizing large quantities of both.[22]

Amidst the embarrassment of arresting a fellow officer, the police took vengeance on SHAC. Officers in riot gear grabbed four prominent campaigners – including Gregg, Natasha, and Heather – and threw them into police vehicles. It was the first time activists were arrested for running SHAC, but it would not be the last.

6
They Think It's All Over ...:
2000–01

Love them or loathe them, SHAC have forever changed the way single-interest pressure groups will wage war against big business.[23]

– Guardian

By August 2000, New Labour had abandoned its promise of a Royal Commission into animal research. Over 100 British MPs signed early day motions demanding it go ahead, but they were ignored.[24] Instead, Chancellor Gordon Brown unveiled a new budget and economic plan, predicated upon growing the research and development (R&D) sector;[25] 23 per cent of that sector was animal research.[26]

The animal liberation movement felt betrayed. In three short years, the UK had careered from potentially phasing out vivisection, to rising through the ranks of the ten most prolific animal testing countries in the world.[27]

ALF activists planted incendiary devices beneath four cars belonging to HLS staff. With the cars reduced to burnt metal and ash, the police and the government sought desperately for the perpetrator. The *Mail on Sunday* reported that Special Branch and MI5 had identified a culprit, but they had fled to India.[28] With leads running dry, and the arsonist proving too difficult to catch, SHAC's founders found themselves serving as convenient scapegoats.

The second issue of the *SHAC Newsletter* had called for activists to take up flyposting, send 'black faxes', and make nuisance calls to HLS' employees.[29] Several subsequent newsletters had followed, all designed to raise eyebrows in certain demographics and fists in others. But for all its tabloid-style rabble-rousing, the newsletter never again called for civil disobedience as overtly as it had in its second issue.

One article featured a cartoon image of Scooby-Doo, accompanied by the home addresses of HLS employees. Scooby declared; 'HLS workers are animal killers, go get 'em', but there was no suggestion this applied to anything beyond lawful letter-writing campaigns and protests. For those intent on prosecuting SHAC, the arson attacks allowed them to paint the article in a rather more sinister light.

Police charged Gregg, Natasha, and Heather with 'Conspiring to Cause a Public Nuisance and Conspiring to Commit Criminal Damage', setting a trial date for the following year. Campaigners suspecting a cynical ploy to paint SHAC as a criminal organisation to justify to a jury PC Manton's violent action against Lynn Sawyer.

It was unclear whether SHAC had actually broken any law. Home Secretary Jack Straw suggested in Parliament that he may need to enact new legislation prohibiting the naming of protest targets in campaign literature. The *Telegraph* reported that his intentions were to quell otherwise lawful civil disobedience:

Mr Straw said yesterday that consideration would now be given to curbing the activities of those activists who stopped short of violent behaviour but made the lives of scientists intolerable.[30]

The government's contempt for the tactic of making protests personal started and ended with SHAC. Jack Straw raised no concerns when *Guardian* journalist Polly Toynbee published Gregg and Heather's personal mobile phone number in a critical article about the campaign.[31] With an immediate circulation of over 400,000 people, Heather began receiving rape threats from people claiming to be HLS employees, while others threatened to burn down Gregg's home.

* * *

Following HLS' licence suspension in 1997, the laboratory resumed a series of xenotransplantation experiments on behalf of their customer Imutran. These experiments involved stitching pig hearts into the necks of baboons and monkeys. An investigator from Uncaged Campaigns initially exposed the tests in 1997:

> A pig kidney was accidentally frozen while waiting to be transplanted into the abdomen of monkey A166M – the transplant went ahead anyway, and the primate died shortly afterwards. Another monkey died when a swab was left in his abdomen following surgery, leading to a lethal infection of the spleen. A series of experimental surgeries performed by out-of-practice surgeons went fatally wrong. Lethal blood clotting and bleeding complications occurred regularly throughout the whole period of research.
>
> If the monkeys and baboons survived surgery, they faced an inevitable, traumatic death from one or a combination of these factors: organ rejection and failure, infections resulting from impaired immune systems, and/or drug toxicity. For example, kidney failure results in an accumulation of waste products such as urea in the blood. This leads to

nausea, vomiting, lethargy, listlessness, swelling, huddling in pain, drowsiness, anorexia, and eventually death.[32]

During this single set of experiments, HLS and their staff breached the Animals (Scientific Procedures) Act 526 times.

Despite having only just returned HLS' licence, the government remained silent. To ensure campaigners did the same, they granted Imutran an injunction against Uncaged Campaigns, preventing them from reporting the scandal.[33] An intense three-year legal battle followed before the report could be published.

With the injunction finally lifted, in 2000, the *Express* newspaper ran several articles detailing the graphic horror of xenotransplantation inside HLS, and evidence of fraudulent science. Animals who died during the tests were retroactively omitted from clinical reports, erroneously implying a low mortality rate. In one report, HLS recorded a baboon as healthy despite it having an implanted pig heart which had swelled to three times its natural size.[34]

Days after their name was splashed across the national media, Imutran announced the closure of their Cambridgeshire offices and fled to North America.[35]

Forced to watch HLS' lawbreaking go unpunished while he was dragged through the legal system for trying to stop them, Gregg furiously declared:

Yet again, HLS has been exposed. How many more times do we have to prove that this place is nothing but a living hell for animals and consistently breaks the law and Home Office conditions? HLS has repeatedly misled the public by saying that the animals do not suffer. We can all see that hundreds of primates have suffered and died inside HLS.

How many times do we have to expose HLS before they are closed down?[36]

The *Mail on Sunday* investigated the Kenyan facility which sourced the baboons. They discovered a highly profitable business which involved capturing primates from their natural lives in the wild, separating them from their family groups, and forcing them to live for weeks at a time in tiny cages, before being shipped for research in the UK and elsewhere. The conditions at the facility were so bad that the Kenyan Wildlife Service immediately closed it and announced, 'What we found was not a pleasant sight.'[37]

Later that year, SHAC received documents from an activist who had walked into HLS' second facility in Occold. Unchallenged, they emerged with video footage and paperwork revealing that workers had been caught taking drugs on-site and conducting research under the influence of alcohol. In perhaps the most bizarre revelation, they uncovered details of a baboon that had escaped the Cambridge site and fled across the A1. The fate of the fugitive primate remains unknown.[38]

On 8 April 2000, Heather organised the first Beagle Day celebration. A giant inflatable beagle dominated Parker's Piece in Cambridge city centre. Twenty-five real beagles – rescued from laboratories – gathered in the park with their new families to show the public victims and survivors of the vivisection industry.

Gamal was also keen to ensure that the dogs inside HLS weren't forgotten. He took action during a protest outside one of their beagle suppliers:

For the whole length of the track, we could hear the dogs barking inside, and it was so upsetting to listen to. By the time I reached the rear gates, I was determined to get inside.

I climbed up and over the razor wire before the police-man who had been standing beside me knew what was happening.

As fast as I could, I ran over to the nearest building and climbed onto the low roof. I stood on the roof for about twenty minutes, as a police helicopter circled overhead. The smell from the breeding units beneath me was overwhelm-ing, and it was all I could do not to vomit. I couldn't take any more and climbed down to explore the site.

As I wandered around, I came to a six-foot wall. I peered over the top and was confronted with eighty or so beagles, who began barking. The condition of the kennels was a disgrace. Concrete, dirty sawdust, and piles of faeces every-where. There was no sign of any bedding or comfort. I felt ashamed to be human. I let all the dogs out into the yard; lots of the younger dogs wanted to play, while most of the older dogs cowered in the corner of their pens, petrified of humans.

I will never forget the look in the beagles' eyes as I let them out into the yard. The thought that these innocent puppies ended up in HLS, alone and afraid, being tortured to death, makes me feel physically sick.

Meanwhile, in the City of London, a new front opened in the battle against HLS' finances.

To blend in with office workers, eleven activists donned suits and walked in pairs through the main entrance of One Canada Square in Canary Wharf – the fifty-storey headquar-ters of one of HLS' top shareholders. Kate Jones was amongst those who launched SHAC's assault on the city:

We went into the Bank of New York, legged it past the bar-riers, and got upstairs into a conference room.

We locked ourselves inside and put a huge table against the door. After an hour a police hostage negotiator arrived to talk to us, asking us what we wanted and whether we had any hostages. We were all laughing because we couldn't believe how seriously they were taking it. We explained our demands; all we wanted was executives from the Bank of New York to watch the video of the puppies inside HLS being beaten and abused, and for them to justify their shares in HLS. The negotiator said he would try to arrange this.

As one person spoke to the negotiator, others were calling the press to get as much publicity as possible. From the window we could see the whole road was sealed off with police tape and a huge crowd was gathering.

After a few hours, the negotiator returned and said two people could watch the video with the CEO of the bank. Two activists left the room with the videotape. As they were walking down the corridor, they turned around in horror as they saw riot cops rush past them. Those of us left inside the boardroom realised what was going on and pushed the table back against the door.

The riot cops smashed the door and brought down the entire wall of the office with it. In a frenzy, they ran in screaming, 'Turn around and put your hands up!' We did as we were told and one by one, we were arrested. We were escorted into the corridor where we were searched on camera. The entire building had been evacuated, with police dogs and riot cops everywhere, and the huge crowd outside was growing. As they dragged us past, we shouted, 'This is what happens when you deal with HLS.' I think the entire City of London got the message.

Although we were all arrested, only two people, who had stuck a couple of stickers inside the office, were convicted of a criminal offence.

The eleven-hour occupation kick-started regular demonstrations in the City of London. Up to 100 protestors regularly marched through the streets or took the tube around the capital to protest inside and outside of HLS' financial supporters. More than once, London Underground services were suspended as the police attempted to keep up. The protests had such an effect on city employees that many became whistle-blowers for SHAC. The Metropolitan Police wrote to every financial institution in the City of London, pleading with them to stop the flow of inside financial information which was being passed to SHAC. Even that letter was leaked to the campaign.[39]

Due to the ongoing protests, one of HLS' stockbrokers, West LB Panmure, contacted SHAC to inform them they would no longer be offering their services to HLS.[40] The situation worsened for HLS as HSBC Bank joined the growing list of companies ditching their shares in the laboratory.[41] Shortly after, HLS' director and fund manager resigned because of the pressure, and as their value fell below the minimum threshold, HLS was dropped from the New York Stock Exchange (NYSE).[42] After a lengthy uphill battle, they eventually listed on the London Stock Exchange instead. As the campaign claimed victory after victory, Gregg told the *Independent*:

> The financial institutions are looking at Huntingdon and seeing it's not worth the hassle. Will the City develop 'backbone'? No, it's only interested in profit. It would sell its granny for a pound. Frankly, they realise that there are easier places to invest money. Huntingdon will close, it's now only a question of time.[43]

The UK's top investment magazine, the *Investors Chronicle*, was no more flattering:

Projecting a positive image is always a challenge when your business is testing new chemical entities on animals. But Huntingdon has shown the rest of the UK plc how not to do it.

The present management team parachuted into Huntingdon after the animal abuse scandal three years ago. They've tried to project a more positive image and invited journalists to come and tour the labs to find out for themselves. But against the newfound power of internet activism, it has proved next to useless ... the anti-vivisectionists have succeeded in painting the company as a multinational empire devoted to wanton animal cruelty.

The failure to counter the image has egged on campaigners to ever more direct action, including gate-crashing drinks receptions at the company's brokers and writing to individual shareholders 'suggesting' they sell their shares.[44]

The day that HLS' loan facility with NatWest was due to end – 31 August 2000 – had come and gone. Every financial specialist agreed that HLS would be forced to close if the loan was not renewed. As the deadline was extended, and extended again, industry insiders reported that the Royal Bank of Scotland (RBS) – who had recently purchased NatWest – were planning to call in their loan to HLS.

In an extreme refinancing scheme, HLS sold their laboratories – and the land they stood on – to a company owned by their own CEO, Andrew Baker, and then rented them back again.[45] It was a bizarre and short-sighted move which benefited only Baker. Now that they didn't own their own buildings, HLS had even less to offer to a future lender as collateral.

Protestors gathered outside the Royal Bank of Scotland's head office in Edinburgh, where the media huddled to film them burning a copy of the bank's ethical policy.

The campaign waited for news, but not in silence. In the run-up to Christmas, 150 activists outwitted the police by declaring a fake meeting point for their protest. As a result, 1,100 police officers waited in the wrong place, at a cost of £250,000,[46] while SHAC carried out 'run-ins' at three HLS' customers. By running into company offices, SHAC campaigners regularly attempted to deliver videotapes and information packages directly to the desks of senior decision-makers. The police caught up by the fourth demonstration at Roche, but not in time to stop three teams storming the buildings.

During the demonstration, one team grabbed several sheets of paper from a wastepaper basket. The papers detailed Roche's upcoming Christmas party at a local pub. The campaign swiftly arranged another protest, and twenty activists with megaphones entered the pub to loudly disrupt the party. The pub happened to be hosting the local police force's Christmas party too. Off-duty officers immediately leapt into action, tussling with protestors as they sprinted for the exit. Frustrated, police arrested three campaigners for stealing the discarded scraps of paper, setting in motion a prosecution which would shock the animal liberation movement.

As the new year rolled in, the financial magazine *Shares* summarised HLS' position in blunt terms:

Even aside from refinancing concerns, Huntingdon's cash position looks increasingly tight. The company reported an operating loss of £718,000 in the nine months to 30th September, but a hefty interest bill blew out the pre-tax loss figure to £5.8 million. At 30 September, the company had just £927,000 left in the bank. With little prospect of raising fresh equity, Huntingdon faces some daunting challenges in securing its long-term future, a fact borne out by its low share price.[47]

Behind the scenes, discussions continued between RBS, the government, and HLS. As senior politicians called on RBS to stand firm,[48] campaigners like Gregg knew this was no time to take their eyes off the prize:

If HLS closes, then our priority will be to re-home all the animals. If it remains open, we will continue our campaign. We are only one year into a three-year campaign. We will financially destroy anyone who funds them.

The government can do what they want – they will not save HLS. It will close.

I don't think most of the medical profession have got a clue about animal testing. Most doctors don't understand what goes on inside the laboratories.[49]

Dr Liela Harvey, from Doctors and Lawyers for Responsible Medicine, shared this view:

Animal testing is evil and totally irrelevant to humans. It is carried out by Frankenstein-like doctors, and we will oppose it until our last dying breath. Closing HLS would send a powerful message to the industry that it has to change its ways. We want a review, so the facts are brought into the open.[50]

With both sides entrenched in their positions, HLS' employees began checking their mortgage protection and local job adverts as the hours ticked down.[51] Finally, RBS confirmed the news; they were cutting their ties to HLS. Against all odds, the campaign had taken on a multinational company and won.

Without their lender, Huntingdon Life Sciences would be forced into administration. Every UK-based bank or financier was aware of SHAC and the protests that would blight anyone willing to prop up the world's most besieged company. No one would be foolish enough to step in. No one, that is, except the British government.

The *Daily Telegraph* reported:

Lord Sainsbury, the science minister, brokered an agreement to refinance [HLS] after the Royal Bank of Scotland withdrew a loan of £22.6 million because staff and customers had been threatened by animal rights protesters.

The minister also arranged a special dispensation with the Stock Exchange for the new backers of HLS to remain secret, breaching the normal trading rules. It is understood that Britain's biggest drug companies, including GlaxoSmithKline – under pressure from the Government – have underwritten the deal by guaranteeing HLS future contracts.

[Lord Sainsbury] said, 'If it had closed, many jobs, including those of 400 scientists, would certainly have gone abroad and some pharmaceutical companies may have decided to do their medical research in another country.'

The new backer is a group of American investors who pledged to match the existing loan and provide 'a significant extra sum' to allow HLS to expand.[52]

Following the 1997 election, biotech billionaire David Sainsbury had given the Labour Party the largest donation in their history. A few months later they awarded him a peerage, allowing him to sit in the House of Lords as Lord Sainsbury of Turville. From there, he was declared the minister for science, without ever having been elected by the British public. From this position, *Lobby Watch* calculated that the third wealthiest man in Britain increased funding to his own biotech businesses – and those he invested in – by up to 300 per cent.[53]

Years later he resigned his position as police investigated wealthy individuals purchasing positions of power,[54] but not before he had wrought havok amongst the animal liberation and environmental movements. Having secured HLS' future, he proposed a government-funded advertising campaign to support animal experiments. His colleagues vetoed the idea.[55]

Despite allowing HLS to pay just £1 to erase half of their £22.5 million debt,[56] RBS insisted that their actions had been financially motivated:

> [HLS] had a track record of huge losses over several years. This is not a refinancing, but a rescue. The only alternative was receivership, and it was only due to the intervention of the Government and pharmaceutical companies that it has survived.[57]

Lord Sainsbury secured HLS a new lender who paid off the remaining £11 million owed to RBS and provided the laboratory with a further £10 million.[58] HLS' CEO Andrew Baker, eager to wring every penny out of his company, loaned them an additional £4 million of his own money,[59] with a hefty 10 per cent interest rate.[60]

He arranged for the new American backer to lend their money through his finance company, FHP Reality, to protect their anonymity, and to add to Baker's ever-growing personal fortune. The deal not only ensured the survival of HLS, but according to Jill Treanor from the *Guardian*, it was likely to increase the number of animals experimented on and killed.[61] SHAC's response to the deal was characteristically defiant:

> We are prepared for a long fight, and while our goal is HLS, we will take on anyone who gets in our way.[62]

As they knuckled down to continue their fight, campaigners like Heather were forced to manage the emotional rollercoaster:

It was such a huge thing, and the government stepping in was completely unprecedented. I was heartbroken, but we just carried on. Full speed ahead. I always remember our philosophy of never being too up and never being too down. When you had a success like NatWest, we were never too jubilant about it. And then when we were knocked back, we were never too depressed about it. Although I'm a very emotional person, especially about this subject, I had to learn to put all emotions to one side because the animals don't care if you cry yourself to sleep at night. There's nothing wrong with doing that, but it doesn't help the animals.

HLS, however, were ecstatic. Employees erected a large sign inside the laboratory's formidable fence declaring 'business as usual'.[63] Natasha answered a call to the SHAC office phone, and on the other end of the line she heard a monkey screaming. A voice asked for some electrodes, and the screaming intensified. Natasha hung up. It wasn't the last time she would have to endure such a phone call.

7

Team America: 1999–2001

We view the UK as the Afghanistan for the growth of
animal rights extremism throughout the world. The movement that we are dealing with in the USA is a direct import
from the UK.[64]

– National Animal Interest Alliance

As a student in the late 1990s, Kevin Kjonaas had been an
active member of the Student Organisation for Animal Rights
(SOAR).[65] Inspired by pressure campaigns in the UK, Kevin
realised that traditional student activism wasn't producing
the desired victories for his University of Minnesota (UoM)
group. So, they changed their strategy:

Our primary target was Marilyn Carroll, who takes rhesus
macaque monkeys and addicts them to crack cocaine
and studies the withdrawal effects. We made flyers with
her picture on and distributed them to her students and
colleagues.

I realised that we were doing a protest against a person
who was doing something wrong. And so we had to make it
personal, and going to her doorstep made it very personal.
She went through the roof, as did her husband. No broken
windows, no paint, just people at her home. It touched a
nerve.

The press never mentioned Marilyn Carroll before we
started going to her house, but then they had to explain why

we were there and what Marilyn Carroll was doing to these primates.[66]

SOAR campaigners held protests at the home of Marilyn Carroll, and chained themselves together at the entrance to her laboratories. One student climbed to the seventeenth floor of a campus tower. They refused to come down until the university administration granted a meeting to discuss animal research.[67]

As Kevin honed the increasingly effective direction of UoM SOAR, other groups took notice. One night, while Kevin was out of town, the Animal Liberation Front (ALF) struck at the Neurological Research Center and the psychology building. According to the FBI, masked activists wearing identical clothing cut through the roof of the building and abseiled into the laboratories.[68] The activists filmed themselves doing flying kicks through doors, and destroying cages and restraining devices in scenes reminiscent of a Hollywood movie.

The activists who carried out the raid rescued twenty-seven pigeons, forty-eight mice, thirty-six rats, and five salamanders from the laboratories.[69] International media converged on the university to report on the largest laboratory animal rescue since the 1980s.

Kevin Kjonaas was a Political Sciences major and his professor had arranged for him to intern with the North American Animal Liberation Press Office (NAALPO). With such a significant action at his own university, Kevin hosted a press conference on NAALPO's behalf. He screened the ALF footage taken during the raid, while fielding questions from the press and police.[70]

The FBI's primary investigator Coleen Rowley sensationally exclaimed:

The impact of an act of terrorism is that it's shocking, that it shocks people. It terrorises. The break in had that impact.[71]

On the FBI's instruction, the Minnesota State Senate drafted a bill criminalising the defence or justification of an ALF action. The law would be retroactive, meaning Kevin would be facing jail time for defending a crime carried out by someone else, under a law which hadn't existed when he broke it. Fortunately for him, by the time it passed through the Senate the law had been watered down to the point of redundancy.

Nonetheless, the FBI sent an armed unit to raid Kevin's house. They tore it apart for over two hours, vandalising and seizing everything they could find. They even confiscated his university coursework. For Kevin, their goal was clear:

This wasn't about solving a crime, this was about sending a message; 'You had better shut up.'[72]

The FBI convened a Grand Jury to investigate the break-in, with Kevin their only lead. He pleaded his fifth amendment right to silence:

At the time of the Grand Jury, I didn't answer any questions. But they can remove your constitutional rights. At that point, if you refuse to answer questions, they imprison you until you cooperate. The life of a Grand Jury is typically eighteen months, but they can just rubber stamp a renewal indefinitely.

The prosecutor told me, 'You've offended the Grand Jury, and we're going to be calling you back with immunity. You will answer these questions.'

And I thought, 'Nope, that's not going to work for me.'

Kevin immediately signed up for an international post-graduate programme. He headed for the UK,[73] where he found a vastly different animal liberation movement:

It wasn't just a bunch of white college kids living an alternative lifestyle. It was a working-class movement. It was a more mature group of people with full-time jobs that were doing this on their weekends or spare time, people who had families but were still coming out to the big rallies and marches.

I appreciated the level of seriousness and the force with which people were demanding changes for animal rights. It was exciting, and it was innovative – these pressure campaigns were a new thing, and they were galvanising people. It wasn't just, 'I hope you go vegan', it was, 'We're going to shut this place down and free these animals, and it will have a knock-on effect on the industry.'

Kevin became heavily involved in several campaigns, including SHAC. Committed to regular protests and civil disobedience, he was arrested several times for public order offences. His final charge – for singing unflattering songs to HLS workers – was serious enough that when he returned to the USA to pay his last respects to his grandfather, he found his way back to Britain barred. While he fought to have the decision overturned, he brought the British style of activism to his home country.

Following Heather's visit earlier in the year, several animal rights groups in New Jersey had carried out intermittent protests against HLS, including the Animal Defense League (ADL) and In Defense of Animals (IDA). Activist Joe Bateman compiled a short newsletter under the name *SHAC USA*. The newsletter collated reports from all the protests and actions being taken against HLS in North America.

On his return to the USA, Kevin Kjonaas resolved to grow SHAC USA into a fully-fledged campaign. He commissioned a website and composed a second *SHAC USA* newsletter on his desktop computer, which he distributed via a large animal rights organisation's mailing list. Kevin's passion was infectious, and he soon found others ready to join him:

> There was a magic to it at that point. People knew all about HLS, and Hill Grove, and Barry Horne. Many of us actively followed the UK, and prior to SHAC, there was cross-Atlantic coordination through email lists. When SHAC USA launched, there was a great deal of excitement and hype about it because US activists needed a victory. Everything had felt so quixotic to that point. We were just tilting at these windmills of social change, achieving nothing, often at great personal sacrifice. This was a time to try new things, and the SHAC model was a very new idea, especially the financial and tertiary targeting.

In September 2000, SHAC USA's first major demonstration saw fifty activists converge upon HLS in New Jersey. During the protest, police shoved four campaigners to the ground and arrested them.[74] In response, activists organised another demonstration. Over 100 activists attended.

SHAC USA established its own dedicated office, began coordinating actions, and launched regular demonstrations against the laboratory.

With news from the UK that a secret US backer had bailed out HLS, everything changed. Kevin rallied the North American movement to his call:

This is coming to the US, and everybody's participation is being sought.[75]

We're a new breed of activism. We're not your parents' Humane Society. We're not Friends of Animals. We're not Earthsave. We're not Greenpeace. We come with a new philosophy. We hold the radical line. We will not compromise. We will not apologise, and we will not relent.[76]

One of those inspired by this call was Josh Harper:

I will never forget the feelings of hopelessness I had watching Michele Rokke's undercover footage for the first time. Here were living, feeling creatures trapped inside a hostile environment with no one there to protect them from their captors. I lived all the way on the other side of the country from the East Millstone laboratory and had no idea what I could do to help these poor souls. The footage tormented me, because in the cries of these animals I heard a plea for help and I thought that there would be none coming. How wrong I was.

Elsewhere in the world, a brave group of people was assembling to become a fighting force for animals. They were not timid like the animal rights groups I had known, and they made certain that animal abusers clearly understood that if they continued to violate the rights of animals, they would be dealt with in a manner that was swift and effective. That group was SHAC UK.

When I heard the campaign was coming to the US, I was elated.[77]

Josh's close friend, Jake Conroy, held a similar view. When one of his friends invited him to travel nearly 3,000 miles from

Seattle to SHAC USA's office on the East Coast, he jumped at the chance:

> I packed up all my stuff into boxes; we flew to New York and then took the train to Philadelphia. Initially, my plan was to spend a few months at the SHAC office and fly back home on September 13, 2001. Of course, the events of 9/11 meant that plan wasn't destined to happen, and I ended up staying far longer. That's where I met Kevin; he was sitting on the floor – because there was no furniture in the house – eating dinner and watching this tiny little television set.

Jake too had followed the British campaign via the animal liberation email lists since Consort. While he had never intended to stay long, he found himself unwilling, or unable, to step away. Soon he saw a way to put his talents to good use:

> One thing I loved about SHAC was the DIY philosophy. We didn't have a bunch of money or resources, but we used our skills, and combined them with each other's, to put together some really interesting and exciting projects. Kevin was such a dynamic speaker and strategist, Lauren Gazola had such a smart mind around legal issues, and I was good at design. Those three pieces combined, allowing us to create this group pretty quickly. It really took off.
>
> I had a conversation very early on with Kevin about how traditionally we would steal advertising banners from McDonald's and then spray-paint our slogans on the other side, or photocopy some crappy flyer that we had made at Kinko's. But it turned out that to make these things look professional doesn't really cost that much money.
>
> We would turn up to big animal rights conferences where everyone else would be asking for bigger cages, and we had

a huge banner with an ALF activist on it holding rescued animals. People were attracted to that, and it felt like the grassroots animal liberation movement finally had a voice that could match these other groups that were saying, 'No, we need to be moderates and we need to pass laws, we need to ask for bigger cages …'

The downside to looking so professional was that the government thought we were well funded. We weren't. We were constantly broke.

Jake Conroy, Kevin Kjonaas, Lauren Gazola, and Josh Harper didn't stand alone. Inspired by the campaign in Britain, and the momentum of the newly formed SHAC USA, activists across the length and breadth of North America began paying attention. And they were eager to get involved.

*   *   *

Inside his imposing twenty-five-storey headquarters in Little Rock, Arkansas, Warren Amerine Stephens was over 1,200 miles from the nascent SHAC USA in Philadelphia, and further still from SHAC in the UK. The CEO of Stephens Inc. was a billionaire who owned four private jets, an expansive collection of rare art, and many of Little Rock's most prestigious buildings – from hotels to golf clubs.[78] He believed the campaign against HLS was a problem for other people, in a place a world away from his own.

With HLS' shareholders swarming to drop their toxic stock, Stephens Inc. had already become the single largest shareholder in the beleaguered firm.

Barely a week after the Lord Sainsbury and the UK government promised HLS' new lender anonymity, SHAC discovered it was Stephens Inc. They broadcast the news around the world via their website, newsletter, and email action alerts. Warren Stephens shrugged it off, claiming, 'I much prefer not to have this fight, but we'll come prepared.'[79]

Almost immediately, protestors picketed Stephens in Little Rock and New York. Activists organised home demos in Chicago and invaded their offices in San Francisco, Atlanta, and Boston. In Seattle, they unleashed powerful stink bombs inside their offices, resulting in five city blocks being closed and three floors of the building being emptied for the day. Police officers in hazmat suits cleared the streets as they attempted to investigate the source of the smell.[80]

Bringing anti-HLS activism into the twenty-first century, a group calling itself the Animal Liberation-Tactical Internet Response Network (AL-TIRN) organised a cyber blockade of Stephens Inc.'s website, successfully taking it offline.[81] It was a technological step forward from clogging fax machines, and Stephens Inc.'s webmaster threatened to quit as a result. Police later arrested an activist named Nathan Brasfield for organising the digital protest. He was sentenced to a year in prison accused of 'Theft of Telecommunications Services.'[82]

In their newsletter and on their website, SHAC USA reported every single action taken against Stephens Inc. and HLS. Kevin based this on legal advice from the campaign's solicitor:

> We wanted to report on many actions, and not all of them were legal, such as animal liberations. We were the go-to resource for anti-HLS news, and we felt people had a right to know the entirety of the actions taken against the laboratory. The legal opinion was that if we picked and chose what we reported on, then we would be accused of advocating or encouraging certain types of actions.

We became a news clearing house, and we reported on everything, even the actions which we found immoral or counterproductive. There were several occasions when we had to sit down and decide whether certain actions should go on our website or in our newsletter, but we always stuck with the same policy: it was not our place to decide which actions should and should not be reported.

As a new form of activism swept North America, the surge of civil disobedience greatly appealed to activists like Josh, who saw a connection to other social justice struggles:

As I dug more into the history of how change occurs, I realised that at every turn, every ounce of progress that we've had towards a more just world has come because there were people who were willing to fight and willing to sacrifice. And really, willing to suffer. Not all of them ended up succeeding in their struggles. But there's something beautiful about a person who has a degree of selflessness that takes them from their comfort and propels them out into the world against great odds, and often ends in tragedy.[83]

8

Mob of 1,000 on Rampage: 2001

A tiny group of activists is succeeding where Karl Marx, the Baader-Meinhof gang and the Red Brigades failed.[84]

– *Financial Times*

While the Stephens Inc. loan inspired activists in the USA, campaigners in the UK felt betrayed by the British government's abrasive U-turn over vivisection. More than a thousand protestors descended on Cambridge city centre to march as a sea of white boiler suits and skull masks. Twenty miles away, 500 police officers waited at the advertised meeting point outside HLS.

Despite mounting frustration, the protest passed peacefully. Nonetheless, Chief Constable of Cambridgeshire Police Ben Gunn told media it was 'only a matter of time before somebody is killed'.[85] For many activists this felt like a threat, which did little to quell the rage that they felt towards HLS, the pharmaceutical industry, and the British state.

People had lost faith in the political system. The government had failed to permanently revoke HLS' licence when Zoe Broughton exposed illegality and cruelty in 1997, and they refused to do anything when the xenotransplantation scandal was uncovered in 2000. Now they had bailed out a company which killed 500 animals every day, and which had broken the law hundreds of times.

The NatWest fiasco had taken its toll on HLS. But as their director, Andrew Gay, noted, without the NatWest campaign

HLS' name would disappear from the high street.[86] Unwilling to let this happen, SHAC sought a new high-profile target.

GlaxoSmithKline (GSK) had underwritten HLS' loan on condition of their continued custom, placing a target on their own heads. If SHAC could persuade them to renege on that arrangement, then the deal would be off and HLS would have to file for bankruptcy.

As well as their pharmaceutical lines, GSK produced staple British consumables including Lucozade, Ribena, and Horlicks. SHAC swiftly distributed thousands of flyers and stickers. They urged people to fill shopping trolleys with GSK products and then leave them abandoned in supermarket aisles or blocking checkouts, covered in campaign literature.[87] In shops across the country, activists plastered GSK products with stickers declaring, 'This product is tested on animals.'

SHAC's organisers had become adept at moving and mobilising large numbers of activists at short notice. With the growing popularity of mobile phones, this skill could be put to devastating use.

On night of 11 February 2001, several SHAC activists visited Chorleywood cricket ground and painstakingly removed dozens of wooden bollards along the edge of the A404 carriageway. The following morning, as a thousand activists headed for an advertised rendezvous at Newport Pagnell service station on the M1, the driver of each vehicle received a phone call redirecting them to Chorleywood.

Hundreds of police officers sealed off the services at Newport Pagnell. They searched and turned away every vehicle attempting to stop for fuel, but the protestors they searched for had congregated forty miles further south.

Undercover officers tipped off their uniformed colleagues about the new location, but it was too late for the hundreds of officers waiting nearly an hour away. At Chorleywood,

SHAC gave the driver of each of the hundred or so vehicles an action sheet. The entire process took only minutes. A single air horn blast signalled for the convoy to leave. The police who managed to scramble to the new rendezvous tried to block the fleet of activists, but with the bollards removed, cars, vans, and minibuses drove across the cricket pitch and flooded onto the A404.

Depending on which sheet they had been given, the vehicles split off into separate teams. Half barrelled west towards Surrey and Hampshire, while the rest whipped north towards Berkshire and Hertfordshire. Each driver did their best to lose the police who had been quick enough to follow, and most succeeded. At exactly 2 o'clock in the afternoon, both teams began their first protest.

'Mob of 1,000 on rampage,'[88] the front page of the *Daily Mail* screamed the following morning. It wasn't far wrong. Protestors, furious that the once anti-vivisection government had conspired to bail out HLS, delivered a clear message.

An activist from one of the Surrey teams relayed their experience, starting at GlaxoSmithKline's Research and Technical Operations site at Weybridge:

Over 100 angry activists surrounded the gates and began to force them open. The one police officer that was present tried to stop them, but it was no good. The gates burst off their hinges and in people went.

Their anger overflowed onto the windows of all the buildings and onto the few workers' cars which were on-site. Activists broke into the building and sprayed slogans everywhere, setting the fire alarms off as they left, and leaving thousands of pounds worth of damage to the premises of one of HLS's most important customers.

As the police helicopter and back up arrived, people moved on to … Eli Lilly's research premises at Erl Wood Manor. Protesters cut through the perimeter fence and swarmed the premises. There was an overwhelming sound of glass shattering as people gained access to the buildings where they had a good look round and left with large amounts of the company's documents.

The crowd went to the final location: Eli Lilly's site at Basingstoke, where the security barrier was brushed aside, and stickers were plastered everywhere. The crowd grew to about 300 and the main gates were broken down and in people went. The office blocks were stormed, and the offices were reduced to a huge pile of broken plastic and scattered documents.

Meanwhile, an intrepid demonstrator had scaled a huge factory building on site and hung a large banner reading, 'Eli Lilly and HLS Torture Animals'. The activist was arrested but then allowed to come down without charge, leaving the huge banner flapping in the wind on the highest building on site.[89]

As one of the first demonstrations that my brother, and cancer research scientist, Dr Joseph Harris, attended, it was a trial by fire. He took part in the protests with his friend Rod Richardson:

Rod drove a car with myself and three other passengers. The first company we stopped at was Bayer. As we all gathered on the road outside the premises, one of the employees rammed their car into the crowd of protestors and knocked a young woman to the ground. People swarmed on the car; it managed to drive off, but it was missing its mirrors, wipers, and several windows.

Someone cut a hole in the fence, and an older guy leaning on a stick waved us through. After entering the grounds people mostly just milled around, but some started throwing stones at windows. Rod entered the building with two other people. He used an axe to smash through a panel next to the main entrance, creating a gap wide enough to squeeze through. After several minutes inside the building Rod came running out. I met him by the fence and we quickly left the scene. He told me he'd caused damage to computers and photocopiers.

As we drove to the various targets, we occasionally saw lines of minibuses which had been stopped by police road-blocks. Around them, hundreds of sheets of paper blew in the wind; the target lists for the day.

We also visited GlaxoSmithKline. I stayed at the front of the company, but Rod climbed the fence and went in with a large number of other people. When I saw him later, he told me he had opened up the valves on large vats of Horlicks, flooding the entire facility. He spent a long time laughing about this. Rod had organised transport to the protest, coordinated the order we visited the 'targets' in, decided when we should leave each one, and was one of the main people responsible for damage that occurred at Bayer and GSK that day.

Rod, it later turned out, was a serving police officer, working undercover to sabotage groups including SHAC.[90] When Home Secretary Jack Straw scoffed in Parliament, 'I have no idea quite how targeting a Horlicks factory can help to prop-agate their aims,'[91] he failed to mention that at least one of the primary instigators was working on his behalf.

Of course, many involved in that protest were not spy cops or agent provocateurs. There was palpable anger against the government, HLS, and everyone who supported the laboratory. The remarkable tactic of the mass mobile demonstration – perhaps the first of its kind in terms of organisation and scale – took the police by surprise, and a thousand angry activists seized their opportunity.

That anger manifested in different ways. Most activists had expected a march around a city centre, and loudly, but lawfully, voiced their protest from outside the targeted companies. They travelled by coach or minibus; easy prey for the roadblocks where police stopped them, searched them, and arrested the occupants en masse. The destruction was caused by a significant minority in cars, who simply bypassed the roadblocks. As a result, virtually everyone detained was later released without charge.

Sweeping arrests of law-abiding protestors caused a feeling of trepidation to seep into the movement. While mobile demonstrations went on to become a staple of the SHAC campaign, they were never replicated on such a scale again.

The next attempt, a month later, was a far smaller affair. SHAC called a protest at HLS' second UK facility in Occold, Suffolk. At the last minute, 100 activists diverted and headed for HLS in Cambridgeshire. With scores of officers protecting the Occold laboratory from a handful of protestors, local press admonished the police for wasting resources. Meanwhile at Huntingdon, just three police officers were present as the bulk of the protest laid siege to the facility, trapping the workers in for hours after they were due to head home.

Following the 'mob of 1,000' mobile demonstration, GSK sent a memo to all of its facilities, warning staff to be prepared for more demonstrations. Yet even as their Coleford factory was having new security fencing installed, several protestors slipped around the construction workers and gained access to the site. They draped a large banner from the roof as protestors on the ground distributed leaflets among the staff. In Grimsby, a group of activists slipped under the fence of Novartis, another customer of HLS. According to a local newspaper:

> Animal rights campaigners stormed Novartis' Grimsby site … The protestors climbed barriers, ran through offices distributing leaflets, and shouted advice through a megaphone to stunned members of staff.[92]

Across the Atlantic, things weren't any easier for HLS. As World Day for Animals in Laboratories approached, protests took place in all ten of the cities where Stephens Inc. had offices. In San Francisco campaigners barricaded themselves into a conference room and used the company's telephone to crank-call other branches and HLS in the UK. Eventually, the police smashed through an internal wall using pickaxes, causing $50,000 in damage.[93] Run-ins took place in Boston, Chicago, and Atlanta. In Las Vegas, animal liberation activist and trauma surgeon, Dr Jerry Vlasak, found himself inside a conference which the police had turned into a semi-militarised zone:

> I went to Las Vegas with my wife Pam and friend Dr Ray Greek. Like me, he used to be an animal researcher but is now an animal advocate. We heard that Stephens were holding an investors conference in one of the big casino hotels, so we rented a conference room in the same building. We planned to set up a press conference about Stephens Inc., and the scientific validity and ethics of animal research.
>
> The night before the press conference, Pam and I went downstairs to the casino and started handing out SHAC flyers to everybody.
>
> I headed back for our room, but right before I got there, these guys grabbed me and threw me on the ground and put

me in a chokehold. They started putting me in handcuffs. I was yelling, 'Who the fuck are you? I have a hotel room. I'm going to my hotel room.'

They shouted back, 'We've heard you have anarchist literature in your hotel room.'

They burst into our hotel room, where Dr Ray Greek was standing in his boxer shorts trying to work out what the hell was going on. They searched the entire room, grabbed every piece of paperwork, and took me to jail. They threw Pam and Ray out of the hotel at 11 o'clock at night and cancelled the press conference room that we had reserved for the next day. They held me in jail for several days, for handing out factual leaflets, but Pam and Ray found another place to stay and another room to host their press conference. Eventually the charges were dropped and I sued them for about $20,000.

In Augusta, another group of protestors were arrested while demonstrating against Warren Stephens as he attempted to enjoy a round of golf at a private club.[94]

Meanwhile, 150 animal activists descended on HLS' laboratory in New Jersey. Several pushed down a barricade and attempted to get into the facility. Police shot pepper spray indiscriminately into the crowd. Tensions rose throughout the day as police assaulted and gassed protestors. At least one activist was hospitalised by police CS gas. Following the protest, an HLS employee had his car flipped onto its roof outside his house.[95]

The reason for the police's over-zealous response occurred the night before the demonstration, as a team of anonymous ALF activists busied themselves inside HLS:

Entry required crossing a canal, at times 100 feet wide. We tied a rope to one of the trees and sent out the boat. At the other shore, the rope was tied to another tree. This enabled us to shuttle each other across the canal in a matter of moments.

We used bolt cutters to create emergency exits every few sections of barbed wire fence in case we needed a quick escape. We knew the precise timing of the security rounds, and we had six or seven minutes.

Climbing up the jungle gym of pipes along the back of the main building, we were able to enter the necropsy room through a skylight. Several operating tables were covered in evidence of painful dissections, with surgical instruments left, uncleaned, to soak in the pools of blood left on the tables overnight.

When we entered the beagle unit, it was eerily silent. The dogs made no noise. Through the darkness, we could see the shining black of the puppies' eyes peering at us with a mixture of curiosity, and an intense fear of humans. We had waited so long for this moment. We ran from cage to cage and flung open all the doors at once. As they saw the first puppy do it, all the others began to understand that they could get up and leave their prison with the slatted steel floor. The puppies ran all over the unit, exercising their newfound freedom to run, jump, and interact with one another. Those who were small enough went into carriers, and for some of the larger dogs we affixed harnesses, to guide them to liberation. We took every living animal we found out with us.

I took two dogs out with me, both the largest dog, and the smallest puppy of the lot. As we ran along a grassy trail created by power lines, the puppy was a ball of energy, and the older dog trotted along at a pace worthy of a Sunday walk. But before we were halfway out, the puppy was getting restless, and he began to cry. The three of us stopped for a moment, and the little one kept jumping up to sniff me as I scratched behind his ears. I pulled him up into my arms, and he began to lick my face through the fabric of my mask. 'I understand Little One, you're tired … You're just a baby here, fleeing for your life …' It was then that I appreciated the steady pace of the older dog. He seemed to know and understand that if he patiently ran and kept moving, he would never have to return to the iron cube he had been in for what was most likely years.

The three of us crossed the canal and knew that we were going to be safe. We were the last ones to meet up with the rest of the group, and as I loaded my new friends up for transportation, all that was visible was a sea of wagging brown and white tails, and bobbing puppies jumping all over, relishing the feeling of contact and play. Within hours, our footprints would be washed away in the mud, and the dogs would be hours away, on the long, well-deserved journey to their new lives. It was a beautiful morning, and it was a brand new day for the animals.[96]

9

Next Time He'll Have a Migraine:
2001

If you go to extreme violence, the chances are you will win.[97]
– Brian Cass, HLS' managing director

In 1991, on a country lane deep in rural Cheshire, Mike Hill lay dying. The eighteen-year-old was with the Merseyside hunt saboteurs, saving foxes from the Cheshire Beagles. As the hunt master loaded his hounds into a trailer to evade the protest, Mike and two other sabs jumped onto the back to prevent it leaving. They wanted to convince the huntsman to concede and go home, but the driver unexpectedly accelerated, leaving the activists clinging on for dear life. Mike tried to leap to safety as the vehicle approached a bend, but the trailer hit him, and he fell beneath its wheels.

Aware of what had happened, the driver ploughed on for another mile. He only stopped when one of Mike's friends smashed the rear window and applied the handbrake. As the passenger rained down blows from a hunting whip, one saboteur ran for help while the other sprinted back to his friend and held him as he lay dying.[98] As he watched his friend pass away, Dave Blenkinsop vowed to avenge Mike and the animals he tried so bravely to defend.

Although the driver handed himself into a police station, he was never charged for any offence. Outraged, activists gathered in protest outside the hunt kennels, and caused extensive damage to the building and several vehicles. Dave was amongst six arrested, and was sentenced to fifteen months in prison.[99]

Nine years later, Dave Blenkinsop was out in the fields of Kent, once more putting himself between wild foxes and those who would kill them. It is impossible to comprehend how he must have felt as he watched a Land Rover – driven by a hunt supporter – plough into another friend, Steve Christmas.[100] As over two tonnes of metal crushed Steve's body, the driver paused, before turning the vehicle around to mock his victim. For the second time in less than a decade, Dave found himself nursing the body of a close friend as their life drained away.

Steve was airlifted to hospital with a crushed pelvis, four broken ribs, and internal bleeding.[101] He remained in intensive care for four long weeks, his life hanging by a thread. Surgeons performed a tracheotomy, fitted a metal plate to his pelvis, and removed over half a metre of his bowel. He eventually pulled through, but not without life-altering injuries.[102]

It was more than Dave could take; he was done with asking, pleading, and screaming for change. He vowed to fight fire with fire.

* * *

On the night of Thursday, 22 February 2001, HLS' managing director, Brian Cass, parked his car outside his St Ives townhouse. As he did every night, he stepped out and locked the door behind him. However, this was not any other night. While the SHAC campaign and the wider animal rights movement convulsed in outrage at the government's support for HLS by storming their customers and American financiers, Dave Blenkinsop and two of his friends carried out an action which sent shockwaves through the movement, and beyond.

Cass was walking towards his front door when two men and one woman approached him, dressed in camouflaged clothing, wearing balaclavas, and welding wooden staves. As they swung the batons towards his body, Cass lost his footing:

> I fell over, and that was when I gashed my head. As I felt a cracking noise on my head, my partner, who realised something was going on outside, opened the door and I stumbled in.[103]

As Cass fell and hit his head, the assailants turned and fled across nearby fields. Two of Cass' neighbours heard the commotion and gave chase, but the perpetrators sprayed one of them with tear gas and vanished into the night.[104]

Whatever was intended, the attack was a violent departure from even the most militant ALF activities thus far. It was, however, an aberration rather than an escalation; there would be no further physical attacks against anyone connected to HLS, and Dave was later arrested and sentenced to prison for his part in the attack. For most animal rights campaigners, motivated by compassion and an intense respect for life, it was a step too far. Natasha made SHAC's opinion clear:

> We unreservedly condemn acts of violence, whether against human beings or animals. I have condemned the attacks, therefore I condemn the people who carried out the attacks.[105]

SHAC's opponents wasted no time capitalising on the incident. The morning after the attack, Brian Cass appeared outside HLS, shaken, with a stitched-up gash on his head. In front of a press scrum, he declared he was undeterred, and called upon the government to implement 'a nationally coordinated strategy to deal with these people'.[106] Within days, Parliament rushed through a new law allowing company directors to keep their personal details anonymous. Two days later, Chief Constable of Cambridgeshire Police, Ben Gunn, seized the opportunity to dictate a new narrative of the event:

> If you hit someone over the head with a baseball bat, it's not by design but by accident that you don't kill them.[107]

Mr Gunn was the senior police officer for the force dealing with the investigation. He knew full well that Cass had slipped and hit his head on the pavement. By falsely claiming he had been struck about the head, Cambridgeshire's most senior police officer appeared intent on inflating the attack to attempted murder.

Policing the Consort campaign had cost West Mercia Police over £1 million, Thames Valley had spent £4.8 million on Hill Grove,[108] and Cambridgeshire Police had already doled out £2 million to protect HLS.[109] To ensure the government paid this bill – which covered wages and resources other forces could not afford – it was essential to portray the entire campaign as extreme, and as politically urgent, as possible. To suggest wider support for violence, anonymous hate mail was quoted to the media. Sober-faced officers read the press quotes such as 'This time he got a headache, next time he'll get a migraine.'[110]

For both HLS and the animal liberation movement, framing activists as an ultra-violent mob served as a double-edged sword. It created a climate of fear amongst companies linked to HLS. Many distanced themselves before a single protest even took place. This was great for SHAC, but terrible for HLS. On the other hand, vilifying the campaign, and the portrayal of animal researchers as victims was great for HLS and terrible for SHAC.

For the police, there was no downside as government money filled their coffers. As time went on, they proactively enforced this climate of fear. Enticed by the allure of new legislation, and eager to spin HLS as victims, Brian Cass altered his version of events in line with the police, telling the *Telegraph*:

> I arrived home in the dark, got out of my car, turned round and there were three individuals with what looked like pickaxe handles already raised above their heads. I protected myself as best I could, but they hit me on the back of my head.[111]

A few weeks prior to the attack, Cass had lambasted the government to *The Times*. After admitting that he didn't have a dog because 'I'm not sure I would be able to look after it properly' – a declaration which 'chilled' the interviewer – he called Tony Blair a 'bastard' for not doing enough to help him.[112] Despite New Labour taking unprecedented action to keep his failing company open, and Cambridgeshire Police allocating forty officers to work on HLS full time,[113] Cass didn't hold back. However, following the attack, the offence he had caused was swiftly forgiven and forgotten.

A month later, the Pharmaceutical Industry Competitiveness Task Force (PICTF) – set up by Tony Blair in 1999 to appease GlaxoSmithKline (GSK) – published their first report. It laid out the industry's power over the government in stark terms:

> Decisions and actions taken by Government will have a major influence on future investment decisions made by the industry and thereby on the contribution it makes to the UK economy … the importance therefore of the PICTF initiative cannot be overstated.[114]

The British government were not willing to risk the £7 billion invested annually by the pharmaceutical industry, particularly since Chancellor Gordon Brown had pinned his economic blueprint on their support.[115] Faced with financial blackmail, the government bent over backwards to sate them, introducing sweeping tax cuts, increasing the price of drugs for the NHS, and relaxing licensing regulation for animal research.[116] The industry demanded amendments to the Criminal Justice and Police Bill (CJPB), the Malicious Communications Act, and the Companies Act, intending to criminalise previously lawful protests; Lord Sainsbury agreed without hesitation. While discussing the CJPB, Lord Jenkin made a contrary statement, which encapsulated the state's attitude – and frustration – towards SHAC:

> The leaders of SHAC have not hidden themselves ... but they have been in receipt of very careful legal advice. They themselves take great care not to fall foul of the existing law.[117]

The government immediately began changing those laws, hopeful that the 'leaders' of SHAC would run afoul of them. They arranged for senior government ministers and pharmaceutical executives to meet four times a year, and invited Brian Cass to Parliament for a private discussion with Home Secretary Jack Straw.[118]

Under intense lobbying from the pro-vivisection Research Defence Society (RDS), amendments to the CJPB passed through Parliament and into the House of Lords. Lord Renton – who had granted HLS' initial planning application – claimed that HLS kept animals in conditions no different to those living as well-loved family members, despite overwhelming evidence to the contrary. Lord Phillips described the new legislation as 'by far the most draconian restriction of peaceful protest ever contemplated for our law'.[119] But with fears for Gordon Brown's economic strategy raised yet again, the bill was enacted into law.[120]

The legislation gave the police authority to disperse home demonstrations. A few weeks later, a director of HLS' largest shareholder received an unexpected phone call at 7 o'clock in the morning. SHAC activists informed him that they had just set up protest on the roof of his house. Mr Powell was on his way to work at the Bank of New York. He hung up the phone and left the police to work out how to remove the activists and their enormous banner.

Over 60 police officers scratched their heads for nine long hours, unable to use their new powers to disperse the protestors. As they searched for a solution, one of Mr Powell's neighbours offered to send up some cups of tea to help keep the protest going. With the entire road cordoned off, police eventually called in a specialist climbing team who carried Kerry Whitburn and Kate Simpson from the roof.

The following month, activists implemented a new tactic at HLS itself. At 4 o'clock one Thursday afternoon, campaigners drove a small fleet of cars and parked them across the gates of the laboratory. The drivers slashed the tyres and left the scene. Ten passengers handcuffed their arms inside metal tubes welded underneath the vehicles. It was a well-rehearsed operation, trialled and perfected in a remote part of rural Wales.

The staff at HLS found themselves trapped behind their own razor wire, unable to leave. More and more police arrived, but six cars, three riot vans, and a helicopter could do nothing. Finally, HLS' security emerged with pruning shears to cut down the hedgerow along the front of the laboratory. Staff squeezed their cars around the blockade and headed home.

With the protest broken up, and those involved loaded into police cars, one campaigner declared:

> We are doing this to highlight the plight of the animals inside HLS. Up to 500 animals are killed every day inside this place, and if this action plays even a small part in closing this place down, then I am happy to be arrested for it.[121]

Lock-ons were not just reserved for HLS. In San Francisco, police smashed through a Plexiglas door with hatchets to remove a group of activists who had D-locked themselves together inside a Stephens Inc. office. Meanwhile in Boston, another Stephens' office lock-on saw three activists arrested and taken to the police station while still chained together. At the station, the police violently cut the locks, resulting in one activist being taken to hospital with a 'deep wound'.[122]

Back in the UK, HLS' shareholder Morgan Stanley Dean Witter (MSDW) became the next target. Four activists D-locked their heads to the main entrance of the company. Another two attached themselves to the revolving doors of a side entrance, and three more chained themselves together at another exit. Other campaigners padlocked shut any remaining doors. Joseph Dawson took part in the action:

> Rather than locking their staff in, we decided it might cost MSDW more money if we locked them out. As soon as the lock-on was underway, the SHAC office issued a press release, and I was ready on the ground to conduct media interviews.
>
> I was near the front entrance, and the activists gave me the keys to their D-locks. Instinctively, I threw them into the Thames so that the police couldn't get them. Eventually a maintenance team unscrewed the door handles and

allowed those attached to the front door to leave. It was great they hadn't been arrested, but they now had D-locks firmly stuck around their necks, and the keys were at the bottom of the river. Oops! We had to search east London for an amiable mechanic who was willing to cut them off.

Removing the door handles allowed MSDW's security to get staff to their desks, but five campaigners were attached to more permanent fixtures and remained firmly in place. The security team placed screens around them as the activists stayed put for several more hours.

When asked for a comment on the incident, SHAC reported MSDW as saying:

> We are sick of hearing about those bloody beagles at HLS. Don't you understand – we don't care ... as long as we make money out of this, I personally couldn't give a shit whether Huntingdon kill 500,000 animals a day, never mind 500.[123]

HLS' financial situation continued to flounder and was set to get worse. NatWest finally severed its last connection with HLS and closed their bank account. HLS suddenly found themselves without banking facilities, and no other bank was willing to help them.

Once more, Lord Sainsbury and the British government galloped to their rescue. In an unprecedented move, the Department of Trade and Industry (DTI) opened a bank account at the Bank of England (BoE) for HLS.[124] They were the first, and perhaps last, company to be given this privilege, usually reserved exclusively for government departments and commercial banks. Mark Matfield, director of the pro-vivi-section lobby group the Research Defence Society (RDS), commented:

This is the perfect solution for Huntingdon's banking problems. Activists can harass the directors of any commercial bank, but I don't think they're going to bring down the government.[125]

10
Give Shell Hell: 2001

There needs to be an understanding that this is a threat to all industries. The tactics could be extended to any other sectors of the economy.[126]

– Brian Cass, HLS' managing director

SHAC campaigned loudly against all animal research, which they denounced as archaic and unreliable, arguing for it to be replaced with future-facing technologies and human cell-based models. They were frustrated by media descriptions of HLS as a 'medical research centre'[127] when they regularly exploitated animals for products including: paint, food additives, glue, and clothes dyes.[128]

In 2001, SHAC uncovered a research paper commissioned by oil giant Royal Dutch Shell. Shell had a shocking history of human rights[129] and environmental abuses,[130] and absolutely no connection to medical research.

The study saw HLS feed PVC plasticisers to pregnant rats, and then to their offspring. The mothers – and later their children – were killed and dissected.[131] In a telephone conversation, Shell informed SHAC that they were a regular customer of HLS, who would test products including food wrapping and detergents on their behalf. Outraged, SHAC declared:

We have sent them the evidence of horrific animal cruelty and staff incompetence at HLS, and they have not even bothered to reply.

It is time for Shell to get a slamming ... Like the NatWest bank, they are a high-profile name that everyone knows. Like the NatWest bank, they have a PR image that they spend millions on every year, and like the NatWest bank they will come to realise that being involved with the animal murderers at HLS means trouble nationwide.[132]

Launching a website called 'Give Shell Hell',[133] SHAC provided their supporters with another highly visible and easily accessible target. The Shell campaign took off immediately.

Fifteen activists from Liverpool occupied and blockaded their local Shell petrol station, forcing the shop to close as they plastered stickers and leaflets over shelves. In Manchester, twelve campaigners toured with a megaphone and a giant bunny costume. Down in Plymouth, thirty activists ran onto a service station forecourt, turned off the electricity to the facility, padlocked the petrol pumps, and barricaded the entrance with wheelie bins. In Newcastle, two protestors climbed onto the awning with a banner. They stayed there for seven hours, creating images which campaigners began to replicate across the country.

Within weeks, protests had launched in every county of the UK, and eighteen separate countries. Shell rushed out a memo to all fuel station managers instructing them to close at the first sign of a protest. In response, twenty activists took over a petrol station in Stoke-on-Trent, where four of them D-locked themselves together at the entrance, preventing traffic from entering: a taster of what was to follow.

* * *

After two hours locked inside a removal van, I was greeted by Sarah Gisborne as she opened the doors with a pair of boxer shorts stretched over her face as a makeshift mask. It was 6 o'clock on a cold morning in 2001, and we were in the middle of the access route for Ellesmere Port Oil Refinery in Cheshire. I leapt out of the van to help my travel companions unload several oil barrels filled with concrete and line them across the road. Sarah hopped back into the driver's seat and disappeared.

Each of the barrels had a tube through it, wide enough to slide an arm in, and in the middle was a metal bar. We each roped a carabiner to one wrist and clipped it to the bar, securing our arms inside the concrete drum. Within minutes we were fastened in place and blockading the entrance. At each access point, a total of thirty-four activists formed human barricades.[134]

I lay on the freezing tarmac dreaming of a warm coat or a sleeping bag. Within minutes, a lorry pulled up behind my head. It was terrifying. We had no idea how angry the driver might be, and were entirely defenceless. If he decided to ram our barricade, we would die. Fortunately, the driver was understanding. After a quiet grumble, he seemed content to wait in his cab.

He didn't have to wait long. As soon as the police arrived, they advised the growing queue of hauliers to turn around and sit out the protest elsewhere. We lay on the cold road for nine long hours – costing Shell a rumoured £2 million – before the police managed to remove us.

As protests against Shell intensified, the *Daily Mirror* ran an article titled 'Sweetener slaughter':

Beagles were among thousands of animals killed in laboratory tests on a new artificial sweetener.

The dogs probably had their throats cut, while marmoset monkeys died from brain damage, and rabbits were poisoned during a twenty-year study into the effects of Sucralose. The sweetener – sold in the United States as Splenda – is expected to be on sale in the UK in a couple of months.

Researchers estimate that 12,800 animals died during the research.

In one experiment at the controversial Huntingdon Research Centre in Cambridgeshire, four beagle puppies were starved before being force-fed Sucralose through tubes. Researchers took blood samples from the animals' jugular veins and examined their urine and faeces to discover the effect of Sucralose on their metabolisms ...

An unspecified number of marmoset monkeys died or were killed after they were force-fed Sucralose at the Life Science Research lab in Eye, Suffolk, now part of Huntingdon Life Sciences. Twelve male monkeys aged under 10 months were examined and force-fed Sucralose for seven weeks. On the seventh day of the study two of the monkeys died from brain defects, a third was killed after four weeks and the remainder of the brain-damaged animals were put down. In another British-based experiment, also carried out at Eye, rabbits were given a dose of Sucralose 1,200 times the expected human daily intake. Many died from trauma. Others suffered extreme weight loss, convulsions, and intestinal disorders.[135]

Three days after the article appeared in the *Mirror*, SHAC received a statement from Splenda's manufacturer, Tate & Lyle, confirming that they would never use HLS again.

Despite the 'sweetener slaughter', mainstream media returned to calling HLS a 'drug testing laboratory' as seamlessly as SHAC returned to targeting HLS directly.

On Thursday, 26 July, a car drove slowly past the entrance to HLS. As discretely as possible, the driver asked two local women who were holding a spontaneous protest to leave. As they made a casual exit, two removal trucks pulled up carrying seven concrete-filled barrels. The lone officer who had been monitoring the small protest watched in shock as a team of activists unloaded the concrete barrels into the road, and the trucks drove away. A relative of an HLS employee – arriving to collect a family member from work – offered to help, telling protestors he thought what they were doing was brilliant. Before the police officer could stop them, ten protestors chained themselves to the barrels and sealed the road. Once more, HLS were under siege.

By coincidence, camera crews from ITV were on-site, filming for the documentary series *Jobs from Hell*.[136] Little could have underlined that title better than staff being barricaded inside their workplace.

Eventually, some staff left the laboratory on foot, escorted towards the main road by police officers. A police helicopter hovered overhead. Inside the foreboding fences, HLS' managing director, Brian Cass, was seen prowling back and forth, unable to hide his frustration that the film crew were interviewing protestors.

After four hours, police located a pallet lift. Ignoring cries that arms were likely to break, they moved one barrel – and the protestors attached to it – to the side of the road. That created enough of a gap to allow workers to squeeze their cars through. Brian Cass was the last to leave at 9 pm.

Pressure continued to mount on the British government. Campaigners handed a petition containing 300,000 signatures, calling for the immediate closure of HLS, to an official at the Home Office.[137] The petition was ignored, and the police later claimed it never even existed.[138]

Concern amongst HLS' customers ran so high that the CEOs of Shell, Glaxo, BP, Bayer, and a host of other companies called a meeting to air their grievances to senior politicians. To ensure the meeting stayed secret, no one was allowed to refer to it in writing; it could only be discussed over the phone or in person. However, at 9:30 am, as the meeting was about to begin, SHAC activists appeared out of nowhere, much to the dismay of the host, Dame Judith Hackett, from the Chemical Industries Association:

It is very disturbing that SHAC has learnt of this meeting. We have no idea how this was leaked, and as you can hear, the noise from the protesters is deafening outside. I really am amazed that they have found this out.[139]

Joseph Dawson helped organise regular protests in the City of London, where increasingly complex precautions were taken to stay one step ahead of the authorities:

The police would turn up en masse to advertised protests and try to stop us legally protesting. After we stopped advertising them, they tapped the SHAC phone line, and we would arrive at an arranged meeting point to find police already there. In the end we developed a system; each tube station had a number, and each day and time had a code. We carried out many successful demos that way without police harassment.

On one such protest, twenty activists stormed the Bank of New York (BNY) building in Canary Wharf. Security rugby tackled and evicted the intruders, shut off the elevators, and sealed all entrances. Despite their efforts, one campaigner dashed all the way to the forty-ninth floor. Other protestors scattered throughout the building, using megaphones and air horns to make as much noise as possible. Outside, someone set off a series of fireworks, and thousands of city employees gathered against the glass walls of their buildings to gaze in shock at the unfolding chaos. As the protestors finished their action and left, police sealed off the front of the building and prevented all London Underground trains from leaving Canary Wharf station.

Meanwhile, protests against one of HLS' brokers, Winterflood Securities, pressured them to abandon the laboratory. The final broker followed suit, leaving HLS with no brokers and in breach of the London Stock Exchange's trading rules. They were kicked down to the Seats Plus system,[140] which the *Financial Times* described as 'a trading system that resembles a lonely-hearts column'.[141]

In the USA, a group calling themselves the Pirates for Animal Liberation took a rather unique action:

In the wee hours of Tuesday, July 24th, we paid a visit to the home of Brian G Rogan, President of Capital Markets to The Bank of New York. 20 holes were drilled in the right side of his 30-foot yacht, and one six-inch by six-inch hole was sawed through the right hull.

Various workings of the boat were also tampered with. As the boat began to take on water, it was cut loose and pushed out to sea. We left before confirming whether or not the boat sank. Both the boat and his personal dock were left covered with painted slogans denouncing BNY's involvement with Huntingdon Life Sciences; the largest reading, 'money means nothing, life means everything'.

Upon escape we cut through his estate to his personal flagpole, his flag was lowered and replaced with the only flag that matters, a pirate flag.[142]

A few days later, thirty SHAC USA activists held a home demonstration outside the same address wearing pirate hats.[143]

As HLS prepared to host its AGM in the heart of New York's financial district, 200 activists waited outside. Eying the activists, the building owners got cold feet. Without notice, they cancelled the event and told HLS to find a new venue. HLS postponed the event, but not a single building in New York was willing to host them. Claiming that the cancellation was due to 'scheduling conflicts',[144] an HLS spokesperson later bemoaned having to host an AGM at all:

> An AGM is supposed to be for shareholders to discuss strategy, but at the last AGM the only people to turn up were animal rights campaigners, who don't want to take the company forward, but want to be destructive.[145]

Without a venue, HLS cancelled the AGM indefinitely, putting them in breach of company law.[146] SHAC took private legal action, and HLS were found guilty, though they were handed an absolute discharge.[147]

SHAC USA teamed up with Physicians for Responsible Medicine, a group of doctors and health care professionals scientifically opposed to animal research. They wrote to all of HLS' customers, explaining the flaws in specific pieces of research, and invited HLS and Stephens Inc. to a scientific debate on the efficacy of animal testing.

HLS and Stephens Inc. failed to respond. Instead, they pooled together $650,000 and used RICO laws – designed to protect small businesses from the mafia[148] – in an attempt to sue SHAC USA for millions of dollars in damages.[149] Jake Conroy was one of those named on the lawsuit:

They wanted to sue us for $12 million apiece, and told us that we could either stop the campaign, or they would pursue – and almost certainly win – the lawsuit.

Kevin, Lauren, and I refused. Finally it became clear that we had pushed this as far as we possibly could. Kevin and I went into the courtroom in our cheap suits, with our one attorney and faced all of HLS and Stephens' attorneys, and executives from both corporations. We came to an agreement we weren't happy with and consented to return a week later to sign the paperwork.

One of the attorneys for Stephens Inc. gave us a smirk as if to say they'd won. It really put me and Kevin's backs up. We returned the following week, with all the HLS and Stephens people there to see us sign this deal and end SHAC USA. We went in and just said, 'No deal.' They were pissed.

Now we had to win before they won their lawsuit, or we would wind up owing them $12 million each. To me that exemplifies the SHAC campaign. We didn't talk about anything except winning, and we were prepared to risk everything. We were going to fight, and we were going to win for the animals.

11

SHAC Europe: 2001

Terrorism is most likely to make the front page, but Animal Rights Extremism is what's most likely to affect your day-to-day business operations in Western Europe.[150]

– US State Department

With SHAC USA in full swing, and international activists acting in support of the Shell campaign, SHAC opened a new front to tackle HLS on a global scale. The most effective place to pressure European pharmaceutical companies was on their home turf.

SHAC's first European tour occurred in the summer of 2001, with twenty activists travelling from the UK to France, Germany, Switzerland, and the Netherlands. Two minibuses of campaigners stormed into the offices of Merial, DuPont, Pharmacia, Novartis, Bayer, and Yamanouchi.[151]

Weeks later came a second tour. Kev, a teenage activist from East Anglia, took part in both:

When I first heard of the cruelty inside HLS, it shocked me to my core. If I did nothing, what did that say about me? I had to act. I jumped at the chance to go on the Euro tour. I told my mum I was going away for a few days with friends. I had no idea what I was getting involved in, and I was both scared and excited.

Arriving in Paris for the first time in my life was a day I'll never forget. We walked into the AGM of one animal testing company with little questioning. We locked ourselves in the boardroom with all these angry men in suits. We put animals on their AGM agenda.

In Lyon, we tried to enter a Merial facility where experiments were taking place. However, the security caught one of us. We stormed their hut, grabbed our friend, and ran. As we left the country, we saw lines of police vehicles rushing down the other side of the motorway towards the laboratory.

We turned up at an animal testing lab in Germany owned by Bayer. I found an open door and in I went. I couldn't have prepared myself for what confronted me. I saw large, beautiful white rabbits in small plastic containers stacked on top of each other and was horrified to see that everything I had heard and read about animal experiments was real. Something had been done to their eyes, which were red and inflamed. It haunted me for a long time, but our action was cut short by the sound of police arriving. I wanted to free them, but the chance had gone.

We tried to get away but were stopped as a police officer barked at us in German. I had no idea what he was saying until he shouted, 'Stop.' I looked back and saw the officer was armed, and I was arrested at gunpoint. We were bundled into a police van and taken to a state detention centre. I was ordered to place my hands on red markers on the dark concrete walls, was searched, and had all my belongings removed. It was great to finally get released a few hours later. The police had taken all our money, but this didn't stop us. We regrouped and got ready to plough on with Europe at our feet and the whole pharmaceutical industry wondering who would be next.

Following the laboratory protests, activists visited the home of Union Carbide director James Robertson, another HLS' customer. They plastered his front door in leaflets and stickers before moving on to the offices of Dow and Arpida in Switzerland. The tour finished in the financial heart of Brussels, where activists used an elevator to travel to the third floor of the Bank of New York. Once inside, they let loose with megaphones, stickers, and leaflets.

Mainland Europe had a proud history of animal liberation activism, but this whirlwind of action felt like something new. The British were invading, and they were bringing one of the hardest-hitting social justice campaigns in the world. In Germany, one local paper anxiously reported that 'militant animal welfare activists' were on their way:

> A certain nervousness exists at the Bayer plant in Leverkusen because something bad seems to be coming from England. Security measures were increased as extremely militant animal welfarist have formed themselves to attack not only Bayer but also other firms that conduct animal experiments. They don't follow the usual method of demonstrating in front of the gates of the firms. Instead, they force their way into their offices, destroy documents, and liberate the animals.
>
> That they have now shifted their activity into France and Germany is a new dimension for the police and of course for the targeted firms in Germany. The Bayer plant has instructed their workers on higher security measures. Nonetheless, a serious trepidation exists.[152]

The UK has long been regarded as the birthplace of the modern animal liberation movement. Formed in 1824, the RSPCA was the world's first animal welfare organisation.[153]

Later in the nineteenth century, the suffragettes were instrumental in pioneering anti-vivisection activism.[154] Radical activists split from the RSPCA in 1924 to form the League Against Cruel Sports,[155] who split again to found the Hunt Saboteurs in 1963,[156] and the Band of Mercy (which later became the ALF) in 1972.[157] When the campaigns against Consort and Hill Grove were waged across the Channel, several activists from mainland Europe visited the UK to help and take notes.

With SHAC taking on a multinational company with a multinational campaign, European activists realised that the British animal liberation movement was coming to them.

Local activists were inspired by the energy and determination of the tours. After the German animal rights magazine *Voice* ran a six-page article about SHAC,[158] activists formed a satellite group in Berlin and another in the west of the country. Within weeks they amalgamated into SHAC Deutschland, and took up the fight against HLS' collaborators in the pharmaceutical heartlands along the Rhine basin.[159]

In Italy, an activist called Claudio seized the opportunity:

I had followed the British campaigns all the way from Consort, and I dreamed of starting something like that. We didn't have the strength to start a proper campaign. But I saw in SHAC the opportunity to do something and be part of a global campaign, even with a small group.

I created a newsletter and set up an email list, hoping to find more activists and become more visible, so we could eventually launch a campaign of our own in Italy.

At the time, Italian animal rights groups were more focused on welfare than liberation. A lot of people needed action, needed to do something new. We gave them that opportunity. Also, there were many people from the environmental and anarchist movements attracted to SHAC's strategies and tactics, so we drew from both groups. They didn't always get on, but we ensured our new group appealed to animal rights activists and political activists, and we ended up with a lot of support.

As SHAC Italia expanded, Claudio visited the UK. Staying at the SHAC office, he learned how the campaign ran on a day-to-day basis and took this knowledge home to apply to his growing chapter.

Groups in Belgium, the Netherlands, Sweden, and the Czech Republic came next.[160] The effect was contagious, and action reports began to appear from as far away as Argentina, South Africa, and Australia.

With SHAC strengthening its global presence, so too did HLS. They were desperate to retain shareholders, and convinced the government to promise new laws to protect shareholder anonymity.[161] However, financial institutions in the City of London baulked at the wider consequences of such measures, forcing the government to do a U-turn.

The state of Maryland in the USA did offer this protection. Unless a person held at least 5 per cent of a company's shares for six months, they were forbidden from knowing who the other shareholders were.[162] This system seemed ideal for HLS. However, it involved moving their headquarters to another country – on paper, at least – and delisting from the London Stock Exchange to join the North American NASDAQ. HLS did not have that kind of money to spare, and so CEO Andrew Baker agreed to invest more of his own cash. He created a new Maryland-based company called Life Sciences Research (LSR), which bought out HLS and became their parent company.[163]

To meet the NASDAQ's criteria, HLS needed to increase their share price, so the move required a consolidation. For every twenty-five HLS shares someone owned, they would receive just one – more valuable – LSR share. Conveniently, this process left 15 per cent of LSR's shares unclaimed, and Baker and Stephens Inc. scooped these up.[164] It was an unpopular move for HLS' other shareholders, but they had no choice but to accept.[165]

While it promised to be a profitable move for Baker, for HLS' managing director, Brian Cass, the whole affair was a major embarrassment. Just six months earlier he had told a local newspaper, 'If we move off the UK exchange to the US, [SHAC] have effectively won. It's a stand that has to be made.'[166]

To minimise scrutiny, and to dodge uncomfortable questions about whether SHAC had now in fact won, HLS made the announcement quietly on Christmas Eve. They knew that most people would be focused on festivities rather than HLS' financial woes.

Even as the move was being planned, activists in North America signalled that the country was no safe harbour for HLS – for the second time in less than a year they rescued dogs due to be tested on and killed inside the laboratory:

We visited Marshall Farms in upstate NY, liberating thirty beagle puppies and ten ferrets. After outsmarting constant security patrols, we scaled the electrified fence, breaking through the door of one of the approximately fifty sheds of animals. Inside, we found hundreds of beagle puppies waiting to be shipped to vivisection labs, destined to be killed.

We packed up thirty puppies and ten ferrets and stole away into the night with them, taking them away from their hellish life, and giving them a life filled with freedom and joy.[167]

PART IV

The Rise: 2001–03

Buoyed by their success, [SHAC] want nothing less than to change the world.[1]

– BBC Radio 4

12

Scooby Says Go Get 'Em: 2001

I think for what they do vivisectionists deserve to be harassed, persecuted and pursued.[2]

– Alexei Sayle, actor and writer

When nineteen Al-Qaeda jihadists hijacked four passenger jets and flew them into high-profile buildings in the USA, everyone felt the change. Outside of Muslim communities, who saw simmering institutional racism explode into visceral public hatred, the demographic perhaps most affected by the fallout from 9/11 were protestors.

I vividly remember my first demonstration after 9/11. Four of us held signs and chanted protest slogans outside a sprawling JP Morgan office complex on the outskirts of Bournemouth. The company held shares in HLS, and we had been conducting regular protests for weeks. This time was different. When the police arrived, they didn't joke with us, nor usher us out of the road and onto a verge. An officer approached me with one hand hovering over his baton. He looked me in the eye and simply said, 'You can't do this anymore.'

Things were never the same after that. It was like a hand had clenched us, and every day it squeezed a little tighter. Protests became about clinging on to the fundamental right to have our voices heard, not just the causes we were fighting for.

Perhaps the most insidious change was increasing comparisons of animal liberation campaigners to terrorists. Industry representatives[3] and lobby groups[4,5] were the first to make this false equivalence, but soon Parliament[6] and the police[7] did so too. For a long time, we laughed off the absurdity of it. The idea that someone chanting through a megaphone, occupying an office, or even pouring paint onto a car could be on a par with a suicide bomber seemed ludicrous. But the years that followed violently eroded our nonchalance.

SHAC USA faced a tough choice. Their country was in turmoil, and over 300 million citizens each tried to grapple with what had happened in their own way. After much deliberation, the organisers of SHAC USA decided to follow the advice of President, George W. Bush, who declared:

> None of us will ever forget this day, yet we go forward to defend freedom, and all that is good and just in our world.[8]

With their commander-in-chief encouraging US citizens to return to normal by going shopping, getting on planes, and heading to Disney World, SHAC USA decided that they too should return to normal as swiftly as possible. Amidst all the turmoil and fallout from 9/11, the poisoning, dissection, and killing of animals inside HLS continued without respite.

With that in mind, SHAC USA continued to plan the largest protest Stephens Inc. would ever see in their hometown of Little Rock. Arkansas police weren't taking any chances. They warned hospitals to brace for an influx of victims of chemical contact – meaning their own CS spray – and prepared for a showdown.[9]

Josh Harper temporarily moved to the city to help organise the demonstration:

> We had to acquire a permit from the local government, and part of that meant providing our planned parade route. I went out one day on my bike to plan the march and got fol-

lowed by local police in an unmarked car for miles. As I was cycling home, they veered towards me, forcing me off the road, and making me crash into the ditch.

Warren Stephens owned many of the buildings in downtown Little Rock. He paid off-duty cops to act as private security at those buildings, meaning that many local officers were reliant upon him for a portion of their income. The loyalty they had for him and the pressure they put on us to leave him alone was intense. By the end of our protest there, I was genuinely scared for my safety. I couldn't wait to get out of town.

Warren Stephens had contacts in higher places than the police force. In the run-up to the demonstration, Stephens Inc. lobbied the local government to implement an ordinance limiting protest.[10] They passed the law overnight without public debate. As a result, when hundreds of activists turned up in the town, police ordered them to stay inside a metal pen, dubbed a 'free speech zone'.[11]

Brenda Shoss was amongst those arriving, and as she approached, a frantic group of other protestors flagged her down:

They warned me, 'Carry the pepper spray antidote; cover your face with a mask or bandanna'. What?! I usually only bring armloads of leaflets, banners, props, and costumes. Surely I won't need to protect myself from the police? Boy, was I wrong.

The first incidence of police brutality occurred outside of Stephens' glass high rise, where protesters pressed against barricades until they toppled over. Police officers and demonstrators became parallel lines, no longer separated by tape and metal. When protesters stepped over the now invisible blockade, police erupted like an overblown balloon. They instantly drew pepper-spray canisters and tear gas as if cowboys in an Old West duel. They sprayed two people in the face. An ear-shattering explosion resonated. I was sure it was a gun but was later told it was a 'sound bomb'. An unfortunate newscaster was knocked down and pepper sprayed. As I surveyed the scene, I observed a young girl on the ground, sobbing and gasping from inhaled pepper spray. A young man's face a watery red mix of fear and anger as he struggled to flush the chemicals out of his eyes.

I saw Josh Harper on the ground, a brutal red welt running down his cheek. When Josh had crossed the police line, one officer said, 'Hit Harper.' Another officer shot a rubber bullet into his face at close range.

Another activist was shot in the eye and rushed to a local hospital. The second wave of disproportionate hostility occurred as we parked our banners and bodies in the middle of Louisiana Street, in front of the Stephens Inc. garage.

A few activists crossed over the police line to sit on the pavement. They linked arms. More joined them. That is when the officers pretty much lost it. I watched as they dragged off activists, hoisting them off the ground like weightless dolls. I saw one young man carted off in an inverted backbend as one cop held his feet, and another grasped his hands. All were limp in an act of passive resistance. Then the cops charged at us. But this time I had no open space before me, only a brick wall. Suddenly I was enveloped in a panic-stricken tangle of arms and legs. I needed to run to the edge. I couldn't think. I couldn't see. Posters and props became confetti in the rush to escape.[12]

Police had identified Josh Harper as an organiser, and pursued him as he attempted to head home:

The cops were following me. I was tackled and dragged into a parking lot where they punched me in the head, knocked my glasses off, put me in a chokehold until I couldn't breathe, handcuffed me, and then carried me down to a bus.

Some of the people who were arrested that day had never been arrested before. In some cases, this was the first demonstration that they had ever attended. Many of them were standing legally on the sidewalk when the cops rushed in and just started snatching people at random. There's something very radicalising about that. They started going back to their communities. They were outraged, and they were angry, and they were raring to go.[13]

Twenty-six activists were arrested,[14] and many more sustained injuries from the police, including a broken wrist, and further wounds from rubber bullets.[15]

To obtain their permit, SHAC USA had been ordered to designate a 'leader' who would march at the front of the procession. That leader was Kevin Kjonaas. But with so many protestors wearing masks, police failed to notice that he wasn't actually there. Kevin was hundreds of miles away, boarding a flight to the UK. His intimate knowledge of running SHAC was needed elsewhere.

In the early aftermath of 9/11, SHAC faced their first major court case in the UK. Over a year after their arrest for inciting a public nuisance with their second newsletter, Gregg, Natasha, and Heather finally faced Judge Zoe Smith from the dock of Basildon Crown Court.

The newsletter had called for people to make nuisance phone calls, send unwanted mail, and cause low-level criminal damage to NatWest property. Many of those on the receiving end of such actions were eager to give evidence, with witnesses lining up to describe the frustration of receiving up to twenty unwanted letters every day or having to spend hours returning unsolicited mail-order items.[16]

The media zeroed in on the 'Scooby says ... go get 'em!' cartoon, complete with the home addresses of HLS' directors and staff. Perhaps, ironically, that article contained nothing illegal. Home demonstrations had been lawful at the time, and there was no suggestion that Scooby was inciting anyone to 'get 'em' through more sinister means.

Calls for fly posting, plastering stickers on cash machines, and mail and telephone blockades were harder to explain. While they maintained their intention was to conduct a 'lawful but vigorous campaign',[17] the three defendants pleaded guilty.

As she handed down a twelve-month sentence – with half suspended – to each of them, Judge Smith stated:

> I accept there is a legitimate debate on whether experiments should be conducted on animals, but there is a proper way to engage in this debate.[18]

She did not offer any insight into exactly how that debate should be conducted, with a government so deeply rooted in the opposing side. Ultimately, Heather, Natasha, and Gregg spent three months in prison. It was far short of the multi-year sentences HLS and the police had pushed for, and the UK campaign – now fronted by Kevin Kjonaas – did little to hide their delight:

> The SHAC campaign had been anticipating the loss of these three great activists and has taken the appropriate steps to make sure the campaign continues even better than before.
>
> Although everyone who cares about the animals suffering inside HLS right now should be ecstatic over the minimal sentencing, we still view this as a travesty of justice. This

sentence is unjustifiable in comparison with the measly fifty hours community service the HLS employees got for punching that puppy in the face. Or the slap on the wrist HLS got from the government for the countless breaches of the Good Laboratory Practice regulations for fraudulent science and their horrendous record of animal abuse.

HLS employees are animal killers. All they know five days a week, eight hours a day, is violence, suffering, and death. They are sick people who need psychological help. Gregg, Heather, and Natasha recognised that fact when they pushed their activism a step further than most and encouraged people (via cartoons like Scooby Doo) to make the job of torturing animals inside of HLS a little harder. Nothing more.[19]

Following the court case, SHAC hired a barrister to check and approve their website on a weekly basis, as well as every subsequent issue of their newsletter. Home addresses were never published again, and comprehensive disclaimers were added, requesting all campaigners remain within the law.

Despite SHAC's defiant statement, it was a dark time for the global animal rights movement. A week before sentencing, on 5 November, veteran activist Barry Horne died on his final hunger strike.[20] However, if anyone thought this would dampen the movement's resolve, they were in for disappointment.

Barry's declaration from his third hunger strike in 1998 resonated once more, becoming a rallying call throughout the animal liberation movement:

The fight is not for us, not for our personal wants and needs. It is for every animal that has ever suffered and died in the vivisection labs, and for every animal that will suffer and die in those same labs unless we end this evil business now. The souls of the tortured dead cry out for justice, the cry of the living is for freedom. We can create that justice, and we can deliver that freedom. The animals have no one but us. We will not fail them.[21]

While most SHAC activists threw themselves into the lawful campaign, others like Sarah Gisborne faced a quandary. Sarah had been working in the SHAC offices, helping with admin and protests, and now watched as her friends went to prison for publishing a newsletter. She decided that if prison was the potential outcome either way, perhaps she should take action that warranted it:

SHAC was a lawful campaign. We were running an office, fundraising on the streets, organising legal demonstrations, and were on the phone a lot. Most people I knew were very law-abiding citizens. They hated injustice, and I think that's what drives all of us: the injustice. I was involved in the day-to-day running of the campaign; I lived and breathed it, but it wasn't enough for me, so I took it upon myself to do other things at night, and sometimes during the day. I thought about it long and hard before I started to do it, and it felt acceptable in light of what was happening in Huntingdon.

Some friends and I went to Cass' brother's house to pressure Cass to stop what he was doing. The idea was to make him think a bit harder about it all. When we threw bricks through the windows of the house, neighbours came out and a chase began. We dove into the car and raced at high speed through country lanes, but the neighbours followed. We hit the main road at speed. In the middle of the night, with no other traffic, we really stood out. About twelve police cars lined up behind us in pursuit, so I cranked up the stereo with some fast music, and thought, 'Fuck it, we might as well enjoy it.' The police chase spanned a couple of counties. We finally got rammed by a police car; some people legged it on foot, and I just sat in the car and put my hands up. That was that.

As police dragged Sarah Gisborne from her car, SHAC's unofficial anthem, 'Sandstorm' by Darude, was still blasting. SHAC USA later used the song in a promotional video, making it synonymous for many campaigners with the lively actions it underscored.

Other activists like Lynn Sawyer continued using less confrontational means to maintain the pressure on HLS:

One day I went to HLS for a protest, but as I arrived, the guards weren't looking, so I drove in and parked amongst the worker's cars. Not believing my luck, I walked about trying doors until a guy opened the entrance to the rodent unit for me.

I knew I would not be able to leave without being caught, so I found a small office and barricaded myself in. I didn't have my phone, so I tried using the telephone in the office to call the switchboard, and they put me through to SHAC's office number. I spoke to someone there to tell them I'd set up the HLS branch of SHAC and then sat it out.

Eventually the security woke up, and so did the police. I stayed put reading through supposedly confidential files which detailed how HLS workers took vaginal swabs from rats and mice every day for ten days prior to mating them. The police and HLS staff rebuked me for reading this as they looked on helplessly. After three hours, a man drilled through the wall enough to allow Sgt Ken Smith to kick it down and arrest me for vagrancy, burglary, abstracting electricity, and criminal damage.

Although Lynn escaped any punishment more serious than community service, as she waited for her court hearing, someone sent her a link to an online forum called Triple I. On this forum, HLS staff discussed raping her. She reported it to the police, but they took no action.

In a bizarre episode, SHAC USA received an unexpected donation of nearly £1,000 from the *Telegraph* newspaper.[22] It was an attempted sting operation, intended to prove that the money would fund criminality. Unfortunately for the newspaper, SHAC USA were not bankrolling the ALF. SHAC and SHAC USA kept accounts detailing all donations, and how they were spent. The *Telegraph*'s money paid for the printing and distribution of the next SHAC USA newsletter and didn't provide the scandalous exposé the newspaper had wished for.

Kevin Kjonaas' presence in the UK had not gone unnoticed. After a few short months helping run SHAC, the British government decided it was time for him to go:

I was at a meeting in a pub one afternoon. Out of nowhere, these people grabbed me, one on each side, ran me outside, and threw me in a car. One of the people I was with tried to stop them, because we didn't know who the fuck they were. It was only because of their intervention that one of these people had to announce that he was a police officer.

The officers locked me in the back of that car, and nobody spoke to me for the entire journey. One of them got a phone call. He just answered it by saying, 'I'm deaf right now,' and hung up. They wouldn't speak in front of me at all.

I got taken to Heathrow Airport detention centre, where I was the only person with English as a native language. I was there for about two weeks before we decided I should leave voluntarily. My best chance of returning to the UK would be to go back to the US and challenge it from there.

13

Insuring Trouble: 2002

Huntingdon had hoped to find sanctuary in the US, having been hounded almost to the point of extinction by Stop Huntingdon Animal Cruelty.[23]

– The *Telegraph*

In the first week of 2002, I was chained to the underside of a minibus outside HLS. I had learned my lessons from the Shell blockade. My right arm was locked inside a metal tube welded to the underside of a small coach, but my left arm was free. I had a sleeping bag, warm clothes, a book, a Walkman, and a pile of bottled water. Katy Brown was locked to the other end of the pipe, and between us we piled a mountain of sandwiches and snacks. We were ready to stay for a week if we could.

At the far end of the road, Don Currie had one arm locked to a car, and the other to a second minibus. He had no way of eating or drinking and had no comfort whatsoever. I've met few people with his determination and knew he would sacrifice those necessities for days if he had to.

When the police arrived, Sgt Ken Smith marched straight up to Don and threatened to release the handbrake on his car and roll it into the ditch, tearing Don's arm off. Fortunately, Smith's colleagues intervened and talked him down.

Police cutting teams tried – and failed – to extricate us. It was going exactly to plan, until one officer noticed a flaw in our set-up. A vital bolt, which should have been welded over, had instead been covered with some tacky gum. They picked off the gum, unscrewed the bolt, dragged us out, and arrested us.

We were devastated. It was all over in three brief hours, but we had attracted significant media attention and more negative publicity for HLS.

To coordinate actions at the gates of HLS, SHAC split a map of the UK into seven regions, and activists in each area had a specific day of the week to organise protests.[24] Staff turnover at HLS remained disproportionately high. Beyond the protests, one ex-employee, and former soldier, explained the emotional toll of working inside the laboratory:

I had seen rough things, but was not prepared for this, and I lasted three days. The beagles never saw daylight. Their vocal cords had been cut. They lived in tiny cages in semi-darkness, on a bare concrete floor and nothing else. Most had scars. Some had eyes missing. Some came to lick my fingers through the bars, tails wagging. Others retreated as far away from me as they could get, shivering and messing themselves because I was looking at them, terrified that I was going to hurt them some more.

Monkeys strapped into chairs, with various attachments linked to various parts of them. Others in cages, a little larger than the beagles', scarred, looking ill and old, afraid, and huddling and clinging or moving very slowly, or just sitting and staring. Even very young ones looked old.

Two horses were in a stall. When somebody asked to be told when the horses collapsed, I walked out to my car without bothering to ask about pay and went home and never went back.[25]

Exhausted by regular protests, Japanese pharmaceutical company Yamanouchi closed their flagship facility in Oxford, and moved it to mainland Europe.[26] However, if they thought this would prevent further attention they were mistaken: ALF activists torched their new offices in the Netherlands the following year.[27]

In February 2002, 1,000 SHAC supporters converged on the town of Huntingdon for a march. Two campaigners scaled the roof of the magistrates' court in support of the many activists who had been tried there. They unfurled a banner reading, 'No Justice, Just Us. Smash HLS.' At the end of the march hundreds of protestors breached police lines and sprinted to the home of an HLS worker for an impromptu protest. As police caught up, activists dashed to another employee's house. Several local teenagers, appalled to learn about their neighbour's employment, joined the protest and were later seen hurling garden ornaments through the house windows. As the police tried to move fifty activists and the group of local youths away from the property, the employee's car got crushed under the garage door, and a police officer had his hat stolen.

Meanwhile, HLS' plan to move their head office to Maryland wasn't going smoothly. They had delisted from the London Stock Exchange[28] but listing on the NASDAQ required at least one market maker to buy and sell their shares.[29] When they departed the UK, they had ten. However, within weeks of being contacted by SHAC USA, every single one deserted HLS. Some withdrew their services after seeing undercover footage from the laboratory, while others had been on the receiving end of intense protests. As HLS found themselves outflanked, they scrambled to enlist a replacement: Spencer Edwards. However, after a handful of protests, including one inside a director's house, they too changed their mind.[30]

Within months of moving their corporate offices to the USA to revive their fortunes, HLS were in limbo, unable to list their shares anywhere.

HLS took another blow during anti-globalisation protests in New York aimed at the World Economic Forum. Despite the attendance of over 15,000 anti-capitalist protestors from across the world, it was a march of 400 people, sponsored by SHAC USA, which garnered the most media attention. According to the *New York Times*:

> A cluster of demonstrators paused in front of a high-rise apartment building at 188 East 76th Street, which some of the protesters described as the home of a certain corporate executive. The building's windows were smashed, and red paint was splattered on the building.
>
> Once property had been damaged, scores of police officers swooped in. Three people were arrested, and the protesters split into separate camps that wended through the East Side streets, chanting slogans to the beat of drums. But no matter where they went, there were police officers in front of them, beside them, behind them – even above them, in helicopters.
>
> A standoff developed. But within a few minutes, the police were wading into the group and making arrests; sixty in all.[31]

The protest, which SHAC USA described as the largest-ever home demonstration, was against Parker Quillen of Quilcap Corp, HLS' second-biggest investor. A week later, Quilcap sold its entire stake in the laboratory.[32]

Amidst their growing crisis, HLS received a glimmer of hope when a venue in Panama, 2,000 miles from New York, finally agreed to host their AGM, a year after they had been forced to postpone.[33]

With HLS shares stagnating, campaigners shifted focus to the shareholders of Stephens Inc. As a result, the Bank of

America once again received protests in London and across the USA.

Just five months after declaring that the 'threshold for pain in the UK was pretty damn low',[34] Warren Stephens changed his attitude. Having been on the receiving end of several SHAC protests – and more militant actions from ALF activists, who covered his home in paint,[35] spent over $100,000 on his credit card, and dug up his favourite golf course – he conceded: 'We were aware of the activists, but I don't think we understood exactly what lengths they would go to.'[36]

Stephens Inc. sold their shares in HLS, and revoked their loan.[37] SHAC activists revelled in their victory. They had taken on a symbol of American wealth and power and won. Josh Harper explained:

I understand why home demonstrations and personal targeting is so controversial, but when you take a billionaire like Warren Stephens, he's got this tremendous amount of comfort and billions of dollars. And on the other hand, there is this group of activists and all they're doing is passing out leaflets and holding signs, money wins. Money wins that situation. But, if you suddenly start clarifying that he has to deal with you, because every time he plays golf; there you are. When he goes out shopping; there you are. And when he comes home; there you are …[38]

That day, activism won. They defeated Stephens Inc. – but HLS were not going down so easily. They had learned their lesson from NatWest and already had a new lender agreed and in place. There would be no begging the British government for help; this time it really was 'business as usual'. HLS struck a deal with the Securities and Exchanges Commission (SEC) in the USA and the Financial Services Authority (FSA) in the

UK, which kept all information on the new lender private.[39] They remained on the brink of closure, but losing Stephens Inc. would not be the finishing blow.

Unable to penetrate the SEC's confidentiality precautions, SHAC needed a new target – one which could offer the ultimate victory.

Gregg realised that a large company could not legally operate without insurance, and discovered HLS sourced theirs through the world's largest broker, Marsh.[40] No Marsh meant no insurance, and no insurance meant no HLS.

With 400 offices in over 100 countries, Marsh was the perfect target for the increasingly global reach of SHAC.[41] The Shell campaign was scaled back as the focus fell fully on HLS' insurers.

Within the first week of the campaign launch, protests occurred at eighteen of Marsh's UK offices. As always, SHAC announced the new campaign target, but local groups and individuals chose autonomously how they wanted to protest. Campaigners stormed buildings in London, Leeds, Norfolk, Leicester, Southampton, and Exeter, demanding to speak to senior management to show them the undercover videos. Megaphones and leaflets informed staff of their company's links to HLS, and at some sites activists unplugged computers and took paperwork. In Newcastle, protestors cut power to the entire building, and in Birmingham, they D-locked the front doors, meaning staff had to evacuate via the fire escape. During a London protest, activists arrived at a publicly advertised demo before the police did. As the protestors flooded the building, police accidentally locked them inside, securing the building against a demonstration which had already begun.

In County Durham, SHAC announced a protest at the grand opening of a pharmaceutical company due to be attended by

Marsh and Princess Anne. The insurance firm were promptly kicked off the billing.

The message from SHAC was simple:

> This is just for starters, Marsh. We've done it to countless companies, and we'll do it to you as well; nobody gets away with involving themselves with HLS.[42]

The protests spread globally. SHAC Deutschland descended on Marsh's offices in Dusseldorf, Frankfurt, Hamburg, Stuttgart, and Munich. Underground activists covered the Berlin offices in painted slogans at night, while SHAC campaigners wielding banners and leaflets stormed inside during the day. Similar actions took place in Austria and Switzerland.

Meanwhile, SHAC Italia coordinated a week of protests outside eight of Marsh's offices. Fifty activists gathered in Rome, and the four offices which didn't receive protests were subjected to phone, fax, and email blockades. It was a pivotal moment for Claudio and his nascent group:

> Marsh really changed the campaign for us. For the first time, we had a target in almost every city which we knew we could win.
>
> Over a full week we travelled from Milan to Naples – over 800 kilometres. We started with eighteen people in two vans and held protests in every city on the way. Halfway, we were joined by another two vans, so we had about forty people protesting outside the offices, from the morning until night, all day every day.
>
> It was really inspiring. We were young, so we could travel all week, and people just jumped in and out of the vans as we went.

In New Zealand, ten protestors occupied the reception of Marsh's office in Dunedin and plastered stickers over the foyer. As the receptionist beat a hasty retreat, activists took her place and answered all incoming phone calls, explaining to the callers why they had seized the office. Other activists occupied Marsh in Wellington, where they ran into the building with megaphones.

North American protests were held at Marsh's offices and directors' homes in San Francisco, Texas, Chicago, and New York. In Texas, Marsh's offices also had their locks glued shut.

It was the fastest, and furthest, protests had travelled against a single SHAC target, dwarfing the previously epic scale of the Shell campaign.

As Marsh felt the full brunt of SHAC, another tactic emerged. In the UK, two activists secured tickets for the BioWise 2002 conference at the London Metropole Hotel. Dressed smartly and disguised as official guests, they attended a discussion about protecting HLS' financial backers from demonstrations. The keynote speaker was SHAC nemesis Lord Sainsbury. As he stood to speak, so too did the two activists. They loudly presented their views to the whole conference and handed out fact sheets as security grabbed them and dragged them from the room.

Invading conferences embarrassed HLS in front of their peers and reminded potential customers, suppliers, and investors of the protests which would follow any decision to deal with the laboratory.

News spread fast. While activists tore down HLS' display stand at a biotech conference in Texas, HLS' director Andrew Gay was banned from attending a symposium on a cruise ship over fears of a protest at sea. In Germany, protestors invaded Bayer's AGM, where an activist took over the podium and gave the packed room an impromptu speech about HLS' animal cruelty and criminal record.

SHAC's more traditional invasions hadn't stopped either. During a mobile protest in the UK, 100 protestors stormed the warehouse of Parkers Fine Foods, who supplied animal flesh for HLS' canteen. As more and more protestors arrived, the police called in a helicopter and finally gained control. As soon as the last intruder was evicted, the entire protest headed for HLS' beagle breeder, Harlan Interfauna.

I joined the protest at Interfauna, arriving a few minutes before everyone else. Walking across fields, my friends and I approached the fence. The barking of the beagles grew louder; a distressing sound as they desperately cried for help which would never come. I eyed up the razor wire, but several police officers appeared and followed us. As I separated from my friends with a lone constable on my tail, I heard over his radio that 100 protestors had just arrived at the front, and he rushed off to help.

Immediately, I scrambled over two sets of eight-foot-high, razor-capped fences, leapt into the compound, and ran towards the beagles. After climbing a roof, I peered into a narrow passageway where I witnessed the terrified animals cowering in fear. I turned and saw the rest of the protestors surrounding the compound, defending themselves against police violence as they tried to reach me. I jumped into the excrement-lined passageway. The shovel of sawdust that had been sprinkled down failed to soak up the urine, which flowed freely through the bars. The smell was overpowering.

The animals' reaction to me made it clear how Interfauna's staff treated them. Most of them ran and hid, whining and shaking at the back of their cages underneath small wooden benches. A few ran up to me, only to bolt back, petrified. An older beagle had desperately tried to chew through the bars, resulting in bloody stumps in her gums where her teeth should have been.

One dog ran up to me and sniffed my hand. She sensed it was safe and wagged her tail as I made a fuss of her. Knowing that soon she would be cut open on a vivisector's table after horrific experimentation is something that will haunt me forever.

I tried to open the cages, but they were locked, and I couldn't get through the bars. Tears poured from my eyes as I reluctantly conceded there was nothing I could do. I approached every cage sobbing, apologising to each dog for being unable to bring them the liberation they so desperately needed and deserved.

I ensured the police saw the dogs as they escorted me from the premises, but they showed no emotion. As they dragged me out of the front gate, a concerned friend tried to reach me, but the police punched him in the stomach and arrested him too. They charged me with aggravated trespass, but after what I had witnessed, four hours in the cells felt like a five-star hotel.

The mobile protest continued on to various locations including HLS' primary taxi firm, the laboratory itself, and several of their employees' homes. At one house, neighbours cheered on protestors as they covered the door in stickers.

A few weeks later, activists attempted another invasion during World Day 2002, at HLS' second British laboratory in Occold. Bolt cutters were strategically hidden in hedges surrounding the razor wire fences, and people charged through the rapeseed fields to get to them. They intended to cut the fence and get into the primate unit.[43]

The rapeseed was six-foot tall, and as protestors and police vanished into it, all that could be seen were fluttering flags, waving placards, and swinging truncheons. As police batons flew, the signs and flags collapsed into the crop. The protestors who managed to make it to the bushes were pulled out and arrested, with only a few holes cut in the fences. Those who gained access were quickly ushered out or arrested.

Later that night, the ALF carried out a far more successful incursion at one of HLS' suppliers:

> A number of us paid a visit to Wrights Breeding Centre.
>
> We got on site, grabbed a crowbar, and began to rip the door off one of the stinking windowless units ... All was going well until the alarms went off – sirens blazing and lights coming on are not what you need in the middle of a raid.
>
> We were determined, and were not leaving without animals in our hands. As others began to smash up the farm's vehicles, we found ourselves in a room full of cages. There was no time to get a good look at these tiny animals and there was no time to take in the full horror of thousands of defenceless creatures boxed up waiting to die. We grabbed as many as we could and vanished ...
>
> Many of the thirty-five hamsters we saved were pregnant and went on to give birth. To look at these tiny creatures mothering their offspring and then to look at the perverts who work at HLS really hammers it home that these people are sick in the head, and we will not stop them with anything short of the full force of our anger at animal abuse.[44]

Desperate to quell the escalation of tactics, police tried once again to topple the SHAC founders. Heather was living with Gregg and Natasha in a house in Surrey:

> I was out one early morning walking the dogs. As I was getting them into the car, Bonny started barking and running up to the top of the lane.

I knew something must be wrong, so I squinted into the darkness and saw a row of what looked like Stormtroopers. There were these men all dressed in black armour, one after the other in a long line. Of course they arrested me straight away. They forgot to check whether I had a phone, so even though they had handcuffed us in the back of the van, I was texting away, telling everyone what was happening.

When we got to the police station, they claimed that when renting our previous property, Gregg lied to the estate agent that he worked with his brother. That was it. The custody sergeant at the police station couldn't believe what was going on. He was looking around asking why there were so many cops and detectives just for that, and then one of the policemen said, 'They're part of SHAC.' The custody sergeant just nodded and said, 'Oh, okay. I understand.'

The whole thing was just a desperate way to have a look inside our house. Obviously, the case got dropped once they'd had a good snoop about.

Despite this inconvenience, SHAC announced a Marsh Office Tour, kicking off five days of action.

Forty protestors occupied the roof and offices of one Marsh's office in Birmingham, causing security at the second branch in the city to panic and lock the staff inside until police arrived to escort them out. In Manchester, activists held protests on the sixth-floor offices of Marsh, while in Norwich, twenty-five people occupied the building, and in Exeter, activists subjected the firm to demonstrations and stink bombs. Some protests became so loud that Environmental Health shut them down.

I joined a group of friends for the London leg of the tour. We met outside Marsh in Cannon Street, a seven-storey building with massive glass doors protected by several security guards.

We headed for a nearby subway, where an underground door into the Marsh building stood unguarded. We slipped through, jumped a turnstile, sprinted up some escalators, and dashed into the foyer. Almost immediately the security guards leapt into action.

As I sprinted towards the lift, they rugby tackled the people on either side of me. I made it to the elevator, only to see two other activists restrained in headlocks. I dodged them and dove for the escalators without even pausing to check if they were headed upwards. They weren't.

I sprinted up seven flights of escalators the wrong way and headed towards the nearest office. Using tables, chairs, filing cabinets, and a yucca plant, I tried to barricade myself inside. My construction proved no match for one member of staff; at a little over five foot, and close to retirement age, she burst through the barricade like it wasn't even there. She snatched the paperwork I was trying to read and began swinging punches. Her manager appeared and calmly ushered her out of the room.

He sat down at the desk and we chatted amiably about the protest and HLS while we waited for the police. When they arrived, they searched me and found a metal teaspoon from my packed lunch. Despite the office manager insisting he had never seen it before, the police claimed I had stolen it and arrested me for burglary. They held me overnight and the next day remanded me into a Young Offenders Institute, where I remained for two weeks, until they finally dropped the charges against me.

Around 3,500 miles away, another teenager at another Marsh protest was enduring an experience even worse than mine. Jen Greenberg was just sixteen when she headed from her home city of Chicago to join a series of protests on the East Coast. She had been politically active for two years, helping feed the homeless with Food Not Bombs, joining pickets at fur retailers, and being as active as she could amongst Chicago's deep-rooted activist community.

Jumping trains and hitchhiking, she travelled with some friends to New York City to join locals for a week of actions against HLS supporters:

Compared to everything else, SHAC felt so organised. It was much more precise, more goal-oriented; it really felt like we were making progress. The demonstrations were so high energy, and our whole attitude was that we aren't asking for change, we're demanding it.

For World Week in New York, we did roving demonstrations. Downtown New York is a mix of the wealthiest people's homes and corporate offices, so anybody who was an HLS business partner would be there.

On one protest, we ran into the ground floor lobby of a Marsh executive's townhouse. We rushed past the doorman, who was very confused, and we held a really loud protest inside the building. There was a video of someone breaking a lamp, and some other things, but you can clearly see me just stood there shouting.

We left the townhouse and made our way to the next protest. Later on, we saw helicopters in the sky above us, and we realised they were looking for us. They caught up with us in front of the Whitney Museum, where they arrested everybody that was on the sidewalk – even some random kid who just happened to be walking past at the time.

I had been used to protests in Chicago, where they basically operated a 'catch-and-release' system. You'd get arrested, released the next day, and then at some point the case would get dropped.

Unfortunately for Jen, she wasn't in Chicago anymore. The previous New York mayor – Rudy Giuliani – had implemented a draconian policy dubbed 'broken windows', under which minor crimes were disproportionately punished to deter more serious criminality. His successor, Michael Bloomberg, had continued this policy.[45] Broken windows, combined with ever-increasing FBI interest in SHAC, led to Jen and several others being indicted on federal charges, including criminal mischief.[46]

Not long after she turned seventeen, Jen found herself in court:

> Even though I hadn't broken anything, the District Attorney used the analogy of a driver on a bank robbery; I was there, I was okay with what was happening, and therefore I was guilty.
>
> The activists I was sentenced with were great. Those relationships with the people that I knew in SHAC really formed my idea of how relationships should be. Ideals like honour, loyalty, and community. The others really felt like if they pleaded guilty, I was going to have a much better chance. Even so, I got sentenced to a year in Rikers Island.
>
> Jail was really, really difficult because it was psychological torture. I would get woken up at four o'clock in the morning, and I wouldn't know what was happening. They just pulled me out of my cell without saying anything and walked me down to the basement where they would leave me for hours. Eventually this guy would show up and ask, 'Are you ready to talk to us now?'

The FBI investigation into SHAC USA's founder Kevin Kjonaas and the 1999 University of Minnesota ALF raid had never gone away. Instead, it slowly shifted, morphed, and evolved into Operation Trailmix,[47] a Joint Terrorism Task Force investigating SHAC and the wider campaign against HLS. The man trying to get Jen to talk was an FBI agent involved in that investigation, and their tactics didn't stop there:

> I have PTSD from being left down there; I can't be cold or else I have a meltdown. I was starving as well; they refused to give us vegan food, and I temporarily lost my eyesight from starving. The FBI told me that if I spoke to them, then they would let me eat. I thought I would be blind forever, but I had nothing to say to the FBI.
>
> Even without the FBI, my time in jail was tough. Rikers is incredibly militarised. The 'boom squad' were the prison SWAT team who would do cell searches. It was a regular thing. They would open your cell at three o'clock in the morning, and the boom squad would be there to search everyone's rooms, and they would just take your personal belongings. They'd turn everything over, and then you had to spend the rest of the morning putting your things back together. At seventeen, it was a hard way to live.

14
Pitching Camp: 2002

SHAC has been remarkably successful with its variety of tactics against HLS.[48]

– The *Independent*

At 11 am on Sunday, 7 July 2002, I attended a new type of home demonstration. Rooftop protests were a bold act of defiance, but they still contravened the Criminal Justice and Police Bill. Activists risked arrest, large fines, and prison sentences. SHAC picked at the new laws until they found a loophole. Protestors had to leave the vicinity of a home if police demanded it. However, there was no mention of how long they had to stay away.[49]

It began with a protest camp on Ightham village green in Kent, near the home of Marsh director Christopher Pearson.[50] My fellow camper, Jenny, explained:

When most people see footage of animals cut open without anaesthesia, people laughing as they punch dogs in the face, and piles of dissected puppies, they have tears in their eyes. The directors and executives of companies like Marsh had dollar signs in theirs.

None of us wanted to be shouting outside someone's home, but if we only wrote polite letters, or protested their offices, the decision-makers wouldn't even know we were there, and certainly wouldn't listen to us.

Everyone should be accountable for the decisions they make in life and in business. There is no ethical argument for poisoning animals to death for Splenda, pesticides, plasticisers, or Viagra.

We had to take it directly to the decision-makers, and we had to give their choices consequences to stop the suffering inside HLS.

The camp was an embarrassment for Mr Pearson and HLS. Established beside the village's main dog-walking path, the campsite – surrounded by banners denouncing Pearson as a 'puppy killer' – drew the attention of his animal-loving neighbours. Local business owners, including the pub landlord, took piles of leaflets to distribute to their customers, and we slipped flyers into every letterbox in the village.

Ten protestors headed to Christopher Pearson's house to hold a noisy protest. The police moved them on and advised Mr Pearson to stay home until the camp dispersed.

As soon as the first protestors returned to the campsite, a second group took their place in a cycle repeated throughout the afternoon and into the night. As darkness fell, air horns and the constant ringing of his doorbell kept Pearson awake.

At 7 am, the campaigners returned to Mr Pearson's gate to greet him as he left for work, but under police advice he stayed home. He expressed his mood to the *Independent*:

It has been most unpleasant. I know greater powers are looking at how they can respond to their tactics.[51]

The 'greater powers' were the British government, who were furious activists had thwarted their plan to end home demonstrations. They set to work tightening the law, prompting veteran liberation activist Mel Broughton to note in the *SHAC Newsletter*:

> The resistance from the animal abuse industries and their friends in Government is an indication of just how effective we have become. HLS would not be torturing animals now without the backing of the Government.
>
> The nearer we get to closing HLS, the dirtier the tactics of our enemies will become. It's vitally important that we all remain resolute and focused on the task ahead.
>
> The struggle for animal liberation is now part of the political landscape, not because we have politicians who care about animals but because we have people who are prepared to act to make them listen.[52]

In a move that his peers dubbed a 'political statement',[53] the government awarded Brian Cass – HLS' controversial managing director – a CBE (Commander of the British Empire) honour.[54] Acclaimed screenwriter Carla Lane returned her own OBE (Officer of the British Empire) to Prime Minister Tony Blair in protest.[55]

A week after the protest camp at Mr Pearson's, we erected a second camp in a park in Buckinghamshire, near the home of another senior Marsh director. We pitched tents and draped banners from nearby trees and lampposts before heading to the home of Hamish Richie. A group of protestors skirted around to the back of his mansion, where they found his swimming pool. Pulling back the cover they took a plunge, leaving before the police arrived.[56]

When I joined the second shift later in the day, an irate Mr Richie charged at us with his umbrella. He screamed about how happy he was to work with HLS.

After a noisy night of protests, we arrived in the morning for another swim in his pool. Surprisingly, the local police didn't stop us, laughing as they radioed our antics back to their colleagues. In the afternoon, we returned again with the press in tow; they photographed us as we bombed and splashed in Mr Richie's pool.

At 4 o'clock the following morning, as we slept in our tents, riot police appeared without warning. With their collar numbers illegally hidden or removed, they smashed and tore up the tents, dragged us out into the park, and gave us five minutes to leave the area, 'Or else.' They didn't specify the threat, but we took the hint and left.

The following week, police demolished a third camp in a similar manner within hours of it being set up. The government were determined to end all home demonstrations, regardless of their legality.

SHAC adapted. Home demos became hit-and-run affairs. Protestors arrived, made as much noise and disruption as possible, and then bolted before the police caught up.

One Sunday afternoon, fifty activists carried out protests at a string of Marsh directors' houses across several counties. It was only as demonstrators were leaving the last house that six riot vans and several patrol cars caught up.

Days later, a second round of identical protests took place, but this time Marsh hired permanent security guards at all their directors' homes. The guards had no legal authority to move anyone on, and watched powerlessly as protests continued unabated.

'For sale' signs began appearing outside Marsh directors' houses, as the company paid for senior staff to jump from one multi-million-pound house to another.

* * *

It had been nearly two years since the Christmas protest at Roche, during which three activists were arrested for stealing scraps of paper from the company's bins. After repeated delays, the trio were brought before the courts and sentenced to a year in prison.[57] If this verdict was intended as a deterrent to a frustrated, emboldened, and determined movement, it did the opposite.

In solidarity with the 'Roche 3', activists in Brussels D-locked Roche's car park gates shut as the workers were due to head home.

Over in Switzerland, protestors invaded the Chemspec conference in Basel. As one activist D-locked her neck to Huntingdon's stand, another pretended to be a potential investor. He filmed an HLS' spokesperson smugly declaring the laboratory was impenetrable and a veritable Fort Knox. The person chained to his table was Lynn Sawyer, who had gained access to HLS twice in as many years.

As more protestors occupied the roof with a banner and air horns, police disassembled the display stand around Lynn and arrested her. They kicked her out onto the streets of Basel with the D-lock still fixed to her neck and no sign of the key.

Weeks later, HLS attended a crop protection conference in Basel. German activists attempted to attach themselves to the exhibition stand, but HLS had learned their lesson; replacing their usual set-up with a collapsible table and two foam chairs without legs. There was nothing to attach to, so the activists handed out leaflets and shouted until security evicted them.

Marsh's managing director, Gareth Hughes, was scheduled to speak at a British insurance conference. As soon as he began his presentation on insurance risks, protestors leapt to their feet and demanded to know how risky it was dealing with HLS.

Like most large companies trying to foster a positive public image, Marsh and their executives sponsored a variety of events and organisations. Disrupting those events struck right at the heart of their high-profile, high-budget self-promotion. The 'Marsh Classic' tennis tournament in Hurlingham was a highlight of Marsh's social calendar. As a group of protestors at the entrance hung a banner and handed out leaflets, I infiltrated the event.

A large oak tree overhung the tall, barbed wire perimeter near the back. I climbed the tree, dropped into the picnic area, and tried to blend in. It didn't work. Everyone was wearing shirts, chinos, and boating shoes, so in my black hoody and shorts, I stuck out immediately. Security gave chase and I crawled under a row of chairs to escape, but they soon grabbed and evicted me.

The following day a group of us tried again, this time dressed for the occasion. I led the way over the tree, but we split up as security arrived. I headed for Court One, expecting to be apprehended, but instead was ushered to the top of the tiered VIP seating. I watched the tennis as I worked out what to do.

As sirens and shouting erupted from elsewhere inside the tennis club, I stood and loudly informed everyone about Marsh's links to HLS. The match abruptly halted, and four big guys stood up, turned around, and jumped me. They punched me in the face, wrestled me to the ground, and threw me down the metal stairs.

Before I could check for broken bones, the security seized me in a headlock and dragged me from the club, leaving my glasses a shattered mess somewhere behind. They hauled me past some TV cameras, and I shouted my protest as I was thrown out onto the street. The police arrived shortly afterwards and arrested everyone still inside the grounds.

With the ubiquitous growth of the internet, a group of cyber activists launched a distributed denial of service (DDoS) attack against HLS. They programmed an online message board, which sent a request to HLS' servers every time someone typed a word. With 2,000 people logging on and chatting, the tsunami of requests forced HLS' website offline and incapacitated their email systems.

Simultaneously, activists stormed into the offices of HLS' service provider WorldCom in Berkshire, where an employee wielding a hammer assaulted one protestor. The protest moved on to Roche in Welwyn Garden City, in solidarity with the 'Roche 3'. Next came a series of home demos, starting with Marsh directors, and ending at the homes of directors of Turner Freight Forwarders, who transported non-human primates for HLS.

SHAC outlined the significance of companies like Turner:

Primates are flown into Paris, then brought by road through Dover. They are brought across the channel by Farmers Ferry and are cleared through customs by a company called Channel Ports. There are numerous freight forwarders who then take the primates on to their fate at Huntingdon. This is a potentially very weak link for Huntingdon.

These companies can never say they don't know what they are doing because they have physically had their filthy hands on the primates.[58]

These imports would become a key focus of the campaign, but first they concentrated on exporting the campaign itself.

15

SHAC Japan: 2002

This is the beginning of an attack on Japanese animal experiments.[59]

– Tsutomu Miki Kurosawa, Osaka University

HLS' Japanese customers provided 20 per cent of their income,[60] and for them the concept of SHAC was alien and absurd. Due to the campaign, Yamanouchi had relocated their Oxford facility to the Netherlands, and a small group of Japanese activists had demanded a meeting with Yamanouchi executives in their home country. However, SHAC remained broadly irrelevant to the company executives in Tokyo.

British activist, Dawn Hurst, decided that had to change:

I flew to Japan with a friend. Unbelievably, and with ease, we gained access to laboratories where experiments were taking place on dogs and primates. We wrote to them in advance pretending to be medical students, and some agreed to let us look around. Other places we just turned up and investigated ourselves.

We wore thick sports tops, with extra pockets sewn in to hold the recording equipment with a pin-hole camera. Over that, we wore smart clothes so we could blend in. We constantly overheated and had to take nearly all our clothes off every time we got back into our hire car, with the air conditioning on full just so we could breathe again.

In a primate laboratory we hadn't got permission to be in, we found ourselves in the basement where vivisection was taking place. To our horror, a worker came in, and we had to hide behind some shelves and hold our breath until he left.

We saw primates with devices cemented to their heads. They were spinning and rocking continuously through mental trauma. There were dogs with electrodes sewn into their heads and pigs with large plugs in their sides. On our final evening, we decided to go back to one of the laboratories at Juntendo University to rescue a small Labrador type puppy we had met in a tiny cage inside. Unfortunately, we couldn't get back in, and we left the country deflated.

Keen to expose the endemic cruelty within HLS' Japanese collaborators, Dawn published a report for SHAC on her findings:

The primates were being used in bone marrow experiments. The researcher said he had been to Huntingdon and their facilities, and the experiments were similar. The cages housed terrified, sad, and totally broken cynomolgus monkeys, which had been caught in the wild in Vietnam.

At the end of one room was a monkey much larger than the others. She was sitting very still, staring blankly into space. They had stopped using her for experiments and had decided to keep her just for a laugh. The researcher laughed in her face to tell her how fat and stupid she was. He decided to use her to show us the method they use for restraining monkeys. He yanked two handles on either side of her cage towards him. This pushed metal bars into her back until she was crushed against the front of the cage. She screamed a high-pitched, terrified scream. He laughed as he released her, telling her to shut up, 'Or his guests would take her back to HLS.'[61]

Following the exposé, Dawn travelled back to Tokyo with several British campaigners and joined a dozen SHAC Japan activists at the CPhI pharmaceutical conference:

> On the first day, we went in with hidden cameras and spoke to the man at the HLS display, Mr Cummings. The second day, we went back with a small group of Japanese activists and started shouting about HLS while handing leaflets out. The police eventually removed us, but the Japanese are so polite that the activists and police were bowing to each other even as they were evicting us.
>
> At the end of our week we returned to Juntendo University, determined to rescue the dog we had been unable to save on our previous visit. With the help of two extremely brave Japanese friends, we bought a bag large enough to put the dog in, found him a home, and asked our friends to be the 'getaway' drivers. I underestimated how big a deal this was for them. It was unheard of, a really huge risk for them, but they agreed. Sadly, I later found out how badly this decision affected them, but at the time it was a very happy day. When we drove away with our liberated friend hanging his head out of the car window and feeling the wind on his face, we were all elated.

As the campaign escalated, a Japanese activist described the feeling amongst the nation's pharmaceutical industry, saying, 'Everyone in Japan is very nervous about SHAC.'[62] The campaign compounded that feeling by announcing:

Our message is simple; we will find you wherever you are in the world. HLS will be dismayed by the formation of SHAC Japan and with more demos planned for their sales offices in Tokyo, this amounts to a major blow to Huntingdon's hopes for new business in Asia.[63]

Nearly 6,000 miles away, SHAC Deutschland held their first national demonstration – 150 campaigners gathered in protest outside of HLS' customer Bayer in Wuppertal. They faced a freshly fortified building, which the company had spent a small fortune protecting. With police pushing protestors away from the new fences, a group broke off and ran to the homes of several of Bayer's animal researchers, where they held noisy protests, declaring:

The movement of people rising up against HLS and anyone who touches them is growing. If you deal with HLS, no matter where you are in the world, it might not be long before people are banging on your front door demanding answers.[64]

In North America, the movement had burgeoned amidst the Stephens Inc. campaign, and now turned its full attention to Marsh. The home demos, office invasions, and phone and email blockades compelled the company to spend hundreds of thousands of dollars trying to bring a SLAPP (Strategic Lawsuit Against Public Participation) against SHAC USA to limit protest activity.[65] SHAC USA founder Kevin Kjonaas found himself on the receiving end of this and a series of other lawsuits:

In total, SHAC USA were sued twenty-three times. For it to be legal, a process server has to physically serve you with the lawsuit. So we were always dodging these process servers. One process server waited outside our house for three days; he had a picnic chair and just sat on the front step, waiting. We were using the back entrance and hopping a neighbour's fence. Finally, they had the police come. They shone a huge spotlight on the house, and got the process server to read the lawsuit over a megaphone. We were served.

The lawsuits backfired for the companies. They wanted to intimidate us; if we lost, we would be sued for millions of dollars. Normal people would say, 'Get me out of this, I don't want to be financially bankrupt.' But they were suing grassroots activists that literally had not a penny to their name. We fought them and we won.

Not all SHAC supporters managed to avoid SLAPPs. Those who fell afoul of one were permanently banned from protesting in the vicinity of the named company. Walking past the company's offices on an unrelated protest or attending the same protest as an employee of the company could result in prison time. Due to these infringements on First Amendment rights, many US states have subsequently implemented anti-SLAPP legislation to protect activists.[66]

Marsh spent a small fortune on litigation, but they had other expenses too. The company paid for twenty-four-hour security outside their employees' homes in the UK and USA.[67] One Texan staff member even insisted that five police officers escort him to work every day.[68]

Using lawsuits to suppress protests not only failed, it actively pushed more activists underground. During a PGA tournament sponsored by Marsh Director Frank Tasco, activists carved, 'Frank Tasco, puppy killer was here' in eighty-foot letters across the greens of Long Island's Meadowbrook Golf Course. Tasco was too embarrassed to return to the club.[69]

In a more dramatic action, anonymous activists in Seattle released two military-grade smoke bombs inside Marsh's offices. The *Seattle Times* reported:

Smoke bombings in two Seattle high-rises yesterday had all the markings of a London-based animal-rights group that targets a British research firm, its American wing and any company that does business with it, say experts and employees of an insurance company that has been a repeated target of the group.

British-based Stop Huntingdon Animal Cruelty or SHAC, denies a connection to the bombings, although it applauded them.

The attacks were described as well-planned and well-timed and occurred within two minutes of each other.

Shortly after 9:30 a.m., approximately 700 people in the Financial Center, Fourth Avenue and Seneca Street, were told to leave the building when what authorities called a military-type smoke bomb was found on the twenty-third floor.

Two minutes earlier, a similar smoke device was set off on the twentieth floor of a building at Seventh Avenue and Pike Street, forcing the evacuation of two floors there.[70]

Attention-grabbing stunts hit HLS thick and fast across North America, including a unique protest during the 14th World Congress of Pharmacology in San Francisco.

Erin Evans had moved to San Francisco's Bay Area two years before. She found herself drawn to SHAC after a protest outside the Bank of America, where activists had lit an effigy on fire outside the building. Due to overuse of water-based glue, the figure had almost failed to ignite, but the visual impact of the stunt struck a chord with Erin, and made her think of a bizarre childhood talent:

> When I was in high school, I did this ridiculous thing, where people would give me money and I could puke on demand. So, at the planning meeting I said, 'Why don't I go in and just puke on HLS' table?' I thought everyone was going to think this was a great idea. They didn't.
>
> I really wanted to do it, but I realised I could no longer puke on command. I got some Ipecac, which you take if you have food poisoning to make you sick.
>
> On the day of the conference, I drank loads of tomato juice and ate a bunch of corn nuts and Amy's noodle soup. I wanted it to be super red, and super chunky; weird and gross was the objective.
>
> When I got there, I headed to the security desk and said, 'Hi, I'm Dr Evans, I'm late and I've got a booth in the back.' Incredibly, they let me in. I headed straight for the bathroom and took the Ipecac, and then waited. It took forever to work. It was horrific having to keep walking around this room full of restraining equipment for holding animals in place to torture them. It was a disturbing and surreal scene, and all the time I was waiting for the Ipecac to kick in.
>
> And then it started happening. I ran up to HLS' display table, screamed, 'Vivisection makes me sick,' and ... bleeeeeeuuuuurrrggh!
>
> As security appeared, there was total confusion, and I took off. Ipecac is nasty stuff. My stomach wasn't right for a good five years after that. I didn't see any of the news coverage, but I heard there was a lot.

The following day, a larger group of activists, including Nik Hensey, held another protest inside the conference hall:

We were all wearing suits or dresses, and we broke up into several groups. I was with a female activist, and we walked over to HLS' booth and started shaking hands with their rep. As we shook his hand, we whispered who we were, and that we knew all about them. My friend yelled, 'Welcome to San Francisco, assholes,' and just yanked the tablecloth off. Their stuff flew everywhere. Of course, we were escorted out, but then half an hour later two other people went in and flipped their table over. After they were evicted, another two went in. They must have thought it was never going to end.

Amidst a wave of direct action sweeping the states, one of HLS' local senators invited SHAC USA to meet him. Senator Torricelli lent his full support to the campaign, telling activists to, 'Give them hell.'[71]

Much of SHAC's intelligence came from whistle-blowers. Some of these were one-off data-dumps; others were more regular tip-offs which provided SHAC with crucial lists of HLS' customers, couriers, suppliers, and financiers.

Eager to grow their web of informants, British SHAC activists set up stalls on high streets in and around Huntingdon. They distributed thousands of leaflets, urging the public to dish the dirt on HLS. As local press spread the message further, police put paid to the scheme, dismantling the stands and threatening arrests under data protection laws.

Fearful of the tactic's success, the government and police rushed to close SHAC's Post Office Box. Thanks to a tip-off from the Post Office, SHAC opened a BM Box as a replacement almost immediately. BM Boxes are a private service, and without the connections to the government that PO Boxes have, they are considered a safer option for controversial protest campaigns. Extreme right-wing hate group Blood and Honour had one,[72] as did groups with IRA connections,[73] and the ALF Supporters Group.[74] SHAC, however, were the exception; within a day of opening their BM Box, the police shut it down.

Long-time SHAC campaigner Lynn Sawyer stepped in to offer her home in Boat Lane, Evesham, as the new official address for SHAC. As a result, the campaign continued essentially unaffected. However, this decision had significant ramifications for Lynn.[75]

Following the whistle-blower outreach stalls, SHAC received information that Cambridge Pet Crematorium were providing services to HLS. One side of the building housed a garden of remembrance for the animal lovers of Cambridgeshire, but the other side – hidden behind a wooden fence – offered a vastly different service.[76]

Gregg and Natasha visited the crematorium to investigate what happened behind the fence:

Believing us to be representatives of a French pharmaceutical company, Mr Richard Pennell, the sales and marketing manager of Cambridge Pet Crematorium, bragged about all the local clients he has.

We filmed him as he discussed working for Huntingdon for a number of years and showed us around ... About 20 yards away were cows and calves just left lying in the yard. Some of them had their heads cut off. It is this work that Cambridge Pet Crematorium carries out for HLS. They cut the heads off cows and horses for HLS and send stem samples back to HLS. Then they burn them in the incinerators.

Before we left, we walked around the gardens of remembrance. There were many headstones with moving inscriptions on them. The sickest part is that most of these people would be totally against vivisection and yet haven't got a clue about the grisly trade going on yards from where their pets are buried.[77]

As soon as their connection to HLS became public, the company cut their ties,[78] forcing the laboratory to build their own crematorium. As more and more suppliers cancelled contracts with HLS, they would be compelled to build their own laundrette, catering department, delivery service,[79] and gas supply lines.[80]

16

Government Insured: 2002–03

Long-term, there is a body of opinion that believes Huntingdon is unlikely to survive.[81]

– Evening Standard

In July 2002, a 4x4 stopped outside the offices of Ian Cawsey
MP. Four shadowy characters yanked balaclavas over their
faces, stepped out of the vehicle, and began painting slogans
across the walls.[82]

This wasn't the ALF. In motive at least, it couldn't have been
further from it. This cell represented the freshly formed Real
Countryside Alliance (Real CA),[83] who militantly declared
war on New Labour's plans to ban fox hunting:

> We've written letters and lobbied, and has it affected the
> politicians or public opinion? Not a jot. Then does there
> come a time when you say, 'Stuff the public', and create a
> war? I don't know … But where are the IRA and Sinn Fein
> now? Round the negotiating table with the government.
> And where are we?
>
> We can be militant, and we can be politicians … and this
> bloke can be an IRA man.[84]

The Real CA warned that they would sabotage essential
services, including Britain's airports,[85] electricity pylons, gas
supplies, and supermarket lorries. They threatened to disrupt
railways and telephone lines, to dump sand into sewers, close

motorways by covering them with spikes, leave 500 suspicious suitcases lying around London, and to pull the plug out of a reservoir so that the City of Birmingham would run out of water.[86]

Amongst the bluster, the Real CA carried out many criminal – and sometimes violent – actions. In a campaign which waged for several years, they rioted and stormed inside the Houses of Parliament,[87] put fireworks through people's letterboxes,[88] nailed dead foxes to opponents' houses,[89] and assaulted politicians[90] and hunt saboteurs.[91] They slashed tyres,[92] carried out arson attacks,[93] and broke into an anti-hunt activist's home, hospitalising him with baseball bats.[94] Their stated aim was to 'unleash a wave of terror on animal rights supporters'.[95]

The official Countryside Alliance (CA) acted as the legitimate face of the pro-hunting lobby. Their relationship with the Real CA reflected that shared by SHAC and the ALF; while they attempted to distance themselves from criminal actions, the CA refused to condemn them. However, the undercover police officers who queued to infiltrate SHAC were nowhere to be seen for the CA.[96] Those arrested for Real CA actions received minimum sentences, rather than the deterrent punishments doled out to ALF activists or SHAC supporters. No new laws were introduced to curb their rights to protest, and police carried out no dawn raids for Real CA spokesperson Edward Duke when he told a journalist:

When it comes to it, we will want to set fire to motorways and Defra offices. We can do naughty things. We don't want to break laws, but we will break an unjust law. That's what pioneers have done throughout history.

We have nutters who are quite capable of blowing up a car, but we can control them.[97]

The duality was stark. When pro-hunt activist Otis Ferry was arrested flyposting Tony Blair's home in Sedgefield, police released him without charge. Months later, when he led hundreds of activists in a home demo at the same address, the prime minister invited him in for a cup of tea and a chat.[98] This was certainly not an opportunity afforded to anyone from SHAC.

There were several reasons for the differing approach, but it underscored the government's politically motivated response to SHAC, and the power of money and influence.

In August 2002, the *Observer* claimed Huntingdon MP Jonathan Djanogly accepted a £1,500 payment from HLS to ask questions on their behalf in Parliament.[99] Mr Djanogly denied this allegation, claiming the money was for tickets to a Conservative Party event, and the *Observer* later retracted it.[100] Nonetheless, just five days after the payment,[101] Jonathan Djanogly stood up in Parliament and asked Tony Blair:

Many hundreds of my constituents working at Huntingdon Life Sciences, its shareholders, and funders are being subjected to a massive campaign of intimidation from animal rights terrorists. Like other terrorists, they organise internationally and use extreme violence to further their views. Does the worldwide international fight against terrorism extend to Huntingdon, and what does the Prime Minister intend to do to stop the violence against my constituents?[102]

While views on what constitutes extreme violence and terrorism vary, it was a stunning declaration by a serving politician. During the entire campaign against HLS, there had been just one confirmed physical attack, for which Dave Blenkinsop was already serving a lengthy prison sentence.

This was the most striking example yet of the 'terrorism' label being thrust upon SHAC, but it wasn't the last. Less than a year after 9/11, Richard Harbon, the police community inspector for Hitchin, unleashed a furious tirade when SHAC supporters changed the location of their protest at the last minute. Rather than a planned protest in Welwyn Garden City, 200 activists descended on Letchworth and the home of HLS' managing director, Andrew Gay; 250 police officers swiftly arrived and moved the protest on. The demonstration was disruptive, but entirely peaceful, and dispersed without incident. Nonetheless, Harbon blasted:

> These people are out to disrupt the peace and damage and destroy property. They are nothing but urban terrorists and this was just a waste of police resources.[103]

No property was reported damaged or destroyed, but that did nothing to dissuade a senior police officer reciting the extreme rhetoric. When law enforcement officers and politicians wield powerful words such as 'terrorism', there can be severe consequences.

Kevin White learned this first-hand when he took a 150-mile trip with his sixty-year-old mother and a friend from Redditch to Kent for a publicised day of action:

> At the meeting point, we met seven other activists in two vehicles. Some of us had met before, but many were strangers.
>
> I didn't know the area, so I followed the other cars to a peaceful demo at the home of a Marsh director. Some protestors opened the gate and walked onto the driveway. My mother and I remained by the gate and shouted, 'Vivisection is scientific fraud!' When the resident security guards

told us to leave, we did so without resistance. The whole protest lasted two minutes. We drove in convoy to the home of another Marsh director, where we held another peaceful two-minute demonstration. I followed the other cars again, but got lost. I found my way back to the second address we had visited and stuck a couple of SHAC stickers on the gate.

Almost a month later, my sixty-year-old mother and I woke to the sound of police raiding our home at 6.30 am. Five people were arrested in total, and the police searched and seized my car for evidence.

In court, we were all remanded to prison. I was sent to Canterbury, and my mother to the notorious Holloway. It was almost a month before we were freed from custody, and another month before the case was dropped.

A year later, the case was reopened, and we were convicted of causing 'intentional harassment, alarm or distress'. We each had to pay £450 costs and my car was crushed. They claimed in court our peaceful protest was an act of terror.

The defendants' solicitor Kevin Tomlinson observed darkly:

I am not one for conspiracy theories, but the whole case against these people stinks of government collusion.[104]

* * *

In August 2002, two young girls, Holly Wells and Jessica Chapman, went missing in Soham, Cambridgeshire, less than thirty miles from HLS. Four hundred officers were tasked with investigating the disappearance, and SHAC called a national pause to protests, to avoid tying up police resources. After two weeks, the search for the missing girls ended in heartbreak, as their bodies were discovered, and their murderer arrested.

SHAC resumed their assault on HLS' finances. Wendy Attwood joined an action in Birmingham:

We climbed onto Marsh's porch-roof at 7 am. The whole town was silent, and I could feel the apprehension setting in as we climbed up. Our driver took the ladder away with him, and we were up on that roof alone with a banner and a megaphone.

As the workers began to arrive, we waved at them through the window behind us. They were not amused. They tried to ignore us, but we kept tapping the window, holding up leaflets about HLS for them to read.

Eventually the police arrived and asked us to come down. We were staying all day. A small but lively protest grew beneath us, and members of the public shouted, 'Good on you!'

When the staff finally left, we called down to them about Marsh's involvement with animal cruelty. By early evening, we agreed to come down. Because we didn't have our ladder anymore, the police called out a fire engine. I was so excited because I'd never gone down a fire engine ladder!

When I got home, I saw we were on the local news, which was great, but also a bit concerning as I'd pulled a sickie from work to do it …

Following this protest came a more dramatic stunt. Heather felt sick with guilt and nerves as she showed her ticket and took her seat in the dress circle at the Mayflower Theatre in Southampton:

One of the most senior Marsh directors was a patron for the English National Ballet, and we had tickets for the opening night performance of their UK tour of *The Nutcracker*. About halfway through the ballet we got up and started to loudly protest. Immediately, the theatre lights came on and we stood there, fully illuminated, just throwing leaflets off of the balcony like confetti, and shouting, 'We don't want to be here. We don't want to spoil your night, but animals are being killed right now. We just need to stop it.' We shouted the name of the person from Marsh and told them it was his fault we were there.

It was amazing how professional the ballerinas were; they just carried on dancing like nothing was happening.

Understandably, the audience didn't take it so well. One man grabbed and shoved me to the floor. I couldn't breathe, and he was crushing me. The theatre staff ran over yelling, 'Let her go, let her go.' They picked me up, and as they led me out an elderly lady came up to me and kicked me. I hated the idea that we ruined people's evening, but animals were dying and we needed people to listen.

People did listen, including the senior management of Marsh. When they realised that SHAC could and would publicly humiliate them, their passion for defending HLS collapsed. The campaign was proving a financial albatross for Marsh. According to FBI affidavits, Marsh made $100,000 per year from their contract with HLS, but were paying $2 million per month on security because of the campaign against them.[105] On 17 December 2002, Marsh cancelled all of HLS' insurance.[106]

SHAC USA activist Aaron Zellhoefer was visiting the British SHAC headquarters:

I truly thought this was like going to be like a huge domino that we had knocked down. I believed this a real death blow to HLS, and I was completely elated, but Gregg just said, 'Okay, on to the next one.'

It turned out he was right; I was naive to think that the British government wasn't going to bend head over heels to protect HLS. I was in the car with Gregg and Natasha when a reporter called and asked Natasha what her thoughts were about the Department of Trade and Industry now insuring Huntingdon. She was stunned.

In fact, the entire movement was stunned. Not only had the British government created historical precedent by giving them a bank account with the Bank of England, but they were also, for the first time in history, providing insurance to a private company.[107]

Gregg summed up the mood when he asked:

What next? Are the army going to guard the gates of Huntingdon Life Sciences? How outrageous that if there is any damage to Huntingdon's lab in America it is the British taxpayer who picks up the bill. The government say they can't afford a wage rise for the fire fighters, but they can afford to insure Huntingdon who kill 500 animals every day.[108]

SHAC's next target was HLS' auditors, Deloitte and Touche. Public companies are legally required to have an auditor file their accounts, so no auditor meant no company.

Following protests outside Deloitte and Touche in Birmingham and Nottingham, a single ALF activist carried out an action which would usher in one of the most intense periods of anti-HLS activism to date. Under cover of darkness and wielding half a paving slab, the masked activist walked right past two police officers, turned the corner, and launched the concrete through the window of Deloitte and Touche in Nottingham.[109] Over the next ten days, ALF activists launched six attacks across the UK, Europe, and the USA, while SHAC held over twenty protests inside and outside offices.

According to the *Financial Times*, SHAC were leaked phone numbers and email addresses for 135 senior staff members at the accountancy firm.[110] SHAC posted the information onto their website, and computer-savvy activists set up an internet message board. They embedded coding into the message board, which caused multiple emails to be sent to Deloitte and Touche staff every time a letter was typed. The emails urged the company to stop dealing with HLS, and within ten days they had received over 200,000. Deloitte and Touche's IT security officer sent a snappy email to the message board's service provider, demanding they end 'this abuse of the internet'.[111]

The request fell on deaf ears. Like Marsh before them – though in days rather than months – Deloitte and Touche stopped dealing with HLS. The news delighted campaign organisers such as Heather, but she wasn't prepared to declare victory just yet:

We were really glad, of course, when both Marsh and Deloitte and Touche pulled out, but honestly, we never really had time to think. We were so busy; it was eighteen hours a day, seven days a week, and we were exhausted. We didn't have time to really think about each victory. We would just say, 'Great, another one down, who's next?'

After NatWest and Marsh, we were really pissed off at the government, and we were more determined than ever to just carry on and get this thing finished.

Indeed, for the second time in as many weeks, SHAC had to decide who would be next on their radar. When asked by the industry magazine *Accountancy Age*, Gregg explained the campaign's position:

We have been talking to the Securities and Exchange Commission (SEC) over this and there are ways and means to find out the next auditor, but there is no legal requirement to reveal their identity until the annual report and we expect HLS to keep it secret for as long as possible.[112]

It would not be as simple as waiting for the next annual report. Rather than bailing out HLS, the UK government simply allowed them to break the law. For the next two years, HLS were the only company in the UK that did not have to file a tax return.[113]

The Animal Procedures Committee advised the British home secretary on matters relating to animal testing. In October 2002, anti-vivisection organisation Uncaged supplied them with a new dossier of leaked information regarding HLS' xenotransplantation experiments from 1999. The committee decided they 'did not wish to take this further'. The British Union for the Abolition of Vivisection (BUAV) also supplied information, detailing suffering caused to marmosets inside Cambridge University which far exceeded the project licences. Rather than addressing the unsanctioned cruelty, the committee concerned themselves with deciding how to tackle 'issues of clandestine investigations and whistle-blowing'.[114]

The committee's fears went deeper than undercover investigations. They expressed concerns that if the wider public became more aware of other primates' sentience, it would threaten animal testing:

There are serious ethical and animal welfare concerns regarding the use of primates in experiments, and considerable public disquiet with regard to such use. These concerns are likely to increase as more is discovered about their advanced cognitive faculties, complex behavioural and social needs, and the difficulties of satisfying these in a laboratory environment.[115]

As SHAC decided on their next priority target, SHAC USA held three days of protests to mark HLS' 50th anniversary. With guest speakers including Black Panther Party co-founder Bobby Seale, UK ALF Press Officer Robin Webb, and Native American eco-anarchist and ALF activist Rod Coronado, they aimed to inspire action. New Jersey law required twenty-four hours' notice before activists carried out home demonstrations, so they scheduled protests at every single HLS employee's house in the state. With New Jersey police sat waiting through the night for the protests to start, campaigners instead headed to neighbouring Philadelphia to protest without interruption.

The following day they arranged a mass mobilisation for HLS' New Jersey laboratory, but the police had an axe to grind. They only allowed a handful of activists to approach the laboratory at a time, corralling the rest at the foot of the path, out of sight and out of mind. Robin Webb tried his luck and skirted around a nearby car park to join the group at the laboratory. He told the police he had become 'disorientated', but was stopped after being directed back to the main protest:

I was suddenly arrested, searched, hands taped together behind my back, bundled into a County Sheriff's van, then off to the County Jail. At the County Jail came the worst indignity, you have to pay $50 for processing through the custody area. At least being arrested in England is free.

Bail on the first night was set at a staggering $50,000. I then received a faxed letter from the Judges office telling me that, unknown to my lawyer or me, a bail hearing on the 30th of November – the day before I was arrested – had reduced the amount to $25,000 but they wanted my passport and birth certificate. Another hearing reduced my bail to $10,000 and when I was finally released after eight days, the press were waiting in the snow and ice for us.[116]

Robin ended up spending nearly six months in the USA, as he waited for his case to be resolved. He spent his time helping in the SHAC USA office and held a coast-to-coast speaking tour, inspiring and recruiting new activists.[117] The tour was closely followed and monitored by an increasingly frustrated FBI.[118]

17

You're Not BBC, You're SHAC!:

2003

We have an animal rights movement in this country which has now become exported worldwide.[119]

> – Brian Cass, HLS' managing director

In 2003, HLS admitted, 'If one or more members of our senior management team were unable or unwilling to continue in their present positions, those persons could be difficult to replace.'[120]

The campaign shifted focus to the company's executives, starting with director John Caldwell. He was Dean of the Faculty of Medicine at Liverpool University and when protestors burst into his office to tell him they would close HLS, he replied, 'I certainly don't underestimate that.' They accosted Caldwell again at a university degree ceremony. As he attempted to sneak in through a side door, activists demanded to know when he planned to leave HLS. This time he turned and fled.[121]

In Brighton, four protestors slipped inside the British Crop Protection Council (BCPC) conference at the Hilton Metropole Hotel after they learned HLS' director Steve Owen was attending with a colleague. Despite a throng of police blocking the entrances, activists convinced the hotel they worked for HLS and were given keys to the company's hospitality suite. Two of them ran into the room, throwing SHAC leaflets into the air and shouting about the cruelty inside HLS. As security flung them out, Owen headed for his booth in the conference hall, where he found the other activists attempting to D-lock themselves to the display. He immediately recognised Lynn Sawyer, who had locked herself to his stand in Basel, and wrestled the heavy lock away from her. He threw it into a crowd of attendees, who had to dive for cover.

Lynn was evicted, but when an employee gave her the keys to HLS' hospitality suite for a second time, she crept back into the hotel. She locked herself inside for over four hours, emptying the contents of HLS' mini bar and preventing them from entertaining potential clients.

Because of the pressure against HLS, research and development spending in the UK dropped by £100 million in a year.[122] According to Brian Cass, much of it would have gone to the beleaguered laboratory:

> HLS has lost orders and is not being considered for future orders as a result of direct and threatened action against some of its customers/potential customers. It is clear from some of the statements made to SHAC by some customers (and privately to HLS) that a considerable amount of orders have been and will continue to be lost due to the intimidatory nature of the activists calling themselves SHAC.[123]

Gordon Brown's vision of Britain as a research and development utopia was cracking. Approaching desperation, two Labour MPs with backgrounds in the vivisection industry launched a debate in Parliament. They urged the government to encourage a more aggressive attitude from the media, to drive a wedge between SHAC and the rest of the animal liberation movement.[124] Their demonisation of SHAC was a convenient distraction from a report by a government select committee. As animal testing continued to increase under New Labour, the report, which was ignored by the Cabinet, stated:

> There is scope for the scientific community to give a greater priority to the development of non-animal methods ...
>
> We consider that the development of scientifically valid non-animal systems of research and testing is important, not just to improve animal welfare, but to provide substantial benefits for human health.[125]

* * *

In North America, the FBI surveilled SHAC USA intensely.[126] FBI agents tapped phones, dredged bins, and followed activists.[127] The agents' identikit outfits and TV-trope mannerisms made them stand out as they staked out houses connected to SHAC USA, and on several occasions activists went out to offer them tea and biscuits.

An activist named Lisa Distefano had been working on and off at the SHAC USA office for several weeks, but was hiding a big secret. The FBI had recruited her to spy on SHAC USA. She reported on the day-to-day activities of SHAC activists and the layout of the SHAC USA office.

Lisa's real motivations were later revealed during a court hearing, but she vanished before she could be subpoenaed to admit the truth: SHAC USA were a lawful protest campaign.

The FBI found no evidence of criminality from their 'covert' monitoring, but they weren't willing to give up. Using Lisa's plans of the SHAC USA offices, in 2003 they mounted a high-profile raid on the property. The raid confirmed what the wiretapping, surveillance, and trash searches had already proved: there was no connection between SHAC and the ALF.

In response to the police break-in, the campaign issued a statement in defiance:

> Never once did we fool ourselves into believing that to the extent we have rattled the cages of the vivisection industry, there would be no consequence.
>
> The Senate Floor is no friend to the animals; the courtrooms will not recognise that animals are not property; and the pages of USA Today are bought and sold to the highest bidder.
>
> Within twenty-four hours of the last FBI agent leaving our home, we had already moved our headquarters to a bigger and better facility. We reordered all our leaflets and obtained new phones and computers. We staged demonstrations at HLS, and the home of its Vice President of Operations. We conducted media interviews and held a vegan outreach dinner.
>
> Unfettered and unfazed – it was business as usual.
>
> Dig your heels in; this raid and our actions over the next few months are going to take this fight to a whole new level. The FBI just disturbed an angry nest of hornets and Huntingdon is going to be stung.[128]

As federal interest in SHAC USA intensified, the grand jury investigating 'Operation Trailmix' continued to subpoena activists. One of them was Lindsay Parme, who found several FBI agents on her doorstep in California. They asked about a lawful protest she had attended months before, and handed her a subpoena to testify in front of the grand jury in New Jersey:

> Knowing the history of FBI repression against social justice movements, I refused to participate in any of the process.

I spent a week and a half in a San Jose jail before the federal marshals drove me to Santa Rita jail near Oakland. Five days later I was transferred into the federal system and was flown on a small private jet with one other inmate to Portland, and then to Seattle, where I spent the night at the SeaTac Federal Detention Center, before being transferred to Oklahoma City. This time it was a commercial-sized plane with a hundred other prisoners – ten of them women. The women sat at the front of the plane, and the men at the back, with armed marshals all around us. Before we boarded the plane, we were strip-searched and given a beige 'transportation' outfit. We had shackles around our ankles, wrists, and waist. I was made to wear a 'black box' over the chain of my handcuffs, so my movement was even more restricted. Normally people who have the black box have assaulted a guard or are an escape risk. I was neither.

At the Oklahoma City Federal Detention Center I was held in solitary confinement before being transferred again. We flew to Harrisburg, where federal marshals drove me for a night through Philadelphia, before going to county jail in New Jersey. After nearly three weeks of prisons and 'con-air', I was finally presented to the grand jury.

I stood in front of over a dozen grand jurors in my prison clothes, and the prosecutor asked me a few dozen questions which I refused to answer. After weeks of travelling, my appearance in front of the grand jury lasted less than an hour.

The FBI led me out of the room and told my lawyer that the government had bought me a plane ticket to get home, which was leaving in two hours. My friends rushed me to the airport and a few hours later I was back in California.

In the UK, Tony Blair received a letter from the Japanese Pharmaceutical Manufacturers' Association (JPMA). They warned that their members would withdraw all investment from HLS and Britain unless the government took immediate action against SHAC. He immediately set up a task force with Lord Sainsbury, to help the companies tighten their security.[129]

In response to the JPMA letter, SHAC campaigners travelled to the largest Japanese pharmaceutical conference of the year in Tokyo. While activists from SHAC Japan handed out leaflets at the entrance, Gregg and Natasha Avery posed as a BBC production team, interviewing companies about HLS. They all expressed apprehension over HLS' future. Eventually, police evicted Gregg and the others:

> As police and security arrived, we managed to manoeuvre ourselves in front of CBC's stall, who own half of HLS's Japanese sales office. The CBC rep who had been filmed earlier on furiously said, 'You're not BBC, you're SHAC. You have tricked me.'
>
> With police trying to snatch leaflets out of our hands and failing as we carried on distributing them, we started shouting about HLS and CBC touting for business for them. Conference goers gathered as the situation escalated and the police, well and truly frustrated by their inability to either move or silence us, finally managed to evict us from the conference as a large audience of people HLS would like as customers looked on.[130]

Following this action, and a string of international protests, CBC sold their stake in HLS, forcing the laboratory to buy out its Japanese sales office completely.

Amongst the other activists leafleting at the conference was Kate Jones, who was arrested alongside Dawn Hurst:

Police and security escorted us to a room. They started firing questions. We acted naive. They wanted our passports, which we didn't have, so they carted us off to a huge skyscraper police station. They questioned me about Dawn. I said I couldn't understand them, so they went and got an interpreter. I didn't know if I was allowed to say, 'No comment,' in Japan, so I said, 'I don't know' to everything. After about eight hours, I was charged with giving out leaflets without a licence, and then released. As I left the station, the cop told me Dawn would be held a very long time for a serious crime. I tried shouting her name, but she couldn't hear me.

Realising they were under surveillance, most of the British activists climbed out of their hostel window, crawled across several gardens, hailed a taxi, and fled the country a day earlier than planned. Dawn's freedom wouldn't come so easily:

Everything was taken extremely seriously because of the connection to SHAC. They accused me of liberating the dog on my previous visit, and stealing videotapes showing experiments, which we had borrowed, copied, and then put back. I was also charged with forgery because of the fake letters we sent asking for appointments to view the laboratories.

I was transported between police holding centres in Osaka and Tokyo while they investigated the allegations. I will never forget using the toilet on the high-speed Bullet Train with the door open, on a leash being held by a police officer, with Mount Fuji in the background.

In Tokyo, I was interviewed three times a day for three weeks. I shared a cell with eight others. There was barely enough room for everyone to lie down, and you touched someone on all sides. I was put right under a hissing strip light that never went off. Luckily, I was held with a woman who spoke English. She was an absolute godsend and kept me sane.

The rules were complicated and strict; there was a 'correct' way to fold our towels and blankets, we had to change our clothes on a specific day twice a week, and I had to learn my prison number in Japanese, which was hard because it kept changing.

I was taken to key places related to my 'crimes'. This began with a search for the shop where I bought the bag to carry the liberated dog in. We drove aimlessly around for several days until we found it. The police took me inside, so I could hold a bag and have my photo taken. Next stop was the laboratories, where I was photographed in front of screaming animals in cages. It was horrifying.

I had to regularly meet with the prosecutor. We were driven on buses with bars on the windows. We were handcuffed and tied together in long lines, before being shuffled along tunnel-like corridors, trying not to fall over each other. One by one our numbers were called, and we were taken to the prosecutor. The office was on a top floor, and I would look at the view over Tokyo while the prosecutor made thoughtful noises. I had no clue what was going on or why I was there.

On one visit, one of my Japanese friends was accidentally put in the same cell as me. She had driven the car we used to rescue the dog and had found them a loving forever home. I was horrified to learn that she had been arrested too and I felt terrible. I told her over and over again how sorry I was, and that she should blame me for everything. The guards heard me and instantly moved her to another cell. She was an incredibly brave and beautiful person. I later found out that she lost everything because of her arrest: her home, her job, her boyfriend, and her family. She was financially ruined, and she received a three-and-a-half-year sentence, thankfully suspended. This was more than some serious crimes, and she was told it was purely because of the SHAC connection.

During Dawn's interrogations, the police revealed they had visited the UK to learn about SHAC and monitored the campaign's website daily. The Japanese vivisection industry was terrified, as HLS' head of science and technology, Dr Frank Bonner, confirmed to the Department of Trade and Industry:

I visited Japan, and every client company I visited is clearly concerned about the environment in this country. They were questioning the appropriateness of conducting research in the UK because of animal rights pressure.[131]

Back in the UK, SHAC activists visited HLS' customer Shin-Etsu's Scottish facility, reporting:

We immediately set about putting leaflets all over the reception area and accessible offices, on desks, on cupboards, units, chairs, tables, inside a jacket – some leaflets even found their way into a photocopier which started churning out copies for the workers – and into the human resources centre whilst another worker was on the internal phone trying to convince someone that, 'Yes, there are protesters in the building; no, it's not a windup'.

Workers gladly took leaflets. In the packaging plant, more leaflets found their way into packages bound for many destinations.[132]

The protest kick-started a global week of action. Activists carried out dozens of protests against nine Japanese customers across several continents. Sankyo's doors were D-locked shut during a protest in London, and Austrian activists publicly screened undercover footage from HLS outside their offices in Vienna. The company sent leaflets to all nearby homes, falsely denying any involvement in animal testing.

Protestors in Sweden snuck into one office via the lift, only to find out that the company had already sent its workers home. SHAC Deutschland carried out office occupations in Dusseldorf and Munich, while SHAC Italia held noisy protests in Milan and Turin, and protestors in New York filled the pavements outside buildings occupied by Japanese customers.

In Japan, it took five gruelling months for Dawn's ordeal to finally end:

When the investigation was over, I was sent to the detention centre. Weak, and about three stone lighter, I struggled to carry my backpack. I thought I was going to fall over with the weight of it, and as I was pushed out across a dusty courtyard, I had this awful feeling that I was going to be marched against the wall and shot.

Of course, I wasn't. They put me in another cell until I was finally taken to court. I couldn't understand any of the proceedings, until eventually my interpreter told me, 'You have been given a three-year prison sentence.' As my world came crashing down, she casually added, 'It is suspended.'

I was placed in an immigration centre for a few weeks, before I was finally put on an aeroplane and allowed to return home.

Back in the UK, protestors resurrected the directors' camps, which had proven so effective during the Marsh campaign.

Lewis Pogson attended one camp near the home of a Yamanouchi director in Surrey:

> Early one Saturday morning we turned up in Shamley Green, an affluent village in Surrey and home to Dudley Ferguson, managing director of Yamanouchi. We pitched our tents on the cricket green. We erected placards and banners denouncing Yamanouchi's involvement in animal abuse and publicised the plight of animals in Huntingdon. It gave Dudley something to think about on his days of rest. We obviously made a commotion within the community, as a local resident and heir to the Born Free dynasty came to speak to us sympathetically. Less sympathetic were the particularly odious police who, despite us not breaking any laws, confiscated all our campaign displays under some spurious idea that they might 'distract passing motorists'.

Activists erected a second camp near Blackpool, against a director of Asahi Glass, who paid HLS to poison beagles with refrigerant gasses.[133] The camp was well received by the public. One neighbour wrote to the SHAC campaign:

> There is obviously a good amount of local concern regarding the issues you address. Protest groups are seen by the popular press as a thorn in society's side, who are unworthy of attention. I however was received with nothing but courtesy and good humour.
>
> The level of research and knowledge involved with SHAC's protest is extremely impressive, the members who attended the Blackpool protest being amongst the most informed members of a movement I have had the pleasure to meet. Your arguments are well researched, well-constructed, and extremely well represented.[134]

In 2003, activists handed another petition into the Home Office. It contained a staggering 1.2 million hand-written signatures calling for HLS to close.[135] This was one of the largest petitions ever handed to the British government and required two carts to be wheeled into the Home Office building. Tony Blair and his Cabinet failed to respond. Instead, Lord Sainsbury went to Japan to 'reassure Japanese investors about the seriousness with which Government regarded the problem [of animal liberation activism] and their determination to deal with it'.[136]

In the USA, an official from the United States Department of Agriculture (USDA) contacted SHAC to inform them of several regulatory breaches in HLS' New Jersey inspection report. Senior officials told inspectors to ignore failings because 'This is political.'[137] The USDA official who contacted SHAC was so appalled that they risked their job to leak the information. Years later, a US judge ordered 1,017 pages of USDA reports relating to HLS be released into the public domain, which outlined the cruelty in detail.[138]

To highlight the endemic abuse in vivisection laboratories, SHAC sent an undercover investigator to HLS' customer Eli Lilly in Surrey, where they exposed experiments into the effects of cocaine:

The activist worked on a programme of disgusting experiments that was scheduled to kill 36,000 rats, mice, gerbils, and guinea pigs per year at the Windlesham site in experiments which are shocking in their cruelty and futility. In some experiments, the animals had various parts of their brains damaged prior to being experimented on, and many had substances injected directly into their brains, sometimes for as long as ninety days, twice a day.

Hamsters and rats were exposed to constant lighting for up to eight weeks at a time. Mice were exposed to high-pitched sound to induce fits and seizures in them: the noise caused wild running, muscle clenching, and then respiratory failure and death.[139]

While SHAC exposed companies connected to HLS, the ALF continued to empty cages. Activists liberated forty-three goats from HLS' supplier, Water Farm Goat Centre, in Somerset, UK. Later in the year, the same supplier found themselves raided for a second time:

This time twenty-one beautiful goats, many of them pregnant, were carefully removed from the hell hole and ferried away to awaiting vehicles. These animals will now be able to live out their lives in caring homes, free from the fear and pain of the vivisector's scalpel.

The British countryside is littered with establishments like Water Farm Goat Centre, and the suffering animals imprisoned inside them are there for the taking. All it takes is careful planning, determination, and the will to save lives now.[140]

Following the raids, Water Farm stopped supplying animals to laboratories. In the USA, a team of ALF activists raided another of HLS' suppliers, reporting:

In the midst of a snowstorm, we made our way to the animal housing units. Using crowbars and bolt cutters, we bypassed alarmed doors by pushing and cutting our way through the windowpanes and wire mesh. After crawling into several barns, we loaded 115 baby chicks into carriers and brought them to safety. Countless animal research facilities commit their atrocities in Maryland, but Merial was targeted specifically because they are a client of Huntingdon Life Sciences. Any friend of HLS is an enemy of the ALF.[141]

Meanwhile, in mainland Europe, ALF activists tried and failed to liberate beagles from HLS' beagle supplier Harlan in the Netherlands. Undeterred, they carried out another raid at Harlan in Germany:

We visited Harlan-Winkelmann gmbh in Borchen-Alfen and liberated twenty-five dogs. Harlan is one of the biggest breeders in the world for so-called lab animals and delivers them also to animal torture places like Huntingdon Life Sciences and Covance in England. In the hell of Borchen, thousands of dogs are imprisoned. Hundreds of kennels filled with sad looking dog eyes, who're not aware of the worst torture awaiting them in animal testing centres. We wanted to take them all. At least twenty-five will have a happy natural life.[142]

18

Never Mind the Injunction: 2003

The number of activists isn't huge, but their impact has been incredible.[143]

– Brian Cass, HLS' managing director

In 1980, punk icon Johnny Rotten received a three-month prison sentence for a bar fight. Despite losing the case, his lawyer Timothy Lawson-Cruttenden used the attention to set up a 'punk rock practice', representing anti-authoritarians such as The Clash and Ian Dury.[144]

In 1997, the 'punk lawyer's' career diverted sharply. The Protection from Harassment Act was intended to protect women from violent stalkers, but Lawson-Cruttenden drafted amendments which led the BBC's *Inside Out* to dub him 'the solicitor protesters love to hate'.[145]

Lawson-Cruttenden now offered HLS a simple solution for dealing with British activists. Due to his amendments, corporations could apply for injunctions under the Act. Unlawful ALF actions were presented to the High Court to persuade them to criminalise SHAC's lawful protests.[146] The *Guardian* reported:

Only one demonstration is permitted every thirty days in the exclusion zones outside [HLS'] two sites in Cambridgeshire and Suffolk. On those occasions, the protesters, who must not number more than twenty-five, must park

more than half a mile away from the sites, and the demonstration must not last more than six hours.

Harassment is also deemed to include any 'artificial music
noise', such as klaxons or hooters.

Breaching the order is an arrestable offence and allows
the police to remove anyone immediately.[147]

While drafting the injunction, Lawson-Cruttenden needed
to name specific groups and individuals. HLS employed a new
security officer, former Cambridgeshire police sergeant, Ken
Smith, to help. Smith used his police experience and contacts
to gather personal information about animal liberation activists. As soon as their injunction was secured, HLS made Ken
Smith redundant.[148]

Dozens of HLS' customers and suppliers attempted to
disrupt SHAC's peaceful protests with a series of injunctions.[149] Each new order brought with it less opportunity for
peaceful protestors to have their voices heard, pushing waves
of activists away from SHAC's lawful protests, and towards the
ALF's more militant approach. Step by step, the government,
the police, HLS, and now Lawson-Cruttenden were exac-
erbating the very issue they claimed to be confronting. The
injunctions saw ALF activity in the UK rise by over 500 per
cent within a year.[150]

Campaigners like Heather were exasperated:

These were only designed to ban lawful protest. It was so
frustrating that big businesses could buy themselves protection from peaceful protests and people asking questions of
them.

Regardless of the illegal actions of others, the law-abiding
public should never be denied their fundamental right to
protest. It became increasingly obvious that you only have

the right to protest until you make a difference, and then you'll be stopped.

The new Anti-Social Behaviour Act allowed police to disperse protests of two or more people, further intensifying the repression of SHAC. Changes to the Criminal Justice Act criminalised office occupations and conference disruptions. The move targeted SHAC[151] but impacted protests by all social justice movements.[152]

HLS' supporters in Parliament became emboldened. Lord Taverne, president of the vivisection lobby group the Research Defence Society (RDS), outrageously exclaimed to the House of Lords:

It is just as important to guard against these terrorists, who are actual terrorists, as against the hypothetical terrorists of Al-Qaeda.[153]

In a more measured speech in the House of Commons, former vivisector Dr Ian Gibson MP highlighted the disparity between the pursuit of anti-vivisectionists and the efforts to replace animal research with modern science:

Money given by the Medical Research Council to look into alternatives to animal experiments has not been taken up. It is not fashionable or interesting, and there is a deep-seated feeling that it will not pay off. I shall now spend a little time telling the Chamber about the pay-off, and about what has been achieved with some of those alternative methods ...

The world is in turmoil over this situation, and the Government now need to go the final mile and tackle the legality of the matter. They need to question scientific methods and induce the scientific community to take alternatives much more seriously than they have done ... The time is right, both politically and scientifically, to move forward.[154]

Other MPs shouted down his voice of reason, and the number of animals killed in laboratories continued to rise. Behind the scenes, the Attorney General, Lord Goldsmith, launched a National Forum for 'the policing and prosecution of animal rights'.[155] The Forum held regular meetings between the Crown Prosecution Service (CPS), court officials, police, and government departments to coordinate their response. They pushed magistrates and judges to deliver sentences based on the totality of animal liberation activism, rather than just the offence at hand.[156] An activist who swore on their first anti-vivisection protest, for example, would receive a harsher sentence than someone swearing on an anti-war protest.

The National Forum became tied to the Ministerial and Industry Steering Committee (MISC), which focused on making the UK desirable for the pharmaceutical industry. Little is known about the Forum, as it is exempt from the Freedom of Information Act.[157] However, private letters between Lord Goldsmith and Home Office Minister Caroline Flint reveal police were encouraged to 'adopt a corporate approach' to dealing with animal liberation.[158] This involved clamping down on all unwelcome protests, regardless of their legality, and those attending the Forum were encouraged to 'identify any further gaps' in legislation to criminalise as much of SHAC's activity as possible.[159] The Forum decided policing animal liberation protests should be 'performance driven ... based on monthly reports of arrests'.[160]

In practice, these changes only affected lawful campaigners. For the ALF they made little difference – unless they were caught, in which case they faced the 'full weight of the criminal justice system'.[161] Most ALF actions passed without arrests, and the new approach did nothing to protect a secret HLS facility near Brighton:

> It is common for the ALF to keep possible targets under close surveillance. When [Shamrock Monkey Farm] closed, ex-employees were always unknowingly under scrutiny.
>
> Their specialist vehicles were followed to France, where it was discovered that they had been purchased by HLS to import primates. The ALF struck again, and the specialist vehicles were destroyed by fire.[162]

The arson attack wiped out HLS' entire fleet of specialist primate transportation lorries. They turned to the only remaining primate logistics company in the UK, Impex. After a single protest at Impex's offices, they vanished and moved to a new facility overnight. SHAC tracked them down, and protests resumed until Impex were forced to move their vehicles inside the safety of HLS itself.[163]

In 2003, a new group who rejected both SHAC's and the ALF's commitment to non-violence formed in the USA. The Revolutionary Cells: Animal Liberation Brigade called for militant action against all forms of oppression, from sexual assault to environmental destruction, but their focus was HLS:

> Volunteers from the Revolutionary Cells descended on the animal killing scum, Chiron. We left them with a small surprise of two pipe bombs filled with an ammonium nitrate slurry with redundant timers.
>
> Chiron, you were asked to sever your ties with HLS, you were told, and yet you continued your relations with them. Now it is time for you to face the consequences of your actions. If you choose to continue your relations with HLS, you will no longer be subject only to the actions of the above

ground animal rights movement, you will face us. This is the endgame for the animal killers and if you choose to stand with them, you will be dealt with accordingly. There will be no quarter given, no more half measures taken.[164]

The dramatic escalation was not a one-off. Weeks later the Revolutionary Cells struck again:

Volunteers from the Revolutionary Cells attacked a subsidiary of a notorious HLS client, Yamanouchi. We left an approximately 10lb ammonium nitrate bomb strapped with nails outside Shaklee Inc. We gave all the customers the chance, the choice, to withdraw their business from HLS. Now you all will have to reap what you have sown. All customers and their families are considered legitimate targets.

We have given all the collaborators a chance to withdraw from their relations from HLS. We will now be doubling the size of every device we make. Today it is 10lbs, tomorrow twenty ... until your buildings are nothing more than rubble. It is time for this war to truly have two sides. No more will all the killing be done by the oppressors, now the oppressed will strike back. We will be nonviolent when these people are nonviolent to the animal nations.[165]

Before the Shaklee bomb went off, a local police officer made a routine vehicle stop on a nearby road. The driver of the car was a young entrepreneur named Daniel San Diego, who had started a business making vegan marshmallows. The FBI named him their chief suspect and placed him under surveillance. When federal agents covertly searched his home, they found 'wire, PVC pipe, batteries, and other material that could be used for bomb making'. To cast these ordinary household items in a more sinister light, they also produced an 'incriminating' ALF t-shirt, identical to those owned by most animal liberation supporters across the world.[166] The day after they searched his home, an FBI team followed Daniel to a BART station (San Francisco's high-speed metro service). He jumped on a train and, whether through guilt or fear, hasn't been seen since.

Whether the Cells seriously designed their actions to cause injury or intended them to be a high-risk publicity stunt remains unknown. While the threat to anyone nearby was real, the devices were only powerful enough to shatter a few windows on an empty industrial park at 3 am. Predictably, the FBI leveraged the attack to enforce their mantra that all animal liberation activists were terrorists.

The police spent a small fortune trying to track Daniel down, searching across the Americas and Europe as they ranked him beside Osama Bin Laden on their most wanted list. They offered a $250,000 reward for his capture, dedicated an episode of *America's Most Wanted* to him, and projected his image on billboards above Times Square.[167] SHAC USA sardonically exclaimed:

> The FBI couldn't catch a cold, let alone an underground liberation activist.[168]

Despite their blasé attitude, they were quick to distance themselves from, the attacks:

> SHAC USA does not materially, vocally, or strategically support the use of violence against any human or animal. SHAC USA does not support terrorism, and as such does support all non-violent actions taken to end the daily terror felt by those sentient animals imprisoned and poisoned inside Huntingdon Life Sciences.

It is important to note that although the message sent by the 'Revolutionary Cells' contains ominous references to acts of violent self-defence on behalf of abused animals, not one single person in the USA has ever been hurt by an animal rights activist. The only violence to have happened is perpetrated by those who work within establishments like HLS, wherein 500 animals are killed daily.[169]

Across San Francisco, plain-clothes FBI agents stopped campaigners in the street and showed them covert photographs of themselves in their own homes. Agents regularly knocked on doors, loitered outside houses, rifled through garbage cans, and followed activists in their cars. More and more protestors were indicted to appear before grand juries. For local campaigners like Banka, even the most mundane activism began to feel like a high-stakes act of defiance:

It made us paranoid. Every person you see, whether on the subway or while riding your bike … you think, 'Is this person watching me?'

I stopped speaking to my mum and my sister on the phone, because I didn't want them to become involved. It all makes you feel like you've done something wrong, when you haven't.

It was a very sobering experience, and many of us came close to nervous breakdowns. At that point we agreed that we should take a step back to let it cool off; it was pretty much the end of SHAC in San Francisco.

As SHAC USA came to terms with the fallout from the San Francisco explosions, a tranche of high-profile leaks piled in from disenfranchised employees of HLS' customers and government workers across the world.

An anonymous whistle-blower in the USA uploaded a year's worth of Yamanouchi's paperwork, containing client lists, employee details, and even visitor logs. In Germany, someone from the tax office released the records of Eisai's employees, and in the UK, paperwork leaked from Japanese drugs giant Daiichi proved that cancer drugs (DX 8951, TZT 1027, and TZT 1027) were killing humans in clinical trials. The drugs had been marked safe during animal tests by HLS. SHAC forwarded the paperwork to over 1,000 of Daiichi and HLS' customers, suppliers, and financial supporters.[170] Around the same time, a government source leaked HLS' Bank of England account details to SHAC.

Meanwhile, an ex-chauffeur for HLS' customer, Eli Lilly, appeared in court. After being sacked, he had passed the details of fifty-three employees to three SHAC campaigners. Eli Lilly accused all four of conspiring to harass the staff members.[171] A few days into the trial, Judge Keith Cutler dismissed the case as there was no evidence that SHAC had harassed anyone, and the chauffeur's actions, though distasteful, weren't actually illegal.[172]

Amidst the leaks, protestors continued to target trade conferences. At the University of Vienna, they disrupted the World Congress on Men's Health – sponsored and attended by several HLS' customers – with megaphones and leaflets. In Germany the CPhI pharmaceutical event saw demonstrations inside and outside the conference hall, with ketchup sprayed over the stands of HLS' Japanese customers. London activists invaded a conference during a speech by the vice president of Chiron; as leaflets filled the air, security ushered the senior executive out of a side door. In Dortmund, a protestor wearing an ape mask doused a salesperson from the world's largest primate supplier with two buckets of fake blood.

SHAC continued to pick the bones of HLS by identifying and removing their suppliers. Companies were abandoning the laboratory at a rate of one per week.[173]

Following a single protest from SHAC and a visit from the ALF, who painted slogans and locked their gates shut with industrial chains, CPS fuels contacted HLS to sever their contract with the laboratory. Not a single company agreed to replace them, forcing HLS to pay over £750,000 having pipes laid to receive gas from the national supply. The company that connected the supply also withdrew from HLS upon completion and refused to service the piping.[174]

During a security conference in London, HLS' managing director, Brian Cass, bemoaned:

> The number of activists isn't huge, but their impact has been incredible.[175]

Shortly after, John Caldwell and another long-serving HLS' director resigned. In a press release detailing their hastily selected replacements, HLS expounded:

> Mr Y. Sesay, an international businessman with an interest in the development of pharmaceutical products, and Mr M. Faruque, Chairman of the Ghulam Faruque Group, have been elected to the Board, effective immediately
>
> Andrew Baker, [HLS'] Chairman, said, 'We look forward to working with our newly constituted Board to help guide us through the exciting future we see for [HLS].'[176]

While HLS sold their new directors as keen and competent business partners, Gregg Avery wasn't so sure. Posing as a journalist from *The Times*, he phoned one of the new directors, and recorded their conversation. It transpired that

Muhammed Faruque was a seventy-eight-year-old cement, sugar, and paper bag merchant from Pakistan with no prior knowledge of, or connection to, HLS.[177] On hearing of the campaign against the laboratory, he resigned as director before he had even signed any paperwork.[178]

In California, campaigners located Andrew Baker's sprawling holiday home in the LA hills. Regular protests began, with his wealthy neighbours split between those horrified at HLS and those horrified at SHAC. When protestors judged it safe, they set effigies of Baker on fire outside the property. While vibrant protests took place during the day, on several occasions the ALF visited the property at night and caused significant damage.

To make matters worse for HLS, SHAC USA also tracked down their transfer agent – the company who kept track of their shareholders – and convinced them to stop doing business with HLS. It was another financial blow as HLS were forced to do the job themselves, at great cost and inconvenience.[179]

In HLS' third quarter report, SHAC's impact was stark. Pressure on their customers saw HLS' turnover first slow, and then freeze. Despite a market value of just $26 million, they were now $84 million in debt, with little explanation as to how they intended to pay it off.[180]

Gregg and Natasha visited several senior bankers in the City of London, posing as investors. Claiming to be a couple named Melanie and Arthur Simpson, who owned horse-racing stables and had just inherited £5 million, they met with two vice presidents of Merrill Lynch, who told them:

Huntingdon Life Sciences are almost impossible to deal in. As high risk goes, you are at the leading edge of high risk. I would stay in cash. If it was my money, I wouldn't touch

[HLS] if my life depended on it ... cheap doesn't mean good. They are cheap usually for a reason: they are crap.

Their next stop was a senior director at UBS Warburg, who confirmed the feeling amongst the City of London's financial experts:

I am a banker. If I was to give you financial advice, I think I would say [HLS] are very, very high risk. I think as a banker I could not recommend those ... stocks to you. Those ... are very, very high risk, off the scale high risk.[181]

* * *

As their national chapter grew, SHAC Italia's organisers launched a new campaign against Morini Farm, a beagle breeder and HLS' supplier in Emilia-Romagna:

Trucks transporting beagles from Morini to a laboratory in Germany were stopped at the Austrian border. There were irregularities with the paperwork, and evidence of cruelty, so several politicians jumped in to try and use it for their own political purposes. As a result, all the dogs were rescued and adopted. Suddenly vivisection was being discussed in Italian media.

We arranged an unauthorised, unannounced demo at Morini, which fifty people turned up to, and we realised that we could start a proper campaign. It was a really great protest and unlike anything that had happened in Italy before; people were so angry.

Following this initial protest, and an ALF raid which saw the rescue of 128 beagles from the farm,[182] Claudio and his friends decided it was time to launch Close Morini. At their first march, over 1,000 activists from across Italy took to the streets.

In the UK, Cambridge University announced plans for the largest non-human primate laboratory in Europe. The laboratory was to be built on protected green-belt land, requiring a planning meeting to determine whether it was in the national interest. The campaign group Animal Aid seized this opportunity to force a debate on the efficacy of animal experiments. They enlisted the help of Dr Ray Greek, Medical Director of Europeans for Medical Advancement (EFMA). Cambridge University refused to provide anyone to stand in support of animal research, instead relying on a note from the government, insisting the laboratory be built.[183]

Dr Greek systematically debunked the research papers Cambridge University supplied to bolster their argument, but the opportunity for a face-to-face debate on the reliability or necessity of animal research was averted. With the government applying pressure, Animal Aid's director, Andrew Tyler, felt he needed something to balance out the 'national interest' argument. He slipped out of the meeting and called Gregg at SHAC from a public phone box.

At Andrew Tyler's request, Gregg Avery and Lynn Sawyer attended the meeting the following day. Outlining the campaign against HLS just a few miles down the road, they suggested the same would almost certainly happen in Cambridge. The police, who did not want another high-profile campaign in their county, eagerly encouraged the narrative.[184]

In his final report, the planning inspector declared that Cambridge University had not submitted evidence to prove their proposal was in the national interest. Concerns over SHAC-style protests took precedence, and he ruled the laboratory should not be built.[185]

Science Minister Lord Sainsbury happened to be a major donor to Cambridge University. On his behest, the government immediately overruled the planning inspector.[186]

In response, Mel Broughton formed Stop Primate Experiments at Cambridge (SPEAC):

> There is no doubt that we were influenced by what SHAC was doing. We had been watching and learning from SHAC, and we used home demos and the disruption of events at Cambridge University to get our message across.
>
> After a big march in Cambridge city centre, some people headed towards the proposed construction site. I jumped into my car to join them but got stuck in traffic. It was completely gridlocked. My phone rang, and I learnt that Joan Court and several others had sat down on the A14 and blocked all traffic in and out of the city.
>
> On another protest, someone got into a university college and took over the lectern from an academic to deliver a speech against the primate lab to shocked students. We disrupted a speech made by Lord Sainsbury on the lawn of the Senate House. Invasions of university colleges were a regular tactic with college porters in bowler hats grappling with activists as they tried to gain entry.
>
> The relentless action drove Cambridge University's security costs up until they decided the project was no longer viable.
>
> It felt incredible to have won such a huge victory. We were elated.

SPEAC's success rippled through the vivisection industry, as primate suppliers across the globe prepared for disruptions, citing 'reservations about the stability of the UK market, in light of recent animal rights activity'.[187]

PART V

The Fall: 2004–07

Investigating and preventing animal rights extremism ... is one of the FBI's highest domestic priorities.[1]

– John Lewis, FBI

19

A Surgeon and a Spy: 2004

Brian Cass tried to make out that staff morale was fine, but when speaking to the workers I was told a very different story.[2]

– The *Independent*

In 2004, Mark Matfield, executive director of the Research Defence Society (RDS), warned that a 'brain drain to the US' was increasingly likely – unless the government created criminal offences targeting animal liberation activists.[3]

At the same time, Trevor Jones, director general of the Association of the British Pharmaceutical Industry (ABPI), claimed his colleagues were drafting legislation 'specific to animal protesters', which they hoped the government would adopt into law.[4]

During a secretive meeting of the Ministerial Industry Strategy Group (MISG) in April 2004, government minister Caroline Flint ruled out the 'problematic' new legislation. In response, Andrew Witty from GlaxoSmithKline announced that the firm 'had decided not to make any further investments in animal research in the UK until and unless the problem of the extremists was resolved'. Tim McKillop from AstraZeneca declared that his firm was similarly minded. He reminded Caroline Flint that they had the power to 'potentially undermine the Government's entire R&D strategy.' She caved, agreeing that the government would 'announce a decision on possible new legislation soon'.[5]

The new laws would take over a year to surface, but other action was already in progress. Amidst claims that Government Communications Headquarters (GCHQ) were monitoring SHAC phones,[6] New Labour set up the National Extremism Tactical Coordination Unit (NETCU).[7] This specialist police unit claimed to combat all forms of radical dissent and extremism. In reality, they targeted SHAC almost exclusively. Unlike most police units, NETCU was established as a private company to ensure it couldn't be scrutinised under the Freedom of Information Act (FoIA). Most of their funding came from the Association of Chief of Police Officers (ACPO), who in turn were financed by the Home Office.[8] They subsidised their income by offering paid advice and other services to private companies.[9]

NETCU made no attempt to veil their bias. Their website 'links' page contained six web pages belonging to pro-vivisection lobby groups.[10] Their focus on SHAC wasn't because the campaign had 'gone too far' but because NETCU viewed their cause as morally wrong. Superintendent Steve Pearl, the public face of NETCU, later became the director of a company which recruited staff for animal testing facilities.[11]

NETCU's first job was to dissuade Securicor from cancelling their security contracts with HLS,[12] because of what Brian Cass described as 'a few ladies with placards and a bit of noise'.[13] They failed, forcing HLS to employ their security guards directly.

In April 2004, the RDS launched a new organisation at a reception in Parliament: Victims of Animal Rights Extremism (VARE).[14] This group, comprised of anonymous targets of ALF activity, intended to emotionally coerce the government into tougher action.[15] Once again, criminal actions were leveraged to supress the lawful protests of above-ground campaigners.

As the government bore down on the animal liberation movement, a lone article in *The Times* pondered an important question. Were the more militant actions a direct result of the government's refusal to enact its pre-election promise to hold a Royal Commission into vivisection?[16]

* * *

World Day for Animals in Laboratories in 2004 was more muted than previous years. Nonetheless, over 1,000 campaigners brought the streets of Cambridge to a standstill.[17]

Events surrounding World Day spilled out and developed into World Week. As activists held demos and actions against HLS' collaborators across the globe, Dr Jerry Vlasak, the North American trauma surgeon, flew to Britain to throw his support behind SHAC UK.

Jerry Vlasak had once been a vivisector himself, having researched arterial hardening in dogs and rabbits at Harbor-UCLA Medical Center as a medical resident.[18] His wife, former child star Pam Ferdin, had encouraged him to read into the issues of animal research. When he did, he came to some stark conclusions:

I had long had the suspicion that vivisection wasn't the magic bullet everyone pretended it was. While I worked in the laboratory, it all seemed to be a political, social, and career game with drug companies taking my wife and me out to fancy dinners and paying for hotel rooms and travel to meetings.

Even though I had grown up with dogs and would have protested that I was an animal lover, I gave no thought whatsoever to experimenting on them in the laboratory. It's what doctors DID, so why should I question it? I wish someone had brought the issue up for discussion with me much sooner, because I hope that I would have listened, thought about it, and changed. But if that weren't effective, I truly believe that they would have been justified in stopping my work by other means.

For the duration of the SHAC campaign, it was incredibly rare for the media to show a debate between a pro-vivisection scientist and an anti-vivisection scientist. It wasn't because the latter didn't exist; a 2004 poll of 500 British GPs suggested 83 per cent of doctors supported an independent evaluation into the efficacy of animal research.[19] The shadow environment secretary, Norman Baker MP, observed:

This is an important survey result which rightly questions the extent to which it is safe to rely on extrapolated results from animal tests. There needs to be a debate about this matter, rather than the sterile one which the media has created, artificially juxtaposing 'animal extremists' with 'men in white coats'. It is wrong to suggest, as the media does all too often, that the scientific and medical community is all in favour of experiments on animals, and that they all feel safe with extrapolating the results. They aren't, and they don't.[20]

Seven years after their pre-election pledge to hold a Royal Commission into vivisection, Home Office Minister Caroline Flint admitted that the UK government 'has not commissioned or evaluated any formal research on the efficacy of animal experiments and has no plans to do so'.[21]

Dr Jerry Vlasak attempted to challenge the narrative by debating scientists from HLS' customers on-camera, but everyone he approached either ignored or refused him. In the end he visited the companies in person to debate with their directors on the ethics and reliability of animal research, particularly at an establishment as notorious as HLS:

Our first visit was to Novartis Pharmaceuticals, who financed the xenotransplantation studies on wild-caught baboons. 31% of the victims died within the first twenty-four hours alone from technical complications. I would be fired and banished from the practice of medicine if I experienced a quarter of that number of complications.

Amidst high security, they kept us waiting for half an hour until a low-level employee appeared, saying only that the company would have no comment.

Next, we arrived at Eli Lilly Pharmaceuticals, or rather their security fence, where the guards took my picture on CCTV while I waited to speak with a company spokesperson. I was again told the company would have no comment.

Our last visit was to GSK, known for their savvy public relations. Their PR man refused to meet me in person, instead conducting a telephone conversation in which he refused to give his name or make any statement as to his company's intentions regarding HLS. He would not arrange a meeting with me and other physicians to discuss the issues around the world's most notorious animal testing facility.[22]

On his return to the USA, Dr Vlasak was asked at a conference whether he thought violence had a place in the animal rights movement. He responded frankly:

I think there is a use for violence in our movement. And I think it can be an effective strategy. Not only is it morally acceptable, but I also think that there are places where it could be used quite effectively from a pragmatic standpoint.

For instance, if vivisectors were routinely being killed, I think it would give other vivisectors pause in what they were doing in their work … If there were prominent vivisectors being assassinated, I think that there would be a trickle-down effect and many, many people who are lower on that totem pole would say, 'I'm not going to get into this business because it's a very dangerous business and there are other things I can do with my life that don't involve getting into a dangerous business'. And I think, from a fear and intimidation factor, that would be an effective tactic.

And I don't think you'd have to assassinate too many vivisectors before you would see a marked decrease in the amount of vivisection going on. And I think for five, ten, fifteen human lives, we could save a million, two million, ten million non-human animals.[23]

Unsurprisingly, the international media leapt on his hypothetical comments. From the USA to Australia, the press publicly denounced him as the doctor who advocated death. He fervently denied the allegation:

I am personally not advocating, condoning, or recommending that anybody be killed. I am a physician who saves lives. I spend my entire day saving people's lives.

You cannot put the animal rights movement in a vacuum. You must put it in a historical context. We are fighting for the right of nonhuman sentient beings to not be exploited, taken against their will, imprisoned, and then tortured beyond anyone's comprehension for profit and bad science.

In looking at other historical movements to end the obscenity and egregious violence and death to innocent lives, including the fight against apartheid in South Africa, the fight to free black slaves here in the US, and the fight for the rights of indigenous cultures, violence has been used and there have been casualties.

I'm not encouraging or calling for this, I am simply stating that the animal rights movement is and has been the most peaceful and restrained movement the world has ever known considering the amount of terror, abuse, and murder done to innocent animals for greed and profit. If by chance violence is used by those who fight for non-human sentient beings, or even if there are casualties, it must be looked at in perspective and in a historical context.[24]

His clarification did little to quell the media hysteria. Despite an impeccable record as a lifesaving surgeon, British Home Secretary David Blunkett ordered that Dr Jerry Vlasak and his wife Pam be banned from the UK. His statement gave them an easy excuse to bar him, but government sources hinted to him that there may be more to their motives. High-profile medical professionals and academics who spoke out against vivisection were not helpful to the government's ambitions.

A second banning order, sent to a respected philosophy professor from Texas, supported that argument. Dr Stephen Best, an outspoken critic of vivisection, had made no violent or incendiary statements. Nonetheless, he was barred from the UK. His ban was temporarily reversed, but the following year the government changed their criteria and tried again. This time they used an excerpt from a speech which Dr Best claimed was taken out of context:

We are not terrorists, but we are a threat. We are a threat both economically and philosophically. Our power is not in the right to vote, but the power to stop production. We will break the law and destroy property until we win.[25]

They accused Dr Best of 'fomenting and justifying terrorist violence and seeking to provoke others to terrorist acts and fomenting other serious criminal activity and seeking to provoke others to serious criminal acts'.[26]

A short while later, the owner of HLS' supplier Newchurch Guinea Pig Farm, John Hall, told a Swedish newspaper:

> If I could only shoot off about thirty [protestors], it would probably be calm after that ... If I could kill a hundred of them, I would be guaranteed to get rid of the problem.[27]

The justice system considered such language tantamount to terrorism when coming from animal rights activists, but when coming from vivisectors, it was an irrelevance. The police took no action against Mr Hall. Aside from the newspaper he initially spoke to, the press failed to report on his comments at all.

Instead of trying to diffuse the outcry, Jerry Vlasak entrenched his position. He created a stark divide between his increasingly pro-violence views and virtually the entire anti-vivisection movement. In response, an ALF cell in North America agreed to be interviewed by *CBS News*. It was a huge risk. They were pressed to confirm their credibility with inside information on specific actions, knowing that the FBI would be analysing every word. They took the risk to convey a simple message:

> [Dr Vlasak] doesn't operate with our endorsement, our support, or our appreciation. We have a strict code of non-violence. Not a single human being in our twenty-to-thirty-year history has ever been harmed in an ALF action; that's not luck.[28]

Meanwhile, despite raids on SHAC USA's offices and the largest wiretapping operation in US history,[29] the FBI were forced to admit there was no connection between SHAC and the ALF:

The techniques used in this investigation, such as electronic surveillance, physical surveillance, record checks, pen registers, trash searches, analysis of telephone toll records, search warrants, federal grand juries, and information received from witnesses and confidential sources have not provided information sufficiently specific as to obtain an indictment or conviction.[30]

Trying a new tack, the FBI infected the computer of at least one SHAC activist by remotely implanting malware code-named Magic Lantern. This virus initiated whenever SHAC launched their PGP encryption software. It captured the decryption passwords, allowing the FBI unrestricted access to all of SHAC's private communications and files.[31] Despite the ongoing 'War on Terror', this was the first time that the FBI attempted such an operation.[32] The encrypted documents revealed none of the salacious criminal connections that the FBI had dreamt of.[33]

Nonetheless, the FBI decided to finish things once and for all. In May 2004, seven SHAC USA campaigners were in for a rude awakening.

At 6 am on a Wednesday morning, SHAC activist Andy Stepanian jerked awake – his mother was screaming at him to run. Before Andy had a chance to leap from his window and descend the garage roof, an officer from the Joint Terrorism Task Force apprehended and arrested him.

On the other side of the USA, the SHAC office in California was three hours behind Andy, and so Kevin Kjonaas was woken less dramatically:

We got a call around 4 or 5 am, from an activist on the East Coast who said that the FBI had arrested Andy and that there were other names on the indictment. I got up and put on court clothes. Sure enough, at 6 am I looked out of the window and saw all these agents in balaclavas wielding a battering ram, with their guns drawn. There were at least a dozen of them surrounding the house, and they all came barging in. They threatened to shoot our dog Buddy because he was barking so much. They had a gun at mine and Buddy's heads; it was horrible.

For Jake Conroy, who was also arrested at the SHAC office, the disparity between how they were viewed by the police and by the judiciary was stark:

There had been fifty or sixty cops to arrest just Lauren, Kevin, and I: non-violent animal rights protestors. I remember sitting in the back of the cop car, surrounded by police in armour. I looked over at one of the arresting officers, who had his balaclava pulled up so he could breathe better. As I looked at him, he looked terrified and pulled the ski mask down. It was all so bizarre.

New Jersey's Attorney General, Chris Christie, called a press conference to declare that they had removed 'seven uncivilised members of an otherwise civilised society'. A couple of hours later we went before a judge who said, 'I don't understand why these people have even been arrested, it doesn't make any sense.' And so, they released us without bail within a few hours.

Kevin shared the judge's bemusement:

> We were back at home by noon. All that hoopla, through all
> that craziness about getting these dangerous people, sending
> in men with balaclavas, and semi-automatic weapons, and
> battering rams – and we're back home by noon eating lunch.

Across the USA, Lauren Gazola, Darius Fulmer, Josh
Harper, and John McGee were also subjected to violent dawn
raids, and arrested for involvement in SHAC USA. The SHAC
7, as they became known, were eventually indicted under the
Animal Enterprise Protection Act.[34] A US senator hinted that
the government could not find the evidence they needed to
stop underground activities, so they went after above-ground
activists instead.[35] The FBI's Domestic Terrorism Section
Chief, Thomas Carey, added:

> We're going to take every tool we have in our toolbox and
> use it. We're going to be as creative as we possibly can to
> charge them with a violation.[36]

When they handed the activists their indictments, Kevin
viewed them with a sense of both bewilderment and relief:

> We knew there had been a grand jury investigating for
> years and so we knew they were going to indict somebody
> or some people on something; we just didn't know what.
> There was too much industry lobbying: a billion-dollar
> industry lobbying the Justice Department to shut these kids
> up. They were pushing really hard to make an example out
> of us because they saw the spectre of our success and what
> that would mean to their bottom line. When we finally got

indicted, we looked at the indictments and thought, 'Well this is ridiculous.'

We felt really confident. It all just seemed so slapdash.

In the UK, Parliamentary Under Secretary of State Caroline Flint privately admitted that the 'American approach' to dealing with animal liberation campaigners impressed her.[37] She arranged for forty-two specialist animal rights prosecutors to be trained in bringing 'difficult to prosecute' animal rights cases to court.[38] In Parliament, MP and ex-animal researcher Jacque Lait declared that Anti-Social Behaviour Orders (ASBOs) should be used against animal liberation campaigners.[39] James Paice MP, who had been lobbied by the BioIndustry Association, supported her call. A few weeks later a judge handed the first ASBO to SHAC activist Kate Jones for protesting on an HLS' customer's property. The order meant she could be sentenced to six months in prison if she protested against, or contacted, anyone connected to HLS. It also banned her from the entire county of Cambridgeshire.[40]

Meanwhile, the National Association of Pension Funds (NAPF) offered a £10 million bounty for information leading to the arrest and conviction of any animal liberation activist.[41] As SHAC supporters across the country considered committing crimes and handing themselves in to claim the cash, the bounty rose to £25 million,[42] higher than the reward the CIA were offering for Osama Bin Laden.[43]

Perhaps coincidentally, at the same time, some of HLS' Japanese customers paid private investigation firm Octaga Security to hire an analyst to research SHAC. Described by former colleagues as 'nearly broke' and a 'fantasist', Adrian Radford wasn't content with passively collating evidence for a fixed wage. He had more elaborate – and more lucrative – plans in mind.

Perhaps eying the immense reward on offer to informants, Adrian offered to go undercover in SHAC under the pseudonym 'Ian Farmer' on behalf of Kent Police.

As former Detective Sergeant Neil Woods explained, the police were desperate to get agents inside SHAC:

I was approached to participate in political work: specifically, to infiltrate animal rights groups. I wasn't interested, as at the time I was wholly invested in catching gangsters. I wanted to make the streets safer and thought that my work did that. So I asked my recruiter, where's the bad guy? Why would I spend months, or even years, infiltrating a group of people who want to rescue beagles?

I was approached again a few weeks later with a more earnest recruitment pitch. My nation needed me, I was told. If the group of businesses that relied on animal testing left the UK, then we could lose 5% of GDP overnight. This would apparently lead to a catastrophic recession. I was disturbed by the idea that police were being directed by political motivations. Or more to the point, that police were being used to protect a specific sector of business and the investments of shareholders.[44]

Interestingly, the political nature of animal rights policing came as a surprise even to the officers who accepted this undercover work. Writing in the *Special Demonstration Squad Tradecraft Manual*, officer DS Coles recounted:

Another strange effect of my tour has been the slow development of my low opinion of uniformed police dealing with animal rights protestors. I suppose that officers in all fields come across police officers who regard political protestors with contempt, but their lack of sensitivity and occasional violent reaction to one as an animal rights activist is often out of proportion to your behaviour.[45]

While dozens of spy cops had been littered throughout the animal liberation movement for years, none of them had uncovered anything linking SHAC to criminal activity. Adrian took a very different approach.[46]

Unjustly dismissed from his role as an army intelligence officer for his sexuality, Adrian had become involved in the gay rights movement, particularly the direct-action group OutRage! In 1998 he stood beside Peter Tatchell as they stormed the pulpit during the Archbishop of Canterbury's Easter Sermon.[47]

Armed with his knowledge of the campaign, a larger-than-life personality, and photos of his protests, Adrian Radford was ready to introduce himself to SHAC.

He made his first appearance at the International Animal Rights Gathering (AR2004), at an animal sanctuary in Kent. He strode straight towards the SHAC stand, mud splashing up his pristine white trousers, as he exclaimed how ghastly it all was. Almost immediately, he struck up a friendship with SHAC co-founder Natasha. He was bright, personable, and mischievous, and a world apart from the multiple undercover police and reporters who were thrown out of the AR2004 gathering over the course of the weekend.

Not everyone was convinced. Some activists including Sarah Gisborne didn't trust him from the outset and made a point of steering clear. Even some newer activists like Gerrah Selby were sceptical:

I was new to the animal rights movement, so I was a little unsure of myself. I was sixteen years old and had travelled to England and turned up alone at the sanctuary with a tent and a sleeping bag. I didn't know anyone and was grateful when I met Adrian Radford at the stalls in the main tent. He was very friendly and seemed like an experienced campaigner.

Despite having initially liked Adrian, I became concerned during the gathering when he tried to convince other activists inside the main tent that the SHAC campaign ought to compare the treatment of prisoners of war in Japanese concentration camps to how Japanese pharmaceutical companies were treating animals. This sat wrong for me, and at the time I spoke out against it. Every other activist there agreed that we shouldn't be exploiting xenophobic sentiments, and nothing ever came of it. Now knowing about Adrian's real motives, I wonder whether he was trying to sow discord around and within the campaign.

A few weeks after Adrian was implanted into SHAC, the £25 million bounty was discretely revoked.[48]

20
Gateway to Hell: 2004–05

At the moment it's not just Huntingdon that is under siege, it's the whole industry, day in day out.[49]
– Association of the British Pharmaceutical Industry

Through his friendship with Natasha, Adrian Radford swiftly embedded himself into SHAC's day-to-day operations. Using what he later described as 'ingenuitive and creative ideas about how to take the campaign forward',[50] he organised a string of attention-grabbing protests.

In a single day, he led a team of activists on twelve demonstrations outside a collection of HLS' suppliers. He declared it a world record and insisted SHAC publicise it on their website.

Next, he arranged an action at the Japanese embassy, which he described in the *SHAC Newsletter*:

Fifteen protestors formed up at Warren St Tube for a demo against the Japanese customers of HLS. Acting as a clever deception plan, they waited, and waited at Green Park, confusing the police, whilst a separate group of protestors silently made their way into the Japanese Embassy itself, past two security checkpoints and into the glass foyer where an exhibition was being hosted. As the deception demo made their way to the embassy, they struck up with their air horns and megaphones in protest. Predictably, the police guarded the doors – but it was too late; we were already in and awaiting our turn to cause mayhem behind closed doors.

The protestors inside struck up shouting, 'Japanese companies are architects of murder ... responsible for the slaughter of thousands of animals at HLS ...' They continued shouting, disrupting the embassy from within. People and visitors were sent scurrying away.[51]

Targeting the Japanese embassy was a new tactic for SHAC, who avoided purely political stunts. Despite Adrian claiming it was 'worth 100 protests', it did not catch on.

His next action took place during a pharmaceutical conference at the Hatton in London. Adrian and two other protestors attended a public meeting in the same venue, before creating a diversion. He detailed it on SHAC's website:

All of a sudden [one of the activists] fell to the floor feigning a sprained ankle. The security guards and receptionists compassionately helped the activist to the seating area, leaving both the main door and the inner door unguarded. [Adrian and the other activist] made the dash through the facility past both security doors and right into the conference. Air horns blaring, they successfully brought the conference to a standstill. As the air horns sounded inside the Gold Room, the security guard on the main door rushed away to assist, allowing the hoard of demonstrators waiting patiently outside to flood into the main foyer.[52]

Inserting activists inside conference buildings before the main protest arrived was a successful tactic, one which Adrian developed with finesse. He later hired hotel rooms inside the buildings to ensure that as police guarded the outside doors, protestors were already securely inside, storming stages and disrupting speeches.

* * *

HLS' draconian injunction didn't simply suppress protest. It offered an even more sinister opportunity for HLS to fight back against SHAC. HLS named several individuals, in addition to the campaign itself, as defendants on the legal paperwork. Former police sergeant Ken Smith had helped select these activists. The handful of names seemed almost random, but there was a pattern: many were people who had personally frustrated Ken Smith during his time as a police officer. Don Currie, for example, had irritated Ken Smith during a lock-on outside HLS' gates, and Lynn Sawyer had earned his ire when he smashed down HLS' wall to arrest her.

Shockingly, the judge agreed to a joint costs order. Don, Lynn, and the other named defenders were liable to pay HLS' legal bills, as well as hundreds of thousands of pounds in damages.[53] They were not accused of involvement in any crime; they just happened to have upset Sgt Ken Smith. Now HLS wanted their houses as compensation and were legally entitled to seize them.

Don convinced the High Court not to take his family home, but Lynn wasn't so fortunate. She battled for seven long years before reluctantly reaching an agreement to save hers. Part of that agreement was that she would never protest HLS again. It was a heavy blow for a campaigner who had devoted and sacrificed so much.

Adrian knew SHAC were a grassroots campaign reliant on donations. Much of their modest income came from outreach stalls and high-street collections. A month after HLS announced they intended to take Lynn's house, the police mirrored SHAC's own methods, studying how to cut their income stream. The editor of *Eye Spy Magazine* introduced Adrian to one of their senior consultants, *Times* journalist Nick Fielding, who reported:

> The police are so concerned about the sums flowing into the coffers of animal rights extremists that they have set up a unit to investigate the funding. Stop Huntingdon Animal Cruelty (SHAC) runs at least six regular stalls – four in central London and two in Croydon, south of the capital. Members of the public who stop to look at the leaflets and other material on the stalls are usually asked to sign a petition against HLS and to make a donation.
>
> Information seen by *The Sunday Times* suggests that each of the stalls raises between £500 and £1,000 a day from members of the public. The money is collected and delivered to SHAC's senior figures, but from there it disappears from sight.
>
> Last night Tim Lawson-Cruttenden, a lawyer acting for HLS, said he had begun to target the activists' financial assets. 'These bank accounts should be open to public inspection so that the campaigns can prove they are bona fide organisations acting within the democratic process', he said.[54]

The amount of money raised, and the allegation that it just disappeared appear to be some of Adrian's first works of fiction. Heather explained the reality:

> It was ridiculous that the police kept trying to spread this false propaganda. They wanted to deter the public from donating to us, but it never really worked. The government and their agents never understood that most people don't want beagle puppies to be tortured to death in cruel exper-

iments. People didn't care what we spent the money on if it stopped that awful abuse.

In reality, SHAC kept thorough accounts of every penny we raised and spent. They were impeccable, because we knew that if there was just 1p out of place, the police would tear us apart. They seized copies of our accounts every time they raided our offices, and trawled them with a fine-toothed comb. Not once did they raise any issues or find any suggestion we were funding illegal direct action, so instead they publicly pretended our accounts never existed.

As Adrian and the police burrowed further into SHAC, other activists continued to wage and win high-profile campaigns. Following their success in Cambridge, SPEAC had rebranded. They changed their name to SPEAK and were pushing to halt the construction of a non-human primate laboratory by Oxford University.[55] After a short but determined skirmish, the main contractors pulled out of the project and the university suspended building work for over a year.

In the Netherlands, a planned primate laboratory in Maastricht was scrapped, following fears it could be on the receiving end of a SHAC-style campaign, while in Spain, an ALF attack permanently closed a monkey breeding facility.[56]

Buoyed by the ongoing successes, Gregg wrote:

These are amazing times and really are the theatre of dreams. If twenty-odd years ago anyone had told me that drugs companies would be threatening to leave the UK due to animal rights pressure, Cambridge University would be unable to build a new primate lab, major high-street banks and hundreds of other well-known companies would publicly distance themselves from vivisection, I never would have believed it.

We are now in the position where we can achieve all those things I previously thought impossible.[57]

Another victory followed. Enduring over 100 protests in five months, HLS' industrial gas supplier, BOC, admitted that the amount they were paying for increased security far outweighed the financial rewards, and they severed their contracts.[58]

The wave of optimism was dampened as the trial of the SHAC 7 got underway in the USA. Although it was swiftly postponed when one of the defence attorneys fell ill,[59] the legal proceedings caused a sense of trepidation across sections of North America. In defiance, activists in other areas intensified their protests. A new chapter sprung up in New York, named Win Animal Rights (WAR), who announced:

What do you do when you learn that the New York Police Department is holding secret meetings in [HLS' CEO Andrew Baker's] apartment? How do you deal with the fact that you are with the only group in the city that cannot get a sound permit to use a bullhorn during a protest? What do you do when you realise that as long as you continue to protest, members of your group will be subjected to police harassment, intimidation, and arrest?

Declare WAR! ... We studied the brilliant campaigns being waged in the U.K. and modelled our efforts after those that we witnessed leading to the greatest economic impact.[60]

Amidst the action, Gregg Avery was having concerns. If HLS admitted defeat, one of their larger, less vulnerable competitors might buy them out. That would be a hollow victory. HLS had initially seemed low-hanging fruit. Due to repeated government intervention, the campaign had laboured on far longer than anyone expected. The movement was largely focused on a single laboratory, rather than the industry as a whole.

Non-human animals are transported to the UK in huge numbers for testing. Some, like certain species of primate, cannot be bred in the British climate, nor in captivity. Others have been genetically engineered by breeders who patent specific strains.[61] Identifying a multitude of bottlenecks which activists could block to end this trade, Gregg co-founded a new grassroots campaign called Gateway to Hell.[62]

Using a decoy protest in Oxford to divert police,[63] the campaign launched with a three-pronged assault on Britain's airports, where laboratory animals routinely arrived in the cargo holds of passenger planes or on private jets. As two teams stormed Terminals 2 and 3 of Heathrow, a third team headed inside Manchester Airport.[64] The protests were loud and visual but intended to win hearts and minds, rather than delaying or grounding flights. SHAC and Gateway to Hell wanted travellers, pilots, ground crew, and aircrew to know all about the countless primates, dogs, guinea pigs, and other animals being transported for vivisection beneath their feet.

Coordinating the Terminal 2 invasion, Adrian was responsible for contacting activists to tell them the protest location. To partially sabotage the action, he waited until the last minute, so it was too late for many to get to the airport.

Adrian had successfully imbedded himself into SHAC, but he had a bigger prize in mind: he wanted to 'infiltrate the ALF'. It wouldn't be easy; ALF activists work alone or in small teams with trusted friends and the friends he had made in SHAC were not part of the ALF.

Unable to infiltrate an existing ALF cell, he created his own. With his police handler's permission, he selected two new activists and convinced them to raid a chicken farm. He later admitted, 'It was myself that set up the operation; nobody would help me, nobody would give me any guidance whatsoever.'[65] The communiqué he released following the action was also remarkably honest:

> Three very novice people went out to find some animals to liberate. It wasn't hard to do; we soon found some chicken sheds, and that was it. We bungled a few times, made loads of noise, but we still managed to liberate nine chickens from their deaths in darkness, which is how they live.[66]

To impress his new team, Adrian purchased a second-hand car, which he parked beneath the sign of an HLS' supplier. He filmed himself covering it in paint stripper. Two weeks later, the Queen addressed the nation during her annual speech:

> The powers the police and others have to fight crime will be strengthened. In particular ... new measures to deal with harassment by animal rights extremists.[67]

It is unknown how many actions the police arranged for Adrian and his new cell to carry out in the weeks that followed, but by January 2005, they had progressed from 'bungling' to highly proficient.

He told his story to *The Times*:

> A Jaguar saloon carrying two animal rights activists and their getaway driver turned into an estate of executive homes in Surrey. Their target: a comfortable, mock-Tudor house behind a screen of trees. Within five minutes, the pair had wrecked three vehicles. They had also daubed abuse all over the front of the property.

The raid in which [Adrian] took part, on the house in Surrey, was the last target of five in what the group called its 'big night'. The owner was an executive at BAA [Margaret Ewing], whose airports were being used for the import of laboratory animals.

Radford remembers buying large quantities of paint stripper and paint at a Homebase store in Croydon, south London, incongruously paying with bags full of coins taken from an ALF stash.

Slogans such as 'scum' were spray-painted over the house. The calling card of the ALF, the letter A inside a circle, was painted on the front door.

Tyres on the three cars in front of the home were pierced with a bradawl and their paintwork wrecked. Expanding foam was sprayed into the tailpipes to wreck their exhaust systems.[68]

Adrian hired a car, purchased the equipment used in the attack, and organised all five of the home visits that took place that night, resulting in significant damage to fourteen vehicles. In one night alone, he was responsible for damaging more cars than any ALF activist has ever been convicted of. The exact number of attacks he organised and carried out over the course of his deployment remains unclear, and his accomplices were never identified or prosecuted.

In an interview for Dutch TV, Adrian admitted that his police handlers selected his targets for a very specific reason:

When the attack happened against Margaret Ewing's house, the director of British Airports Authority, and they were attacking Heathrow Airport. It then became political … If it gets political, more resources are dedicated against it.

And eventually, or very quickly, you'll see people getting rounded up.[69]

A year after GlaxoSmithKline and AstraZeneca had pressured the British government into agreeing to 'legislation specific to animal protesters',[70] Adrian's activism gave them the excuse they needed to roll it out. Amongst those arguing for it in the House of Lords were former vivisector Lord Soulsby and biotech CEO Lord Drayson. They didn't just criticise criminal actions like those carried out by Adrian Radford, they wanted to outlaw all effective protest. Lord Drayson complained, 'These extremists are adept at exploiting the freedoms that our democracy provides.'[71]

The proposed new laws were draconian. As well as changing the Police and Justice Bill to finally ban home demonstrations completely, Sections 145 and 146 of the Serious and Organised Crime and Police Act (SOCPA) introduced even harsher restrictions.[72] Under the Act, any civil or criminal offence which 'interfered with the contractual relationship of an animal research organisation' carried up to five years in prison.

Under the proposals, age-old protest tactics such as lock-ons, or even walking through the car park of a company handing out leaflets, could be punishable by years in prison. If you chained yourself to the gate of a chicken farm, you would face a small fine. If the chicken farm bred hens for animal testing, you would now be looking at jail time.

To fend off civil liberties concerns, the Research Defence Society (RDS) arranged a meeting between human rights organisation Liberty and the Victims of Animal Rights Extremism (VARE).[73] Once more, ALF actions were used to persecute SHAC. Following the meeting, Liberty refused to speak with SHAC and have never publicly discussed the controversial laws.[74] The only person to speak out against them was social justice advocate and environmentalist, George Monbiot:

> Protest is inseparable from democracy. Every time it is restricted, the state becomes less democratic. Democracies such as ours will come to an end not with the stamping of boots and the hoisting of flags, but through the slow accretion of a thousand dusty codicils.
>
> By the time we have lost our freedoms, we will have forgotten what they were.[75]

This was perhaps the most significant assault on the right to protest since the miners' strike. Nevertheless, the laws passed.

For many activists, like Sarah Gisborne, the new laws were irrelevant. Following her release from prison, she had slowly moved away from SHAC and focused on ALF activities, until the police caught up with her once more:

> When you start protesting with banners and leaflets, and they're not listening to you, you have to think about what you can do so they might listen a bit more. And that's when people like me start doing home visits. When something affects you personally, you tend to listen harder.
>
> I got caught because I got carried away. I just happened to be passing the house of a couple who have worked at HLS in primate toxicology for years. On the spur of the moment I thought, 'Oh, fuck it, this needs to be done.' Even though I parked a little bit away, new cameras had been installed, and they picked up my number plate.
>
> When I took my car back to the rental place, a plainclothes police officer came up to me and said, 'Sarah Gisborne?' and that was that.

I was landed with a six-and-a-half-year prison sentence because I just couldn't resist getting those people while I was in the area. I knew I shouldn't; I was unprepared. But they torture monkeys to death daily in the most perverse way, and someone has to defend those innocent individuals who are facing the worst kind of violence imaginable. You can't be lucky all the time, I got caught, and I have no regrets about anything I did. I still feel it wasn't enough.

Sarah's lengthy prison sentence was for damaging eight vehicles belonging to HLS staff and associates,[76] six fewer than Adrian Radford confessed to attacking. Despite having no evidence to connect her to other ALF attacks, the judge was asked to take into consideration a folder full of similar actions at sentencing. It is likely that at least some of those attacks were carried out by Adrian Radford. When she was released from prison, in an attempt to humiliate her, Sarah was informed that she had to sign the Sex Offenders Register, as the cars she had damaged were parked outside homes where children might have been living. In disgust she refused, and the matter was quickly dropped.

Facing a growing mountain of injunctions and with the new SOCPA legislation criminalising anything but the most ineffectual protest, more and more frustrated protestors felt compelled to follow the same path as Sarah.

At the other end of the spectrum, John Curtin – a key figure during the Huntingdon Death Sciences camps – attempted the opposite tactic. Under the banner of 'Meditate to Liberate',[77] he gathered a group of religious and spiritual activists to try something different:

I'd been to India and met a Buddhist monk. We told him about HLS, and he said he felt sorry for the people who worked there. His first sympathy lay with the animals, but he also pitied the people who worked there. It gave me an idea that just for one day we should send love and kindness to the staff.

We had Christians, Jews, Sikhs, Buddhists, Native Americans, and people from a huge variety of religious and spiritual backgrounds.

It was a serious idea, but it was done with a sense of humour to throw their heads out. As the staff drove in, we called on them to turn around and go home, but did not yell at them.

For one day, instead of people screaming and shouting, there were Buddhist monks in their robes, in total silence, with candles. It was never meant to be the new kind of activism, but I'm sure having this quiet and peace for one day would have thrown them.

SHAC continued to demonstrate almost daily outside company premises, but injunctions forced them to stand far outside, out of sight and out of mind. SHAC campaigners with specialist knowledge of the law acted as legal observers to ensure that the police didn't overstep their already far-reaching powers. SHAC also embraced another strategy with a more global reach.

Repeating the success of European tours in 2001, SHAC made excursions to the continent a staple part of their approach. British activists who could no longer protest effectively against companies in the UK teamed up with colleagues across mainland Europe.

They found the European police's initial laissez-faire attitude a stark contrast to the militancy of their British counterparts. With little restriction on what they could or could not do, some protestors tested their luck, becoming increasingly mischievous and emboldened, and occasionally pushed the police into action. Theresa Portwine attended a protest at HLS' customer, Sanofi Aventis, in Paris:

We got past security and into their offices. We ran into every single room to cause maximum disruption. All their paperwork was dragged out and thrown everywhere. We explained to Sanofi's employees why we had been compelled to come and defend animals, but all the staff were just running around, and no one knew what was going on. We heard police sirens coming, so we all ran off in different directions.

I remember getting to the crossroads and seeing the police. I'd already taken my jacket off and tied it around my waist, and I saw this kid waiting by the lights, so I helped walk him across the road. It worked, and the police drove past. I hid in a public toilet, and as I stood there, I could hear the police going past with dogs.

What felt like hours later, I left the toilet and made my way back to a park. I had no cash on me, and no phone to contact anyone, but luckily another activist turned up in the same park at the same time.

As Theresa made her escape, Heather found herself cornered by the police:

We had all scattered, and it was funny to see the police walking right past everyone. Pam and Jerry were kneeling next to a grave, pretending to cry. Somebody else was hidden in a bush, but they found and arrested me and a few others. They locked us all in a cell together. It was horrible, like something from the Wild West with bars from top to bottom.

It turned out we hadn't broken the law, so they let us go. As I'd already been arrested and released, I flew home as planned, but Jerry bought everyone else tickets for the Eurostar.

As I landed in the UK, there were loads of men in suits on the other side of the barriers, but I didn't think anything of it, and gave my passport to customs. He looked at it, turned around, and handed it straight over to a man in a suit.

All these Men in Black characters suddenly surrounded me. They confiscated my rucksack and took me into an interview room. I refused to speak to them, and they kept saying, 'If you don't answer our questions, we can hold you for forty-eight hours.'

I was exhausted, so being able to sleep for forty-eight hours sounded quite nice. They kept asking where the others were; I found it hilarious that the others were already back in the UK and they had no idea.

They let me go after a few hours.

Police detained Heather under Schedule 7, a law intended for questioning and searching potential terror suspects as they enter the UK. As part of the 'War on Terror', these powers fall outside the usual police framework, and allow officers to hold anyone for up to nine hours without 'reasonable suspicion' of a crime, and without a lawyer.[78] Being stopped under Schedule 7 became routine for anyone travelling home to the UK after a SHAC protest.

The British government were frustrated that the French authorities hadn't done more to counter SHAC's disruptive protests. They contacted all the EU countries in which SHAC operated and pleaded with them to act 'hard and efficient'.[79]

Perhaps as a result, police arrested several activists on the next SHAC tour in Scandinavia.[80] One of the British activists who took part remembers:

Without all the restrictions we had in the UK, we finally felt free to protest again. As always, we were peaceful and non-violent, but we did go a bit wild. I remember as we drove away from one office in Sweden we were followed across the country and as I turned around and looked behind us, I could see a convoy of police cars. It was like the OJ Simpson pursuit. Eventually they put up a roadblock and arrested us. I stayed in prison for about a week before they let us go. We were really annoying, but we hadn't actually broken any laws so they couldn't charge us with anything. They basically said, 'As long as you leave the country we don't really care.'

We went to Finland, and loads of us got arrested there too. Again, we hadn't broken any laws, they just didn't know what to do with us. At the police station, I was taken to have my picture taken, but I refused and hid my face. An officer pulled my hood off so I pulled faces so they couldn't get a proper photo. They yanked my hair, and it really hurt, so I started screaming. Everyone else had been released by this point and were waiting outside, but they heard me screaming and thought I was being tortured, and suddenly someone outside threw a rock through the window!

As I was being released, everyone else was being brought back in for smashing the window, just because I was being stroppy.

Our protests were certainly disruptive, but I always found it strange when the media or the British police described them as 'violent'. We all abhorred violence. That was the whole point. We hurt no one, and we were never violent. We were just really annoying.

21

Operation Kick Ass: 2005

I'm dismayed and shocked. To go right to the heart of the financial powerhouse of the world in that way is very serious indeed.[81]

– Simon Festing, RDS

SHAC's European tours came fast and furious. Protests in the Netherlands were followed with an excursion to HLS' Swiss customers, and then a road trip around Italy. Megaphone-wielding protestors invaded Novartis in Basel, as others stormed Roche's laboratories in Milan. In Paris, demonstrators set off sirens in offices and flung paperwork into the air.[82]

With British activists feeling pushed out of their own country, their determination fuelled the energy of existing European groups. Gerrah Selby was one of the British activists who travelled to the continent:

I grew up in France and was used to a culture of lively and vivacious protesting. When I moved to the UK to attend university, I was baffled by the heavy-handed way in which animal rights protests were policed in England. On my first demonstration in Britain, I was arrested and held in a police cell for twelve hours, but I hadn't done anything other than stand silently on the side of a pavement with a photo of a vivisected animal. It felt like protesting had been made impossible.

It felt important to demonstrate in mainland Europe, where we could take our protest into the offices and onto the doorsteps of the corporate decision-makers who were signing away animals' lives. I would play them the tapes of the beagles screaming inside HLS, as I was convinced that being confronted with the horrific reality of their business decisions would compel them to want to sever their ties to HLS.

There wasn't the fervent irrationality from the police which was found in the UK. A megaphone wasn't seen as a weapon. Of course, we would be evicted from offices, and we got pushed around a bit, but it was seen for what it was: a non-violent disruption, nothing more.

Activists were regularly travelling, not just from the UK to the continent, but also within Europe and even from across the Atlantic to work together. Local ideas, tactics, and passion were spreading exponentially, and crossing borders to launch a protest became as normal as organising one in your own town.

Laura Broxson was a teenage activist from Ireland who joined activists from SHAC UK and USA when they visited Dublin:

The SHAC style of activism was something I hadn't seen before. Events in Ireland were passive, irregular, and lacked the tactics and determination needed for success. SHAC changed everything. It was the first time I took part in office occupations, and it was the first time I had even heard slogans chanted on megaphones. The knowledge, time-keeping, and efficiency were awe-inspiring. The cama-raderie was wonderful, and as a young teenager not only did they look out for me, but they treated me as an equal and made me feel part of the team.

SHAC visited Ireland several times, and the protests were always so effective in shaking things up. Most of the time we protested, the buildings went on lockdown and the Gardai [police] were called. Every target took SHAC so seriously.

While campaigners like Laura greeted SHAC's continued expansion enthusiastically, HLS' managing director, Brian Cass, was less impressed:

We have an animal rights movement in this country which has now become exported worldwide. Actually, I think the government in this country is doing well to begin to at least control the activities and put in place both laws and police resources to tackle them. What's happening is it's now being pushed abroad, so other countries now need to look at what's happened in the UK and learn from it.[83]

Despite the new SOCPA laws, SHAC's impact on pharmaceutical R&D spending in the UK continued unabated, as spending dropped by a further £100 million.[84]

To compound HLS' problems, throughout 2005 they lost one supplier every three days: more than twice the rate of 2003.[85] Every single company sent termination statements to SHAC, such as this from Penn-Century Inc., who supplied HLS with medical research equipment:

In light of recent publicity about Huntingdon Life Sciences and its research practices and the recent suit against HLS by the New Jersey Society for the Prevention of Cruelty to Animals, I had already made the decision that I would no longer do business with them.

Your e-mail message reinforces this decision. I want to assure you and others who will read this that I will never sell my products to HLS again.[86]

SHAC's approach of taking the message into a company's offices was highly effective, as Theresa Portwine found:

We walked into Britvic's head office because they were supplying vending machines to HLS. Someone asked if they could help, so I told her, 'I want to speak to the most senior person in this building. Don't bring me anyone else.'

The owner of the entire company was brought down to talk to us. He turned to his staff and said, 'I'll be in the boardroom with these people. I don't want to be disturbed.'

We sat around this huge table, and I started telling him about the violence and horror inside HLS. I told him about the puppies that were punched in the face; the primates cut open while they were still alive; and the countless animals poisoned, injected, mutilated, and dissected. I also told him how much money HLS owed Britvic, since HLS were never able to pay their suppliers on time. It always surprised companies when we knew stuff like that. After a while, the Britvic owner interrupted me and said, 'This is my business. I deal with tens of thousands of people, and I couldn't even tell you who's on my books, but let me tell you now, if we are dealing with a company that is involved with animals like this ... I don't need them in my life. What would you like me to do?'

They cancelled their contract with HLS immediately.

SHAC and Gateway to Hell launched a new offensive against the vivisection industry's supply lines. They targeted specialist couriers, who transported clinical waste or live animals, as well as pressuring basic mail services. The proved so successful that HLS removed their company signs and used the pseudonym 'Paragon Global Services' – a dormant subsidiary of HLS established in 1994 – so that they could receive post from companies who had blacklisted HLS.[87]

Activists planned a march for World Day 2005 in Dover, a major British port through which thousands of laboratory animals are transported each year.[88] March organisers, council officials, and the police agreed a route, but at the last minute, on police orders, the Chief Executive of Dover Council blocked the protest entirely.[89] In response, protestors launched a new plan called 'The Real World Day'.

What began as a simple march around Dover became three days of unannounced protests across Cambridgeshire and the home counties. With cars weaving back and forth in different directions, police struggled to keep up as protestors popped up at one target after another. Eventually, police contained protestors outside HLS' beagle breeder, Interfauna, where a sit-down protest blocked the road for over an hour. As more police arrived and a helicopter circled overhead, activists moved on to the secretive Babraham Institute. There, they filmed dissection tables through laboratory windows.

In July 2005, at the International Animal Rights Gathering in Kent, a dozen activists from across the world launched a series of protests against HLS' collaborators around the M25. Dubbing the protests 'Operation Kick Ass', campaigners from outside the UK ignored the SOCPA legislation and protested as they would at home. Buoyed by their enthusiasm, their British friends, including Theresa Portwine, followed suit:

> To be honest, the demos were pretty run-of-the-mill, or at least they would have been a couple of years before. Mostly we stood outside, and at some places we would wait for an

employee to go inside, and all run in before the door shut. We made as much noise as possible, and sometimes some paperwork might get thrown around. After a while someone would shout, 'It's time to go', and we would all pile out.

Following one protest, the police caught up with the car Theresa was travelling in. She found herself faced with Sections 145 and 146 of SOCPA:

Suddenly the police were behind us, and they swarmed around the car, banging on the windows, and shouting that we were under arrest.

They were really angry and shouted, 'Get out the car or we'll smash the window and pull you out.'

We were taken to a police station where the custody sergeant asked what we had been arrested for. He was told, 'Section 145, 146.' The custody sergeant looked blank. The arresting officer shrugged and admitted he had no idea either. Eventually our solicitor came down and spoke to us, and he told us that none of the police officers knew what was going on.

Theresa was charged alongside Mark and Suzanne Taylor, and the trio were hauled before a magistrate. The police remained unsure about how the new law worked, or even whether it had been broken. The magistrate gave them two weeks to make sense of it or they would dismiss the case.

Under legal advice, Theresa took a step back from activism. But for Mark and Suzanne, the incident seemed such a farce that they continued to protest as they always had. Over the next three months they carried out twenty-three demonstrations between them,[90] mostly shouting outside offices and occasionally attempting to run inside. Without Theresa or their international cohort, most of their protests involved a handful of people and only lasted a few minutes.

Their case passed from local police to specialist national units. Amidst confusion over the law's application, it was more than a year after 'Operation Kick Ass' that Theresa, Mark, and Suzanne were called before the Old Bailey, the country's largest criminal court.

Most of the trial evidence for the 'Operation Kick Ass' case relied upon CCTV and the activists' own video footage. While prosecutors described disruption to 'lawful' companies,[91] they failed to mention that these companies included firms like Monock Freight, who had a criminal conviction for allowing seventy-nine beagle puppies to suffocate to death in their vans.[92]

As the trial ground on, Theresa resigned herself to her fate:

In court, a police officer admitted under oath that I wasn't actually at the protests which formed the crux of the case. They had a photo of a guy with very short, cropped hair. He couldn't have looked less like me. It was ridiculous. Nonetheless, the judge said to the police officer, 'She was there as far as I'm concerned, I think you've made a mistake.' And that was it. He found me guilty. And that was basically the entire case against me.

I was just thinking, 'I can't have been in the right case because I've just been sentenced for something I didn't do.' One of the guards put their hand on my shoulder and said, 'You shouldn't be here. We've been following your case; you should not be sitting in the cells right now.'

Passing sentence, the judge explained he intended to provide a 'deterrent to others'.[93] However, his actions could only deter those protesting vivisection; no comparable law existed to disrupt any other form of social activism.

Mark was sentenced to four years in prison, Susanne to two and a half, and Theresa to fifteen months.[94] Just months before, their protests would have been legal. Nonetheless, the press labelled Mark as a 'terror plotter'.[95]

The prosecution took so long to build their case that before the trial started, another activist, Dr Joe Harris, was arrested for ALF actions and became the first convicted under Section 145 SOCPA.

* * *

Not to be outdone by their British cohorts, activists in Philadelphia smashed the daily protest record by holding an extraordinary forty protests in a single day.[96]

However, with the SHAC 7 trial approaching in the USA and SOCPA legislation being enforced in the UK, HLS felt confident the worst was behind them. They had worked hard behind the scenes to return to the New York Stock Exchange (NYSE) five years after being kicked off. With a loyal market maker, Legacy, HLS were ready for their listing. They finally had something to celebrate.

Their top team flew to the USA for a champagne breakfast with executives from the NYSE. Counting down the minutes until their listing went live, Brian Cass, HLS' managing director, explained what happened next:

We were ushered into a private room within the exchange where we met up with representatives from the exchange who welcomed us. There were signs everywhere saying, 'Welcome Life Sciences to New York Stock Exchange.' We were given our small, engraved brass badges, with our names, titles and 'first day of trading; Thursday seventh September.'

The Head of the Exchange came along after about half an hour and said she had something she needed to discuss with us, and then said that the trading was going to be postponed for a period while they considered various issues.[97]

The move was unprecedented, and the NYSE offered no explanation. In their entire history they had never changed their mind about listing a company less than an hour before trading, but HLS' lawyer, Mark Bibi, reflected the theories of many:

It was patently clear to me that the only reason the NYSE postponed our listing was because of concerns about the SHAC campaign.[98]

With protests hamstrung in the UK, and key activists facing lengthy prison sentences in the USA, SHAC had managed to publicly – and embarrassingly – sabotage HLS within the most powerful institution on Wall Street.

More bad news came for HLS in their third quarter results for 2005. SHAC's campaign against HLS' customers had slowed, stalled, and finally reversed HLS' orders.[99] The supplier campaign had doubled their operating costs. With lost income and increased expenses, HLS needed the NYSE listing as a chance to recapitalise.

To ensure HLS stayed off the NYSE, SHAC USA continued to target the laboratory's market makers and shareholders. In California, Nik Hensey hired a bus to take the show on the road:

I rented a party bus, and we drove around to different locations in Los Angeles with a huge crew of activists who would storm into offices and have a wild protest. Then we'd hop back on the bus and head to another location where things would get lively again.

One girl brought snacks for everybody, sandwiches, popcorn, and stuff like that. It was lovely of her, but most of the popcorn ended up being thrown all over these offices.

Eventually the police caught up and arrested a dozen of us. I was representing myself and was the de facto voice for us all at trial. I seemed to impress the judge, and I had a rapport going with him, right up until he saw a video of me taking someone's Beanie Baby off their desk and just chucking it. He was so disappointed.

22

The SHAC 7: 2006

We don't have a bank, we don't have a listing and everybody views us as a pariah.[100]

– Andrew Baker, HLS' CEO

On the far right of the Republican Party, Senator Jim Inhofe was repeatedly voted the most conservative member of Congress.[101] As a climate change denier who believed global warming was a hoax,[102] he later encouraged President Trump to leave the Paris Climate Agreement, while racking up a small fortune in donations from oil industry lobbyists.[103] He opposed gay marriage, refused to acknowledge homophobia as a hate crime,[104] and boasted a lengthy record voting against civil rights bills.[105]

For a man like Inhofe, the SHAC campaign was an anathema; the welfare of non-human animals could never outweigh corporate profit. Flexing his political muscles, he initiated hearings in the US Senate to introduce new legislation:

Its level of violence and propensity for harm has led the FBI to include SHAC, along with the Animal Liberation Front and the Earth Liberation Front, as the most serious domestic terrorist threat today, having committed over 1,200 acts of terror and over $200 million in damages. There is a need for tighter yet concise legislation to curb this criminal activity that, up to date, has been impervious to law enforcement authorities. Such legislation will close the gaps in the criminal code that have allowed SHAC, working with multiple other animal rights groups, the freedom to terrorise people.[106]

For a movement that had never seriously hurt – let alone killed – anybody, it was a confusing claim. Since the conception of SHAC USA in 2001, far right extremists had killed six people in the USA, but because such murders didn't impact America's economy, Inhofe and the FBI deemed them less of a threat than animal liberationists and environmental activists.[107]

Senator Inhofe called Skip Boruchin from Legacy Traders to the Senate as an example of a law-abiding citizen 'terrorised' by SHAC. As the owner of HLS' only market maker, Skip had received a home visit from the ALF, who poured paint on his house. Predictably, Inhofe blamed SHAC. Presenting the trader to the Senate, Inhofe withheld the fact that Skip was under investigation for illegal trading – a crime which later saw him banned from the securities industry,[108] and his company fined $1 million.[109]

Skip's character raised other red flags. In recorded phone calls to SHAC, Skip was reported as saying, 'I would trade in child porn stocks if it were legal.'[110] During the same call, he offered a complete list of HLS' shareholders to SHAC if they would allow him to remain HLS' sole market maker.[111] This deal would allow him to charge HLS an extortionate premium. SHAC called Skip's bluff by accepting the shareholder list but refusing to offer anything in return.

Inhofe's Senate hearings aimed to escalate the existing Animal Enterprise Protection Act (AEPA) into the Animal Enterprise Terrorism Act (AETA). As well as convicting animal liberationists as terrorists, the new law would increase sentences, and make it a crime to cause economic loss to any company connected to an industry which exploits animals. Having lined their pockets from industry lobbying, Inhofe and other lawmakers wanted to build a compelling case. They called a single animal liberation proponent, Dr Jerry Vlasak, to make the hearings appear balanced. Forbidden from showing any images of animal testing, Dr Vlasak began his speech:

> There are thousands of physicians like myself worldwide who realise there is no need to experiment on animals in order to help humans ... in a country where 45 million people have no access to medical care, in a world where 20,000 children are dying from lack of clean water every single week, there is no reason to waste hundreds of millions of dollars experimenting on animals. Huntingdon is the poster child of an abhorrent, unnecessary, and wasteful industry that not only murders millions of innocent animals, but dooms countless humans to their own unnecessary suffering, because scarce health care dollars are wasted on useless animal research and testing. The struggle for animal liberation needs to be seen in an historical context, like the Boston Tea Party ignited a revolution, like Nelson Mandela and his fight against apartheid, like the suffragettes, and John Brown, all of these noble and historical figures fought the governmental powers of oppression, slavery, and exploitation. Today, groups like SHAC USA and other SHAC activists around the world fight legally to end these needless atrocities and the ALF and other groups fight underground for the same purpose. This struggle will go down in history as one of the most moral ever fought.[112]

Senators and the press predictably ignored Dr Vlasak's explanation of the motives driving SHAC and the wider anti-

HLS movement. They focused instead on his previous violent rhetoric.

When the AETA finally passed, it happened in the middle of the night under an obscure procedure called 'Suspension of the Rules'. This allowed the Senate to usher it through quickly and quietly with only four or five lawmakers in the room to avoid objection.[113]

Lawmakers pushed AETA through the Senate by claiming it was essential to stop SHAC USA. However, the SHAC 7 were already on trial facing AEPA charges. Lawmakers and law enforcement had failed to communicate with one another and were working from very different playbooks.

SHAC USA were lucky to have their trial before the new bill passed, though it was the only luck they'd have. The court ruled against their defence at every turn, and even prevented them from choosing their own attorneys. Instead, the court allocated them advocates who had no prior understanding or experience of protest cases, let alone one as complex as this.

SHAC USA had become an incorporated company so organisers could avoid personal liability from endless lawsuits. As such, prosecutors added SHAC USA to the indictment as the seventh defendant, alongside Kevin Jonas, Lauren Gazola, Jake Conroy, Josh Harper, Andrew Stepanian, and Darius Fulmer. The case against John McGhee was dropped. Discussing their case and the AEPA laws, civil liberties attorney and politician, Barry Silver, remarked:

How dare they suggest that allowing people to know what's going on within these facilities constitutes terrorism? There is grotesque extreme violence going on within these facilities, and that should not be protected; the speech should be protected that lets people know what's going on. If that law was in effect when Martin Luther King was engaged in his activities, then he and all his followers would have been in jail for the rest of their lives because they brought down a lot of powerful interests and caused economic damage to people. It is a horrendous law; it's too vague, unconstitutionally vague, it's infringing on First Amendment rights. They haven't killed anyone, they haven't committed violence, but they're being bracketed with terrorists. That's what's unfair about the law; it segregates them out because the government doesn't particularly like their message or their cause.

This country used to be dedicated to the proposition that civil rights, the right to speak, is a paramount right. Now, the right to make money is the most important right. Now, corporations get protection, and the First Amendment gets very little.[114]

The SHAC 7 stood accused of inciting criminal activity by posting protest and direct-action reports on their website, as well as announcing and publishing details of campaign targets. Nothing suggested that any of them had committed – or organised – any specific crime, and nothing they had done or said breached any existing precedent for First Amendment rights to free speech.

The prosecution had been compiling their case for years. Unable to accuse anyone of anything specific, they devised a different strategy to convince the jury to convict. Their opening case statement began:

On a summer day in suburban Dallas, Texas, Sally Dillenback, an employee with Marsh incorporated, was home with her young son. The doorbell rang and Mrs Dillenback walked through the house to answer the door. When she got to the door, she saw her young son cowering behind the door with a kitchen knife. He was cowering behind the door that day, ladies and gentlemen of the jury, because he thought that the animal people were coming to get him … And that fear, ladies and gentlemen, is why we are here today. The animal people were coming.[115]

None of the defendants had attended that protest or had any contact with Mrs Dillenback and her son, but that was irrelevant. The tone was set: this trial would see victim after victim wheeled out to deliver tear-filled testimonies to an aghast jury. The defendants were banned from mentioning what happened inside HLS, as it might prejudice the jury and convince them that the protests were justified.

While the prosecution executed a well-rehearsed plan of action, the court-appointed defence lawyers were still scribbling their opening speeches minutes before they were due to be delivered.

A key witness was Brian Cass, who recounted how he had been attacked five years before. The prosecution brushed over the fact that his attack happened before SHAC USA had formed, on a different continent, and by an assailant with no direct affiliation to SHAC or SHAC USA.

Andy Stepanian saw where things were heading:

The jury felt the need for someone to be prosecuted for what was happening around the country, and we were the only people the government were providing.[116]

They did not convict based on the law; they did not convict based on the merits, or the constitution, but rather based on their disoriented emotions.[117]

All six defendants were found guilty, even though the prosecution couldn't connect a single one to any specific criminal act.[118] Accused of running the campaign, Kevin received six years in prison, and Lauren received four years and four months. For designing the SHAC USA newsletter and website, Jake received four years. Josh and Andy, as regional coordinators – organising demonstrations, and speaking at concerts and events in their hometowns – received three years in prison while Darius, who had barely any contact with his co-defendants, received a year.[119]

Andy spent six months of his sentence in a secret prison called a Communication Management Unit (CMU),[120] which was set up as part of George Bush's 'War on Terror':

> The CMU exists to fully restrict and vet an inmate's ability to communicate with the outside world … Each inmate must register their family or acquaintance with the Bureau of Prisons, and if approved can only make a single fifteen-minute phone call a week. Families are limited to a two-hour visit each month. Visits must be behind glass. Both the inmate and his visitor must comply with a search, and the visits occur with the oversight of a live monitor and a monitor listening in via telephone from Washington, DC.
>
> Unlike most prison compounds, there is no yard. Instead, there are three outdoor cages exposed to open air. Light passes between the cage tops, which are layered with razor wire, and there is a catwalk that surrounds the three cages. The catwalk is the only area where you can look up and see open sky without the intrusion of razor wire, concrete walls, or towers.[121]

Over the years that followed, the SHAC 7 pursued every possible course to win an appeal, but the justice system would never be on their side. One appeal rejection document claimed Lauren had participated in a bombing.[122] In reality, a radio station had interviewed her as a SHAC USA representative following the Seattle smoke bomb attack, which she had refused to condemn or condone. Meanwhile, the appeal judges concluded of Josh Harper that:

> Harper's personal conduct does not cross the line of illegality. To punish him simply on the basis of his political speeches would run afoul of the Constitution.[123]

Nonetheless, they upheld his conviction, insisting that his lawful actions paradoxically proved he was part of a wider conspiracy.

The SHAC 7 drew attention and support from social justice and human rights groups worldwide. The 2019 documentary based on their story, *The Animal People*, was executively produced by Joaquin Phoenix.[124]

San Francisco-based activist Banka felt her heart shatter as she watched the trial:

> There is no way to describe what it is like to see your friends being nailed to a cross for something you know they haven't done.
>
> We didn't hurt anyone, we didn't kill anyone, and yet these people, who ran a lawful campaign, were sent to prison. The Animal Enterprise Protection Act targets animal rights activists because we are effective. If you aren't effective, the FBI don't fuck with you, it's as simple as that.
>
> I ended up leaving the US mainland. I didn't trust the system there to protect my right to protest.

North of the border, SHAC Canada had been growing, and as the SHAC 7 trial ended, they found themselves on the receiving end of similar repression.

The Canadian campaign had carried out sporadic protests since 2003. It became a full-time campaign in 2006 when Gabriel Villeneuve visited the UK:

> I stayed in Britain for a few months and was really impressed with how passionate the protests were. Seeing people campaigning full time was really inspiring, and not something I had seen before.
>
> I got back in June 2006 and was really pumped. I was stopped at the airport by the police who asked, 'Okay, so what are you going to do now?' Well, I was going to start campaigning for SHAC full time, of course.
>
> It was a very intense campaign, with home demos every week. For us, it didn't matter at all that HLS was in another country; their New Jersey laboratory was a seven-hour drive away, and in Canada that is nothing. It felt like it was right next door.

As some of the wealthiest members of Canadian society, SHAC Canada's targets mostly lived in Quebec's luxurious suburb of Westmount, where residents boast an average net worth of nearly $4 million.[125] For those inhabiting the mansions which littered the neighbourhood, the black-clad activists descending on their exclusive community were abhorrent.[126] An article in the *Westmount Examiner* lamented SHAC's actions being protected under the Canadian Charter.

The Mayor of Westmount delivered a leaflet to everyone in the area and called a meeting to 'share what we know about the cause of these demonstrations and what we can (and cannot) do to prevent and/or control them'.[127]

Following the meeting, residents hired private detectives to trail activists from each demonstration, and local police were put on full-time alert.

Despite their protests remaining lawful, police infiltrated the organisation and subjected them to video surveillance and wiretaps, and bugged their homes and cars. In October 2006, police searched their houses, seizing and destroying personal property and campaign materials. Police illegally blocked access to Westmount, disregarding Section 2 of the Canadian Charter, which preserved the freedom of peaceful assembly.[128] Before one publicly announced protest, police arrested several SHAC Canada activists at their homes and at work.

Amongst those detained was Gabriel:

We were arrested before a Halloween home demonstration we had planned. Although the protest was going to be legal – and the police had no reason to think otherwise – we were charged at the federal court for virtually every protest and action which had happened in Canada.

Unfortunately for us, just a few years before, the province of Quebec had invested billions of dollars in the pharmaceutical industry, encouraging companies to move their headquarters there. So, there was a lot of political pressure to silence us.

There was no evidence we had done anything illegal, but the police claimed that some things we shouted on protests were threatening, and we therefore must be behind everything else that happened too. It was enough to allow the police to ban us from protesting against most of our campaign targets.

With SHAC USA decimated and outlawed, and SHAC Canada under increasing pressure, UK activists refused to be swayed. They continued as they always had. Activists like Heather assumed the strike back was confined to North America:

What happened to them was horrific, but honestly, it seemed so far away, and we were so busy with our activism that we didn't stop or change in any way, because it was different governments, different authorities, police, and laws ...

I was constantly exhausted and had no time to think. It would definitely have helped to have had time to stop and think a little bit, but it always felt like a race against time. At the end of each day, 500 more animals were dead inside HLS. 500 animals I hadn't saved. The next day, another 500 dead ...

Heather had no way of knowing the secretive Ministerial Industry Strategy Group (MISG) was hatching a plan at that very moment in the Old Library at Whitehall's Richmond House. Government officials and pharmaceutical executives were in attendance. Addressing the room, unelected Minister of Science Lord Sainsbury outlined his 'five strand approach' for 'eliminating the threat' of animal liberation activism, which he promised would 'solve the problem by the summer'.[129] Any mention of his plan was redacted from official documents, and no government department holds any written record of what exactly the 'five strands' were. Beyond its existence, all details of the plan remain a mystery, but its ramifications would come to shatter a movement.

23

The Calm Before the Storm: 2006

No group is more dangerous and determined to end animal testing than the Europe-based Stop Huntingdon Animal Cruelty.[130]

– Journal of Life Sciences

The SHAC 7 trial aimed to end HLS activism in North America. The government had removed people with varying involvement in SHAC USA, sending all activists a clear message: 'This could be you.' The threat of even tougher sentencing under the Animal Enterprise Terrorism Act (AETA)[131] hung the sword of Damocles above the head of every animal liberationist in the USA.

Growing trepidation pushed many activists away from the frontlines of animal liberation activism. However, parts of the US movement saw the state's fightback as proof of their success. Jake Conroy observed from prison:

If a handful of idealistic teenagers armed with nothing but big mouths and bigger hearts can move on to wrecking irreparable harm on the fur and vivisection industries, then any of us can. And must.[132]

Although SHAC USA had been ordered to end and remove their website within forty-eight hours of the trial ending, a new campaign appeared almost immediately. Close HLS' sleek and professional newsletter echoed the tongue-in-cheek hubris of its predecessor. Their first editorial was a direct call to action:

Martin Luther King Jr. famously stated that 'The arc of the universe is long, but it bends towards justice.' That wasn't empty rhetoric – in 1957 King was federally indicted for his part in the Montgomery bus boycott on charges of conspiracy to hinder and prevent the operation of business without 'just or legal cause'. The modem civil rights movement was still in its early years, and it would have been easy for King to give up hope. Though the absurd charges and arrests kept coming ... King maintained perspective on how long the fight for racial equality has been and will continue to be.

Now more than ever we must strengthen ourselves for the journey ahead. Now we must make the choice between giving our all to the struggle, or giving up in hopelessness because we wanted instant gratification and easy victory.

While SHAC USA has had to (temporarily) shut its doors, the campaign to shut down Huntingdon carries on as strong as ever.[133]

The debut *Close HLS* newsletter carried just a single protest report, covering a biotech conference in Chicago at which activists harangued HLS from the opening banquet to the closing ceremony. The second issue, released a few months later, featured reports from Ohio, California, Washington DC, Utah, New York, Pennsylvania, New Jersey, and Massachusetts.[134]

* * *

With Legacy refusing to abandon HLS as their last remaining market maker, SHAC discovered a weakness. Clearing brokers act as a 'middle-person' between the market maker and the stock exchange, and without them no trading can take place. HLS had been banished from the major stock exchanges and were trading on the Over The Counter Bulletin Board (OTCBB), but they still had further to fall.

Gregg Avery seized the opportunity:

Maybe Legacy who were in Hicksville USA, and who had shown two fingers to the animals inside HLS, were now vulnerable.

With a bit of research, we discovered that the clearing broker for Legacy was a company called Sterne Agee. We sent out an email action alert with details of Sterne Agee and [Close HLS] prepared to carry out demos against them.

We noticed some odd goings-on [so] we contacted the OTCBB and they said HLS had been bumped off on to the Pink Sheets.[135]

Even on the Pink Sheets, the lowest form of stock exchange,[136] HLS needed market makers. On the promise of anonymity, two small firms stepped forward. A mole inside the SEC revealed the new market makers were Seaboard Securities and Vertical Trading. In New York, Win Animal Rights (WAR) staged several protests outside Seaboard's offices. The company's president, Anthony DiGiovanni, warned WAR they would find 'the FBI crawling up your ass'; unfazed, activists distributed 5,000 flyers listing the companies' convictions for stock fraud.[137] When Close HLS and SHAC UK began targeting Seaboard's and Vertical's clearing brokers, both market makers withdrew their services from the laboratory. HLS were kicked off the lowest rung of the stock exchange into the murky world of the Grey Markets.[138]

The Grey Markets have no website or organised structure. They work like an auction, and few people find, let alone buy, shares there.[139] To be reconsidered by the NYSE, HLS needed a new market maker and to keep their share price above $8. Wallowing in the sub-depths of the financial markets, HLS repeatedly purchased their own shares at inflated prices to maintain any chance of re-listing.[140]

Right-wing lobby group, the Center for Consumer Freedom,[141] rallied to HLS' defence. They commissioned a full-page advert in the *New York Times*, costing $150,000, which showed a figure in a balaclava declaring, 'I control Wall Street.'[142] As HLS tried to convince investors that the situation was under control, the advert sent a fresh wave of fear through the very financial institutions they were trying to win over. Despite the adverse reaction, the Centre for Consumer Freedom paid another $150,000 to run the advert again two weeks later.

The advert coincided with a SHAC march through the City of London, dubbed 'March Against the Money Men'. Describing the demonstration, Gregg recalled:

> On April 28th during World Week for Lab Animals, SHAC held a march through the City of London to get the message across that to invest in HLS is financial madness ... In January when we planned this demo there were fifteen targets in the City of London yet as we approached April 28th these targets started to rapidly disappear.[143]

With few targets left in London, the march became symbolic; over 100 protestors wearing blood-splattered lab coats marched slowly past dozens of companies who had renounced HLS. The protest came to a halt in America Square, where speakers addressed the small but determined crowd, before several minibuses pulled up alongside. Activists piled into the vehicles and split into four teams, springing surprise protests at HLS' customers around London and the home counties.

Two weeks later, a new organisation called Campaign Against Huntingdon Life Sciences (CAHLS) posted letters to each of GlaxoSmithKline's (GSK) 167,000 shareholders, urging them to sell their stake. The letter read:

Holding HLS accountable means holding GSK to its promise not to use HLS ever again following the TV documentary 'Countryside Undercover', showing workers punching beagle puppies.

The only way to hold GSK to its promise is to target its financial vulnerability. We are therefore giving you this opportunity to sell your shares in GSK.

Over the next two weeks, every shareholder of GSK will be receiving this letter. If you have any doubts over the effectiveness of this action, then keep a close eye on the GSK share price and watch it plummet.

Should you choose not to sell your shares within the next fourteen days, your details will be publicised and within weeks a website will be hosted with all remaining shareholders listed.

The choice is yours.[144]

Although there was no specific threat, one shareholder branded the letter an act of 'terrorism'.[145] The *Financial Times* unintentionally highlighted how diluted the label of terror had become:

Whether its action is legitimate seems to turn on the motivation of its activists: are they practicing terrorism-by-proxy, identifying the shareholders as legitimate targets to other animal-rights activists with a record of violence? Or does CAHLS sincerely believe that publishing shareholders' names would shame them? If so, it is acting in a rather mainstream way.[146]

In response to the letters, a new police unit, the National Domestic Extremism Team (NDET),[147] launched an inquiry. Newspapers including the *Guardian* urged recipients to seal their letter in a plastic bag without touching it so that it could be forensically analysed.[148]

CAHLS had signed the letter, but the media accused SHAC. With the government already considering tightening shareholder anonymity, Gregg insisted SHAC had no interest in such an action,[149] and a campaign spokesperson was clear in their response:

We think it is perfectly acceptable to contact Glaxo shareholders to politely inform them of this connection. However, SHAC does not support the publication of individual shareholders' details.[150]

Amidst the excitement of the 'terrorist' letter-writing campaign, Tony Blair unveiled a new policing body called SOCA (Serious Organised Crime Agency), dubbed the 'British FBI'.[151] Like the anti-protest police units NETCU/NDET, SOCA reported directly to the Home Office,[152] and were set up as a QUANGO,[153] exempting them from any form of scrutiny. Their primary focus was international criminal gangs and according to New Labour, that label fit SHAC. Tony Blair commanded SOCA to be 'ruthless', suggesting they use their unaccountability to go further than Britain's uniformed police could:

My impression sometimes is that the system is struggling against a presumption that you treat these crimes like every other type of crime and that you build up cases beyond reasonable doubt. I think we have got to look at this.

To require everything beyond reasonable doubt in these cases is very difficult. I think people would accept that within certain categories of case, provided it's big enough, you don't take the normal burden.[154]

SOCA's role was not to arrest nor prosecute people. It existed to gather intelligence and work behind the scenes to concoct methods of breaking and dismantling criminal networks. Following SOCA's formation, encounters with mysterious 'men in suits' became increasingly common among British SHAC activists.

Meanwhile, another activist who had lost faith in the path of lawful protest was being sent to prison. Don Currie, the former psychiatric nurse whose family home had nearly been seized by HLS, was spotted by the director of PDP, one of HLS' specialist couriers, as he planted an incendiary device under her car. Don sprinted away, hiding in a dark telephone box just metres from his getaway bicycle. As a police car approached, the traffic lights beside him turned red, causing the vehicle to stop. An officer happened to peer into the phone box and saw Don hiding.[155]

Police connected him to a second arson attack outside the home of a GSK executive and remanded him into custody. He pleaded guilty to both counts and was sentenced to twelve years in prison. Judge Zoe Smith also handed him a life licence, which means if he ever breaches any of his licence conditions – which are rumoured to include not talking to another vegan – he could spend the rest of his life in prison.[156]

Another arrest quickly followed Don's. In the middle of the night, I received a phone call. My brother, Dr Joseph Harris, informed me he was in an Oxfordshire police station, and had been arrested for sabotaging companies connected to HLS. As a research scientist specialising in gastro-oncology, he felt compelled to save lives, both human and non-human:

My day job was developing a cure for gastrointestinal cancers using humane research. I also caused over £20,000 of damage to companies involved in supporting animal experiments at HLS. Experiments I view as wrong on every level. I am embarrassed when fellow scientists say that the testing of household products, agrochemicals, food colourings, artificial sweeteners ... on animals can be justified in the name of progress.

I hold a PHD in pre-clinical oncology and I've worked alongside vivisectors. I've experienced the inherent flaws of animals as models of human disease and the pressure on scientists to test on animals. I was not prepared to sit back whilst I knew that two floors above me animals were being needlessly sacrificed on the altar of human greed and curiosity.

I was imprisoned for three acts of economic sabotage against companies supplying Huntingdon Life Sciences. I slashed tyres, painted buildings and vehicles, super-glued locks, destroyed air conditioning systems, and in one instance flooded a building with a hose pipe through their letterbox, causing part of the ceiling to collapse.

At one company I triggered a motion-activated camera. The police arrived, so I made a run for it. Vaulting an eight-foot spiked fence, I was chased by ten police cars, and the officers took it in turns to jump out and pursue me. Eventually they got the better of me and I was brought to the ground under a volley of truncheon blows.[157]

When my brother was arrested, the 'Operation Kick Ass' activists were still awaiting trial. So, when he entered a guilty plea, Dr Harris became the first person ever convicted under Section 145 SOCPA. When passing sentence, Judge Ian Alexander said:

I am sorry that your conviction and the sentence I impose will seriously damage what was a very promising career. It may well be that your future inability to continue your research into gastrointestinal cancer will be a great loss to those who suffer that disease. The seriousness and objective of your offences must be marked both as a punishment and as a deterrent to others.[158]

Detective Superintendent Larry Ennis, of Northamptonshire Police, elaborated on why the deterrent was required:

This was not just a case of a few smashed windows. Harris's actions were ultimately affecting businesses and the wider economy.

The government used the case to prove their 'tough new measures' were effectively targeting the ALF, rather than suppressing otherwise lawful protest. In doing so, they failed to acknowledge the irony. With a guilty plea for Section 145 SOCPA, three years was the maximum Dr Harris could receive.[159] Criminal damage charges would have allowed a far higher sentence, such as the six and a half years awarded to Sarah Gisborne.

In an attempt to win hearts and minds, HLS allowed Channel 4 to film dogs undergoing experimentation. The puppies were slowly poisoned and killed on prime-time TV.

The programme showed the public HLS on their very best behaviour, and it made for chilling and harrowing viewing.[160]

Following the TV coverage, a mother and daughter contacted the SHAC campaign, desperate to tell their story:

'Animal technician, must be animal lover,' the job-ad read. I rang and asked for an application form.

I met my team leader. She was in the middle of doing a bleed with another member of staff ... Her left hand was used to hold the dog's muzzle upwards so that the neck was clearly visible to the technician taking the blood. The dogs were struggling and whimpering as the needle was stabbed and plunged in and out of their necks.

Every time I have to get the dogs out for something, I'm just thinking I don't want to do this. They think every time I come out of this cage, I'm going to have something done to me, and they are.

One study I was working on was an anti-cancer drug. When I got there in the morning, there was blood everywhere. I was shocked but told to write each dog up as having red-stained faeces. When I went in the next day, one of the dogs was dead in his pen.

Some dogs were not happy to be bled, and they would struggle and not sit still. I saw co-workers grab them by the scruff, shout and swear at them, swing them by the scruff and slap them. One [person] I worked with would go in and out about five times with the same needle, not hitting the vein. The amount the same needle could be used was two. I reported this to my team leader, but nothing was done.

There was a study that made dogs grow warts. These dogs had procedures done by a gun-like instrument, which they shot onto six sites on the stomach ... One female dog had warts in her mouth, and on her face, legs and paws ... and a male worker used to call her 'dirty bitch', 'slag' etc ...

When bone marrow was to be taken, the dog wasn't to be dead when it was taken but nearly there. The dog was laid on its back and the bone marrow taken from the chest bone. I was always told not to cry; they were doing their job; the dogs are bred for a purpose, and now they'd done their part and they had to go. On a night out, someone from necropsy was boasting about cutting the head open and sawing through the bone to get to the brain and how the smell of blood made them hungry.[161]

The police had planted listening devices inside the SHAC offices, and so were alerted to the whistle-blowers. Two Scotland Yard officers visited their homes to pressure them to stay quiet.

When the women's testimony was published, the Home Office accused SHAC of lying and claimed the mother and daughter denied making their statements. HLS declared they were going to sue SHAC, but the campaign had two tape-recorded telephone interviews and two videotaped face-to-face meetings. They were ready and prepared to expose the laboratory in court. Before they could, HLS went silent on the issue and refused to mention it again.

Regarding the employees themselves, Gregg surmised ruefully:

I can see the picture ... Cass sat on their sofa with a senior police officer telling them that unless they retracted what they had said they could go to jail for two years (which they could under the Animal Scientific Procedures Act) whilst these vulnerable people sobbed on their sofa and were bullied by the state.[162]

24

Eliminating the Threat: 2006–07

We are in a situation where anything that could be done to normalise our business practices would be welcome.[163]

– HLS

With SHAC fighting an increasingly uphill battle, the British police liaised with the FBI, hoping to replicate their success.[164]

The government's campaign to secure 'the elimination'[165] of anti-vivisection activism began with the arrests of four activists from Save the Newchurch Guinea Pigs (SNGP).[166] SNGP launched in 1999 to close a guinea pig farm which supplied animals to vivisection laboratories including HLS. In 2006, the farm conceded defeat and closed, but the activists were charged with 'conspiracy to commit blackmail'.[167] They were alleged to have played a part in, agreed with, or had carried out an 'unwarranted demand with menaces' against Darley Oaks Farm in Newchurch. The demand was 'close down your farm', and the menace was any or all criminal actions which had taken place against it.[168]

With a litany of ALF actions laid at their feet, the four pleaded guilty. Three were sentenced to twelve years in prison, and the fourth received four years.[169]

Buoyed by their success, the police moved swiftly on.

Dubbed 'Operation Tornado',[170] riot police battered down the doors of twelve campaigners from Stop Sequani Animal Testing (SSAT) and arrested them under SOCPA legislation. Sean Kirtley was amongst those arrested:

The door on my house had been so violently battered that there were only two shards of wood hanging from the remaining hinges. Police arrested me and spent nine hours searching the premises while my partner remained in the house; not pleasant at all. A megaphone, banners, thousands of leaflets, mobile phones, computer, digital camera, clothes, letters, and discs were all seized as evidence of my involvement in the campaign against Sequani animal testing laboratory in Herefordshire.[171]

While the Newchurch campaign had been synonymous with direct action and ALF attacks, the Sequani campaign was very different, as *Corporate Watch* observed:

What the defendants were accused of amounted to nothing more than a public, legal protest campaign. Nothing the average person would perceive as illegal occurred. No acts of direct action were relied on by the prosecution and no physical damage had been done to Sequani or any other company (except for one window broken by accident).[172]

Following a four-and-a-half-month trial costing the British state over £4.5 million,[173] Sean Kirtly was found guilty and sentenced to four and a half years in prison. His 'crime' was maintaining a website which reported lawful protest activity. After a sixteen-month battle, he appealed his case from his prison cell and his conviction was quashed, but not before the government and the police had made their point: if you were involved in organising anti-vivisection campaigns, you were in big trouble.

Tony Blair publicly displayed his personal views when he signed a petition declaring unwavering and unquestioning support for animal research.[174] Despite his grand gesture in front of a throng of journalists, which he acknowledged was highly unusual for a serving prime minister, the petition attracted less than 22,000 signatures,[175] a far cry from the 1.5 million thus far gathered by SHAC.

In a series of protests dubbed 'The SHAC Shakedown', HLS' customers and suppliers received protests outside their homes and offices across the globe. New groups formed in Denmark, Israel, and Croatia.[176] Protest tours around the UK and Europe continued with new energy and enthusiasm.

One tour saw fifty-two hours of protests over five days in the UK, with just one day of rest before the activists travelled to mainland Europe, where they joined activists from seven other countries.[177] They covered over 4,000 kilometres to protest against the head offices of HLS' customers and suppliers in four countries. British police asked their counterparts in each of the countries for permission to attend and monitor. European police forces unanimously refused the request, insulted by the implication they couldn't do their jobs.

However, following the tour, activists launched a string of home demonstrations against Novartis vivisectors in Switzerland, and at the luxury apartment of a Sanofi Aventis director beside the Eiffel Tower in Paris. As a result, the French and Swiss governments banned the next SHAC tour.

Frustrated, British campaigners travelled unannounced to the Netherlands for a five-day campaign trip with local activists. Taking an entirely different approach, the Dutch police posed for photographs with protestors. The only person arrested was a Novartis security guard who tried to throw rocks at protestors from the roof.[178]

To resume protests in France, SHAC obtained a permit from the Paris police and hired a French lawyer to accompany them. The French police gave just one stipulation: don't trespass. The protests were passionate but remained firmly within the law.

As SHAC maintained their presence in Europe, so too did the ALF. They rescued eleven beagles from HLS' supplier Harlan in Germany, and raided another Harlan facility in Italy, taking twenty-five monkeys and 1,000 mice to live out their natural lives at animal sanctuaries.[179]

The grim reality of life as a research monkey was revealed when the British Union for the Abolition of Vivisection (BUAV) released their findings from a twelve-month investigation into Vietnamese monkey farms which supplied HLS. Investigators filmed macaques crammed into tiny, dirty cages, compelling internationally renowned primatologist Stephen Brend to observe:

> The very scale of the operation gives cause for alarm. The whole feel is of an intensive 'farm' which, as with battery chicken farming, is designed with the quantity of output given priority over quality and welfare.[180]

In June 2006, undercover operative Adrian Radford attended the international Animal Rights Gathering in Kent. With deliberate irony he ran a workshop on security and surveillance, during which he dismissed activists trying to discuss lawful protest, focussing instead on avoiding criminal detection. He appeared intent on riling international activists into more militant action across mainland Europe.

Following the gathering, Adrian told the activists that he was closest to, including Theresa Portwine, some devastating news:

> One day we were sitting down, and he blurted out that he was terminally ill. I was so upset. Of course, I told him I

would support him, and that I would be there for him no matter what.

He started crying, and as we hugged, I told him that he was so dedicated to animal rights, but it was like he was lost between two worlds. He was putting so much of himself into animal rights, but I told him he should devote that time to his partner now.

The tears, like his illness, were fake. Adrian was not terminally ill, but the police had instructed him to extract himself from the animal rights movement.

After leaving SHAC, Adrian worked as a private investigator with surveillance firm ISS. According to former colleagues, he was tasked with tackling a major criminal gang and assembled a four-man team to provide logs, photographs, and witness statements related to alleged gun crime. ISS forwarded his evidence to the Crown Prosecution Service.

A year later, ISS informed the police they believed Adrian had provided falsified statements. They claimed Adrian had carried out the job with one other operative, not three; he'd submitted fake witness statements to pocket the wages of two imaginary operatives. The criminal trial against the gang collapsed, and police launched an eighteen-month investigation into Adrian's conduct.

The CPS informed ISS that they intended to prosecute Adrian for perverting the course of justice and obtaining money by deception. Instead, the police quietly closed the case, deciding it 'would not be in the public interest' to pursue charges. According to a source in British intelligence, a 'higher up' likely shut down the case to avoid Adrian's real name, photograph, or dubious reputation being brought to SHAC's attention.

* * *

The fissure caused by the SHAC 7 trial remained open in the North American animal liberation movement. For many, the deterrent worked as the FBI had hoped. For others, like Jeremy Beckham, it provided yet another reason to continue the fight against HLS:

The greatest gift we could give the SHAC 7 in their jail cells was HLS shutting down. We decided to hold a protest tour to let HLS and everyone know that SHAC in North America was not over.

The tour covered a huge area along the East Coast. In New York we protested outside the home of someone who transported animals for HLS. The police arrived and leapt out of their cars, shouting that we were all under arrest and ordering us to sit on the curb. One by one they led everyone to a police car, except me. Eventually I caught the attention of one of the cops and asked if I was being arrested too. He told me to shut up and sit still. So, I did. One by one the cops all got in their cars and drove off with my friends, leaving me sat alone on the curb. It felt like a trap, but I eventually stood up and just walked away.

At another protest, I was protesting inside an office in the usual way, shouting about HLS and handing out leaflets, but then I turned around and saw someone throwing computer monitors around. We all started running and split up into little groups. Me and two others were chased by two security guards. We ran all the way through downtown DC, the fastest I've ever run in my life. We sprinted right in front of the White House, pursued by these two guys in suits who had now been joined by two other cops, but somehow they didn't manage to stop us. We reached an intersection, where we piled into a taxi, and my friend screamed, 'Go, go, go! My psycho ex is chasing me.' The driver floored it, and we got away. We got dropped off at a Starbucks where some friends met us. They gave me spare clothes and told me to get changed and take off my glasses. As we were walking back through DC, we walked past a police officer, and I heard my description come through on his radio; they described everything I had been wearing, but this cop didn't have a clue.

North of the border, SHAC Canada continued to face harassment and repression from police in Quebec. Protests which once drew up to a hundred activists were now supported by just a handful. To evade the persecution, they attempted to move 3,000 miles across Canada to Vancouver. However, West Vancouver Police and the Royal Canadian Mounted Police (RCMP) were waiting for SHAC Canada the day they arrived. With police confiscating leaflets and arresting anyone who attempted to protest, SHAC Canada found its existence increasingly untenable. Gabriel and the other activists were forced into a difficult decision:

The intimidation became so bad that anti-police brutality organisations were reaching out to support us and writing articles about us.

I once got arrested for jaywalking and was taken to the local police station where the Canadian Security Intelligence Service were waiting to interview me. Another time, I was arrested for shouting threats at a protest that I wasn't even on. In the end, I spent a month in jail before I was able to prove I wasn't there. Again, they were just trying to tire us out, waste our resources, and prevent us from protesting.

It got to the point that we were involved in something we didn't sign up for. We wanted to fight to end vivisection, but we were just fighting to protest at all.

SHAC Canada's co-founders still faced charges from their arrests following the SHAC 7 trial. Facing an impending court case and constant pressure from the police, SHAC Canada renamed themselves Montreal Friends of Animals (MFA). The trick worked briefly, but soon enough, police subjected MFA outreach stalls and protests to the same persecution.

After lengthy delays, Dominique, Gabriel, and their friend Frederic were finally taken before the courts. Dominique was found not guilty of every count, while Gabriel and Frederic were fined and forced to obey strict conditions for three years. While protests continued sporadically, many of those involved found themselves forced into other forms of activism.

Despite police all but squeezing SHAC Canada out of existence, the situation did little to help HLS. Paying extortionate interest rates to their anonymous lender, they shouldered a long-term debt of over $70 million.[181] As they continued to languish on the Grey Markets, weeks would pass without a single HLS share being bought or sold.

A mysterious auditing firm called Hugh Scott stepped in to file HLS' accounts with the SEC.[182] Something about the new auditors felt odd to Close HLS. It soon became apparent that for the first time in history, the US government had set up a fake auditing firm to prevent a commercial company from going out of business.

Simultaneously, the US and UK governments pressured the NYSE to slip HLS quietly onto their newly formed ARCA exchange. ARCA was electronic and supposedly anonymous. To ensure the listing stayed secret, it took place on the last day of trading before Christmas, with a brief press release at

4 am.[183] There were no champagne breakfasts or bronze name tags this time.

SHAC were immediately alerted to the listing, which coincided with the NYSE merging with the Euronext stock exchange in Amsterdam, Brussels, and Paris. While HLS had escaped the Grey Markets, SHAC could now target their stock exchange on both sides of the Atlantic.[184] Gregg declared:

> If the NYSE humiliated them in 2005, why would Huntingdon want to list their shares on there at all? The simple answer is that they have to for their very survival.
>
> If they get kicked off the NYSE [again], then they are in the financial wilderness forever. Brian Cass and Andrew Baker are not scientists, they are trained accountants, and they are both fast approaching 60. If HLS are kicked off the NYSE, they will have spent the last 10 years for nothing, and all their plans will be in ruins. We will not back down from this fight, no matter how long it takes.
>
> No HLS means no 500 animals dead on their cage floors every day. Don't forget that. We will not fail them.[185]

With SHAC maintaining pressure on HLS' finances, the British government and police continued to do the same to SHAC.

Campaign groups of all leanings held regular outreach stalls on high streets throughout London and across the UK. Activists tended to stand behind a pasting table with posters, leaflets, and petitions highlighting their cause. Prior to social media, it was the main avenue for grassroots activists to present their case to the public.

Campaigners were legally required to have a council licence to collect money, but there had long been an unspoken understanding that this stipulation was reserved for large charities focused on aggressive fundraising, rather than small groups who kept a discrete collection tin on their table. For SHAC, that was about to change.

Two years after Adrian Radford encouraged his handlers to target SHAC's income, the police acted. On a single day, they arrested twenty-one SHAC supporters on street stalls across central London. While police press releases prompted headlines, such as 'Twenty-One "Illegally" Collected for Animal Rights Terror', when pushed, Detective Chief Inspector Tim Yarrow could only go as far as 'They may well be funding criminal activity.'[186]

The police had no evidence to suggest the money was being used for illegal actions, let alone terror. Gregg Avery retorted:

> Of course we raise money on the stalls. People know exactly who they are giving money to. They support SHAC and our objectives. This is a dirty tricks campaign.[187]

His accusation was well founded. Police press releases claimed that the petitions they seized were a sham and sent nowhere. They failed to mention the 1.5 million signatures already handed to the Home Office. They later seized petitions containing a further 2 million signatures from SHAC's offices; activists had hand counted every page and sorted them into numbered boxes, ready to deliver to the government. Even then, the police pretended that SHAC simply discarded them. The 'dirty tricks campaign' continued two weeks later, as Gerrah Selby was fined for Obstruction of the Highway during a street stall on Oxford Street:

> Further along the road from us was a Socialist Workers Party stall who were collecting donations, and the police

didn't even look at them. I went to court, received a fine, and learned my lesson the hard way.

A month or so later, I did another collection, but this time I received a licence from Camden Council. Nonetheless, police came and threatened to arrest us. They told us our licence was fake and refused to phone the council to check. We didn't want to be arrested again, so packed up and went to Hammersmith. We hoped the police there would be more reasonable, even though our licence was for another London borough. A few minutes after we set up we saw a huge group of police forming, so we packed up. However, we were arrested for Section 5 of the Public Order Act, accused of showing photos of vivisected animals which they alleged were 'offensive, alarming or harassing'. If they found it upsetting, you would think they would want to help us stop it. Instead, they arrested us and locked us in filthy, unhygienic cells. My seventeen-year-old friend was strip-searched.

The police dropped the case, but two months later gave Gerrah a subtler indication of their interest in her:

I had been out all day at a publicised day of national protests against GlaxoSmithKline. When I returned home with some of my friends, my key wouldn't fit into the lock. I looked closer and saw a long bit of broken metal stuck inside it.

The door was open, and it was obvious someone had broken in. We had no idea who it might be, so we all crept into the house and searched everywhere just in case.

Nothing appeared to have been stolen, but it was clear someone had been inside my house. I cannot think of anyone who would have broken into my house but not stolen anything other than the police.

At the same time, Jason 'JJ' Mullen encountered a very similar experience:

The front door of my flat on Holloway Road in London was communal. It was a Saturday night and, unusually for us, my partner and I were home. At 10 pm we heard someone trying to open our front door with a key, so I jumped off my sofa and grabbed a saucepan. My partner called the police while I shouted through the door that I had a weapon. I could hear the person running up the stairs towards the third floor. A police van arrived moments later, and they ran up to my flat, and then pursued the person up to the third floor. There was silence for a few moments before they came down and told me it must have been a neighbour. My neighbours were a very nice, quiet family with a young child, and certainly wouldn't have tried to burgle me. To this day I believe that whoever was upstairs must have shown the police some sort of ID which stopped them being arrested.

Another break-in took place at the home of acclaimed composer Edwin Roxburgh and his wife Julie. The septuagenarian had kept SHAC's accounts for several years. As the couple returned home one day, they spotted a figure dart out of their house and through a bush, seemingly making their escape in a police car.

With the police attempting to stifle SHAC's income and breaking into activists' homes, Tony Blair and Lord Sainsbury had initiated their endgame. During a protest at Little Creek Kennels – which cleared dogs through customs for HLS – the owner gloated that the police had claimed the protestors were all going to be locked up. Activists dismissed it as bluster and continued their protest unabated.

Tony Blair was so confident in his plan that he held a meeting with the US president, George Bush, to discuss his 'war on animal rights extremism'. He hoped it might encourage more American pharmaceutical companies to invest in British research.[188]

25

SHAC Attacked: 2007

A handful of animal extremists had succeeded where Osama bin Laden had failed.[189]

– Mark Bibi

I remember the noise as a roar of violent activity. A splintering crash, immediately followed by shouting, stamping feet, and smashing doors. I scrambled for my glasses, but before I could get them to my face, a police officer in full riot gear launched himself through the door and swan-dived on top of me as I lay in bed.

'Police! Don't move!' he screamed into my face. I couldn't physically move whether he yelled at me or not.

I was in the spare bedroom at the SHAC office at Little Moorcote in Eversley, ready for a protest tour in Europe. If the police had arrived an hour later, we would have been gone, safely boarding a train to France. As it was, they caught Natasha, Gregg, and me as we slept.

The dogs who lived at the SHAC house were screaming. Amidst the confusion, and somewhere beyond my bedroom door, Natasha shouted desperately back at the police. The noise subsided as the police relented and loosened the extendable nooses they had used to ensnare the terrified animals.

As they marched Natasha and Gregg from the house, I promised I would look after the dogs and phone their solicitor. This was just another speculative probe into the SHAC offices; of that, we were certain. As much as the government hated us, we were a legitimate campaign and none of us were doing anything illegal.

Suddenly I was alone in their house with two dozen police officers.

A detective demanded my name and confirmed I would be free to leave as soon as they completed their search. However, twenty minutes later he returned to arrest me on suspicion of committing blackmail. I was shocked, but assumed it was a ploy to prevent me from alerting Gregg and Natasha's solicitor.

They drove me to Alton police station and led me past an interview room, where Gregg sat in silence. I waved at him and he waved back before the door was swiftly swung shut. Instead of being booked in, they led me out of the building, put me in another van, and drove me down to Fareham police station. I was eager to call my partner, Nicci Tapping, to let her know that we had been arrested and I was likely to be home a lot earlier than planned.

However, as I walked past the cells at the police station, I spotted a pair of Nicci's shoes sitting outside one of the thick metal doors. My heart sank.

Nicci had been abruptly awoken at exactly the same time as Natasha, Gregg, and I:

On the evening of 30 April 2007, something didn't feel right. After dropping Tom at the SHAC HQ, an unmarked police car followed me home. Tom and I were founders of the Southern Animal Rights Coalition (SARC), and I was staying in the UK to continue our campaign against Royal Navy experiments on goats.

At sunrise, I awoke to what sounded like an explosion. I was disorientated, and I could hear heavy footprints stomping up the stairs in unison. Fearing I was being robbed, I sat up in bed panicking that I didn't have any money or valuables to give them. What if they had guns?

A swarm of black-clad men in body armour with masked faces burst into my room. They were screaming at me to put my hands up, and they towered over me with batons drawn.

One of the masked men asked my name, so I gave my details, and was told I was under arrest for blackmail. I was told I had the right to remain silent, but I waived that right.

'Who have I blackmailed?' They ignored me, so I asked over and over, 'Who have I blackmailed? How have I blackmailed?' The arresting officer told me he didn't know, and I would find out at the station. They handcuffed me and led me through my house, which was swarming with black-clad Stormtroopers, all with their faces covered. Everywhere I looked they were there, rooting through my property.

I wasn't allowed to get dressed and was led onto the street in my pyjamas in front of a *BBC News* camera crew. The police drove me to Fareham. The officer who was guarding me in the van told me that the whole thing was over the top. She said she loved animals, that we had done nothing wrong, and that at times like this she was ashamed of her job.

Once I checked in at the police station, I was refused my legal right to a phone call to family and was barred from my solicitor for over two hours.

Just a few miles away from the SHAC office, eighteen-year-old Gerrah Selby's world changed forever:

The sound of glass shattering woke me up. Before I could register what was happening, police kicked my bedroom door down. Half a dozen officers piled into my bedroom, screaming at me to put my hands up. I will never forget the dilemma I faced in that moment: whether to hold up the bed sheet to cover my naked chest from the aggressive, hostile eyes of strange men who had just broken into my home, or to obey their orders. After what felt like an eternity, I dropped the sheet, embarrassed at my own vulnerability and intimidated by the demands being shouted at me. I was afraid that if I refused them, I might get shot. I recognised one of the police officers in my room from our demos. He was smirking at me. They informed me they were arresting me for three separate offences, carrying a combined sentence of twenty-four years' imprisonment. I assumed it must be a case of mistaken identity, as I knew I'd never blackmailed anyone. After they allowed me to get dressed and then handcuffed me, they hauled me to a police cell. There, my shoelaces were removed in case I should try to kill myself, and when I couldn't bring myself to eat, officers threatened to send me to hospital where they insisted I would be force-fed.

Across the UK, Belgium, and the Netherlands, 700 police officers busted down doors and dragged dozens of people from their beds.[190] Kent police had been working from an abandoned police station recommissioned especially for this purpose,[191] spearheading a government-led plan to destroy SHAC dubbed 'Operation Achilles'.

Many activists were alerted by a battering ram breaching their front door. But others, such as Jason 'JJ' Mullen, found out a different way:

I hadn't been involved in the animal rights movement for a few months as my mum was very ill. I was at her house on 1 May 2007, when I woke up, ready to celebrate my twenty-ninth birthday.

I happened to check the *BBC News* website. The top story was nationwide raids on activists linked to the campaign against HLS. It was shaping up to be a pretty crappy birthday.

I phoned my ex-girlfriend, who lived at the last address the police had for me. Someone answered her phone, and I heard male voices in the background before the line went dead. The police were there.

I'd done nothing wrong, but was concerned about the two cats living at my ex-partner's flat, so I jumped on a train to Finsbury Park. I walked past a line of police vans and went through what remained of the flat's communal front door. I ran upstairs where a police officer asked if he could help me.

I replied, 'Yeah, I think you're looking for me.'

They immediately arrested me and drove me to West End Central Station. The custody sergeant asked who I was, and when the arresting officer told him, the whole room started to applaud.

Heather Nicholson had also temporarily slipped through the police's fingers:

I happened to be staying at a friend's house, and I turned on the TV to see Gregg and Natasha being led out of their house by the police. All I could think was 'Are the dogs okay?'

I phoned my solicitor, who told me that the police wanted to talk to me. I called the police to ask if the dogs were okay. They said, 'They're fine, come and get them.' They refused to say whether I would be arrested.

One of my friends collected the dogs, and I met them at a service station in Wales. We stayed with my mum and dad, assuming the police would show up at any moment, but they didn't. Two days later I handed myself in, after the police told my solicitor that Gregg and Natasha would be released on bail if I did. It was a lie, of course, but I couldn't just stay on the run, because what kind of life is that?

In that moment I lost the campaign, my family, my friends, and my partner. I lost my whole life in a single day, and the worst part was that I never got to see my dogs again.

Remarkably, despite intense surveillance and a two-year investigation, the police also couldn't find Debbie Vincent:

Even though I hadn't been there for eight months, around fifty police officers raided Freshfields Animal Rescue searching for me.

Ignoring the sanctuary volunteers, who offered them keys, police broke locks, doors, and windows to access every building. They released vulnerable dogs from their kennels, some of which were missing for over a week. As the large animal manager attempted to stop police leaving gates open that would lead to pigs escaping, the police broke his collarbone.

A trainee vet was arrested and held in the back of a van for hours, along with about six others, all of whom were later released with no further action. For several hours they refused to let anyone in to care for and treat the hundreds of animals, until finally they agreed to admit one sanctuary employee under police supervision.

The police seized the charity's computers, telephones, CCTV unit, and paperwork, affecting their day-to-day running for months.

When I heard about the raid, I phoned the rescue to see if I could help. I was told that my name was the only one on the search warrant. I voluntarily handed myself in to the police on 9 May 2007.

Many of those raided had little if any involvement in SHAC. Undercover agent Adrian Radford had compiled a list of Heather, Gregg, and Natasha's friends, and the police had rounded them up indiscriminately. A covert camera outside the SHAC office ensured any recent visitors were drawn into the raids, and HLS selected other targets themselves.[192]

One of Radford's allegations was that an activist named James Gorman was SHAC's primary source of funding. This claim had no substance, but on Adrian's tip-off, Nick Fielding from *The Times* had interviewed James for a sensationalist article he theatrically titled, 'Vegan bodybuilder funds animal extremists'.[193] The piece failed to offer a single example of any extremists he had funded.

This baseless accusation was enough to secure a warrant for James' arrest:

I received a phone call from the police, who asked me to come and talk to them. I hung up. Twenty minutes later they called back, and said, 'We have your ex-partner at the police station in Gosport, and she's not going to be released until you come and speak with us.'

I didn't have a choice but to go. I drove past the osteopathy clinic where I used to teach on my way, and I've never seen anything like it. The whole road was blocked off with more police than I've seen on even the biggest protest.

I carried on to Gosport, where police arrested and interviewed me. Eventually I was released on bail, and had to attend a police station in London, where I was put in a glass cell like a serial killer. They were threatening me with a twenty-year sentence for all these financial offences because they said I was sponsoring SHAC. It was all based on Adrian Radford's lies. But even if it had been true, how could donating money to a lawful campaign deserve this kind of treatment?

The scary thing was the power the police seemed to have. It didn't feel like I was in England anymore. It was like I had been taken to some dictatorship where they could just do what they wanted.

I'd done nothing wrong, and so eventually I was released without charge, but not before they had frozen my bank accounts and tried everything they could do to destroy my reputation and my finances.

Having been arrested, we were subjected to regular interviews over a period of up to thirty-six hours. They interrogated me on six separate occasions, for about an hour each time. I remained in total silence as the police fired question after question. Something felt strange: not even one of those questions related to me committing a crime.

During almost all my interviews, they placed photographs of completely peaceful and lawful protests in front of me and asked if I was in the pictures. I almost certainly was, though I didn't look at the photos. Nicci did look at the ones shown to her and couldn't believe what she saw:

They'd point to a random woman who had been circled to ask if it was me. None of them were. They weren't even the same person. How could I possibly be five-foot with short blond hair one week and then five-foot-six with long brown hair the next? Some photos were from protests in countries I'd never even been to.

The interview questions were vague, and I wasn't asked about criminal activity or blackmail. I answered, 'No comment,' to every question, and my solicitor raised his eyebrows and impatiently sighed every time another photo was presented. Even the interviewing officer looked awkward, as he clearly knew none of the photos were of me, and it wouldn't have mattered if they were. They were just peaceful campaigners stood on the streets holding posters. No violence, no blackmail, not even confrontation, just people exercising their right to protest.

I didn't know why I was there. I had nothing to do with SHAC at an organisational level, most of my time was spent on campaigns for the Southern Animal Rights Coalition, which Tom and I had founded.

The following day I was released onto the streets of Fareham, still in my pyjamas. I had no money, no phone, not even a key to my house.

Nicci and I returned to a home which had been entirely gutted. They'd stolen computers, clothes, and entire filing cabinets full of campaign and personal paperwork. Virtually all that remained in our bedroom was a box in the middle of the floor, once full of Nicci's childhood memories. Police had smashed irreplaceable ornaments, unspooled and broken demo cassettes from her first band, and torn and scrunched up photographs. They deliberately removed several nails from our back gate. It wasn't immediately noticeable, but allowed our dogs to escape. Still terrified and traumatised from their ordeal, the dogs took hours to find. Our neighbours were surprisingly supportive, considering the police had brought sniffer dogs into our house and falsely told onlookers they were searching for bombs.

Every major newspaper and television news channel displayed photos from a random selection of actions which we had never seen before, and which police hadn't mentioned in our interviews. The police in charge of the investigation remained vague when speaking to journalists, but threw around buzzwords like 'extremism', 'climate of fear', and of course 'terrorism'. This seemed to dissuade any deeper analysis.[194] They made much of the fact that they had seized £100,000 in cash from those arrested,[195] but didn't mention this was mostly the life savings of an older lady who was never even charged.

Those of us who were released were the lucky ones. Of the thirty-two people violently arrested, police charged ten with conspiracy to commit blackmail. Most appeared to have been picked almost at random. The evidence presented to them was no more damning than the evidence presented to those who avoided charges, as Gerrah recalls:

> In the interview room, police repeatedly showed me photos of my friends and myself attending lawful protests. I couldn't understand why I was being charged with a crime I hadn't committed. My solicitor was surprised too, and told me he hadn't been presented with evidence that anyone had been involved in a conspiracy to blackmail, let alone me.

Gerrah Selby, Dan Wadham, Dan Amos, Gavin Med-Hall, Grace Quantock, Linus Harrison, and Trevor Holmes were released on bail, pending a hearing at Portsmouth Magistrates' Court a few days later.[196] Gregg, Natasha, and Heather were transported in handcuffs directly from the police station to the court hearing.[197]

If the case outlined to the court constituted a blackmail conspiracy, it criminalised virtually every protest group in existence. SHAC published contact details of HLS-affiliated companies via their website and newsletter, alongside disclaimers insisting all correspondence remain polite and lawful. Since 2001, SHAC had engaged a barrister to approve the website and the newsletter regularly. The police insisted those involved in the day-to-day running of SHAC were liable for every individual who chose to ignore their disclaimers.

The magistrates referred the case to the Crown Court, where the judge reviewed the evidence and indicated he was minded to dismiss the case there and then. Campaigners witnessed two men in dark suits ask to speak with the judge in private. On his return, the judge denied bail to Gregg, Heather, and Natasha and remanded them to prison.

In the USA, the FBI published a triumphant press release, hinting at their involvement:

> [These] arrests send a message that criminal activity is not protected on either side of the ocean. The FBI continues to address this kind of criminal activity as a high priority and has forged strong partnerships with our international law enforcement counterparts. When necessary, and to the full extent the law allows, we will share and exchange information with them to target these criminals.[198]

FBI supervisory special agent Phil Celestini went a little further when he informed the BIO International Convention in Boston that his agency's involvement was a direct catalyst for the arrests. He also warned, 'You can bank on there being more [arrests] to come.'[199]

HLS themselves were jubilant, vociferously proclaiming their troubles were now over.[200]

PART VI

The Ending: 2007–18

If HLS was brought down by animal rights extremists, they would merely move on to another organisation. The domino effect this would have would be a matter of serious concern for the government.[1]

    – Ben Gunn, Chief Constable of Cambridgeshire Police

26
SHAC Is Back: 2007–08

There is still a perception in the financial community that
we are radioactive.[2]

– Brian Cass, HLS' managing director

The police raids appeared to be an aggressive and desperate
attempt to disrupt SHAC through 'shock and awe'. Nonetheless, remanding SHAC's founders into prison put the campaign
in a desperate situation.

Emma Phipps, who had joined the SHAC campaign just a
few months before, was caught up in the aftermath:

I was staying with friends when their house was raided. As
a guest in their house, the police seized my phone, camera,
and several personal items before they let me leave.

I used a phone box to try and call other friends, but no
one answered. It was only when I called my parents, who
were watching the raids on the news, that we realised the
scope of the police operation.

Another activist and myself made our way to the SHAC
office to see how we could help. The place had been ransacked. Police had taken all leaflets and merchandise …
Even the landline phone had been taken.

We bought a new telephone and tidied up, trawled
through dozens of answer-phone messages, took calls,
updated other groups and individuals, and began to piece
together what had happened.

With Emma and her friends maintaining the office, myself and three other activists felt compelled to save the campaign. Although the police had arrested us, they had not charged us with any offences. To make sure SHAC survived, we devised a new decentralised structure until we could hand the campaign back to the core team. We wound down the SHAC office and distributed each of its key roles between us.

Nicci and I were coordinating our own organisation, Southern Animal Rights Coalition (SARC). We combined a lot of the SHAC duties into our existing workload. We managed the *SHAC Newsletter*, email action alerts, merchandise, and resources. Debbie Vincent updated the website and responded to supporter enquiries, while Sarah Whitehead took on the SHAC phone line, postal address, and admin.

We had to replace our computers, redirect phone numbers, open new bank accounts, gain access to the website and email servers, and purchase megaphones, placards, leaflets, and everything else required to run a protest campaign. For some reason, all the police left in the SHAC office was a single eMac computer. Desperately in need of computers, I took it home as a spare.

To the outside world it must have looked like the end of SHAC, but behind the scenes we were frantically pulling everything back together. It took nine days before we could access the SHAC website again.

Our first five posts covered protests in the UK and Europe which predated the police raids. We hoped to send a sign to the global movement that SHAC wasn't dead yet. The message was heard, and the floodgates opened. Activists from St Petersburg in Russia formed a new SHAC chapter and protested outside GSK. Campaigners in Paris held three consecutive days of action. Los Angeles, New York, and the Netherlands all took to the streets. SHAC global was alive and well.[3]

In the UK itself, it took a little longer. For only the second time in seven and a half years, SHAC demonstrations in Britain halted for nearly two weeks. The protest which broke the drought took place outside Novartis in Horsham, under the severe restrictions of the company's injunction. Protestors informed the police in advance, and exactly six people stood behind a black screen erected by Novartis so employees didn't have to look at our photos of vivisected animals. Megaphone use was limited to fifteen minutes per hour.[4] Despite the constraints, when a senior member of staff saw the protest, he muttered under his breath, 'The police said this would all be over.'

Emma helped reignite protests in London:

It was the general consensus that we needed to get back out there and carry on with protests. We needed to show the vivisection industry and the government that we did not need leaders to tell us what to do, and that we would be much harder to get rid of than they believed.

I ended up moving to London, where SHAC protests became a weekly occurrence. Often, we'd carry out protests four days a week, travelling to numerous targets each day.

While the police insisted that they had targetted SHAC to disrupt the ALF, the reality proved very different. As we struggled for nearly two weeks to return SHAC to an even keel, the ALF barely blinked – just days after the police raids, they torched the head office of HLS' cage supplier Tecniplast in Limonest, France.[5]

* * *

HLS' loan was due to be repaid in 2011, and we were determined to make that impossible. We compiled a new list of HLS' shareholders and launched a fresh wave of protests against them. It seemed HLS had spoken with every company we visited, insisting they were now a safe investment. As protests resumed, the false sense of security vanished. Following a week of protests across three continents, Allianz Bank were the first to drop their 600,000 shares in HLS.[6]

Echoing HLS' staff after they narrowly evaded bankruptcy in 2001, the first issue of the *SHAC Newsletter* after the raids carried the headline 'business as usual'.[7] In the short period between the newsletter being written and it being printed, every shareholder listed inside had sold their stake in the laboratory.

From her cell in HMP Bronzefield, Heather wrote:

For the last eight years, I have worked so hard and put my heart and soul into the campaign to close Huntingdon Life Sciences because what they do is wrong, it is unscientific, and what they are guilty of completely breaks my heart. The atrocities they commit behind the razor wire and soundproofed walls makes me so angry it can hardly be expressed in words.

Our show trial next June will be a straightforward battle between good and evil, mercy and misery, compassion and cruelty. They can imprison us, but they can never change the fact that we are right. I will be immensely proud to stand up in court and expose HLS for the callous, money grabbing sadists that they are.

I would happily stay in prison for the rest of my life if it meant this hellhole would close right now, for good.

I will never, so long as I live, understand how those monsters can do what they do to those beautiful animals. I will never, so long as I live, understand why so many people in the Government, the police, the courts, the media, and Brian Cass himself could hate those animals so much that they want their agony to continue, and in some cases find it funny.[8]

While we did all we could to ensure 'business as usual', campaigning in the UK changed noticeably. Lia Phillips was involved in SHAC protests immediately before and after the SHAC shutdown:

I became involved in SHAC in March 2007, when I was sixteen. To find that there was a group of people who were just as passionate as me was incredible. It felt like a family.

I jumped in at the deep end, and my first protests had been a three-day trip to France. It was a whirlwind; we drove to Paris, and before I knew it, I was protesting in front of huge companies with a placard in my hand and felt like I was where I was supposed to be. The next couple of months I went to every SHAC demo I could. I loved being out there, feeling like I was doing something to make a difference. I loved the people I was surrounded by; I was inspired by their determination and compassion.

And then the raids happened. I remember it, probably in the same way that others remember tragic historical events. My dad telephoned me to tell me that some animal rights activists had been raided and arrested. I secretly tried to call several of my friends during my maths lesson, and every single number went straight to voicemail. During my lunch break I learnt that all of my closest friends had been raided and arrested.

I refused to back down. HLS were no less immoral just because the police were defending them, so we picked ourselves up and dusted ourselves off. The biggest change was that different people were organising protests, and a lot of new people began to take part.

In many areas of the UK a generational divide appeared. Veterans of the animal liberation movement had witnessed the increasing resistance to SHAC and feared what might follow. Seasoned activists – from both SHAC and the ALF – turned their attention to other issues or disappeared from the movement completely.

Many younger activists viewed the mass arrests of peaceful protestors as an attack on their own democratic rights, which had to be resisted. While pockets of the SHAC old guard stood firm, groups of youngsters who had attended few, if any, SHAC demonstrations before the police raids were responsible for many of the British protests which took place after May 2007. They were inexperienced, but every bit as tenacious and passionate as those who had come before.

Andy Silverwood was amongst the new wave of protestors:

The SHAC campaign defined my teenage years. I had always been taught what was right from wrong, but it was only through meeting people in the animal rights movement that I learnt I could take action and change the things I disagreed with.

For a couple of years, I spent every single day off from college at protests and organising campaigns. We spent every moment thinking about what we could do to save the animals inside HLS, and we arranged full days of driving from protest to protest to voice our objection. Our protests were loud, no-nonsense, and hopefully very annoying, but within the minefield of anti-vivisection protest laws, they were always legal.

Nonetheless, a bloc within the police had clearly decided that viewing us as the 'enemy' justified pretty much any behaviour towards us, and they did their best to make our lives intolerable. They followed us, bugged our phones, threatened us, and regularly pulled over our cars. They once took me aside and asked if I'd snitch on my – law-abiding – friends.

How could they defend the bad guys in a society that was so in love with their cats, dogs, rabbits, and other animal companions?

A decade later, my brother got a job working for the government, and in an interview, he was asked about my involvement with the ALF. I only took part in legal SHAC protests, and was never active with the ALF, but the British government saw no distinction.

With the police harassment and the shadow it left behind, would I have done anything differently? I couldn't have. I couldn't have done *nothing* knowing what I knew about HLS.

Across Britain, SHAC protests were once again a daily occurrence. As she was discharged from hospital following a car accident, Sarah Whitehead joined regular demonstrations outside Novartis in Horsham. She insisted that her wheelchair be parked blocking the gates with the brakes firmly applied.

In the USA, *United Press International* ran an article commenting on the impact of the SHAC 7 prison sentences:

Despite the FBI's efforts and a new law passed at the end of last year that allows for stiffer penalties ... animal-rights activists have been carrying out legal protests as well as vandalism of labs, facilities and even the homes of executives of pharmaceutical firms. Jacquie Calnan, president of Americans for Medical Progress, a group that is supported by the pharmaceutical industry, told *UPI* she hasn't seen a decrease in the activities of animal-rights activists or an increase in arrests or prosecutions. 'I haven't noticed any higher or lower level,' Calnan said, 'It's pretty much a continuum of where we were last year.'

'The whole thing is meant to chill free speech,' Camille Hankins, spokeswoman for Win Animal Rights, told *United Press International*.

Hankins said actions seeking to limit public protests will only serve to drive some activists underground to commit illegal activity.

'It's a lot easier to do something at night, to do something anonymously,' she said. 'Those people are not being caught. It's the above-ground activists that are being targeted.'[9]

In the UK, the new generation were drawn to SHAC, but far fewer seemed drawn to the ALF; just a handful of unlawful actions took place throughout 2007. However, towards the end of the year, the Animal Rights Militia (ARM) carried out a string of contamination hoaxes against Novartis and GSK, which forced mass recalls of products including Savlon,[10] Lipsyl, Lucozade,[11] and contact lens solutions from pharmacies and supermarkets across the UK and France.[12]

During an international animal rights gathering in the Netherlands, activists from around the globe stormed the NYSE Euronext exchange in Amsterdam with megaphones and leaflets, before security and police evicted them. Protests continued across the UK, France, Italy, Poland, Venezuela, Spain, the USA, Switzerland, Germany, Israel, and Belgium. An exasperated Brian Cass pleaded with the financial industry:

I still struggle to know what it is going to take to get back to normal relations. We are an important and successful part of the animal research community. All we are asking is to be treated the same way as other firms and be given the same commercial services that they are given. The most important thing is to be given a normal bank account because that will open other doors.[13]

His plea fell on deaf ears. But his advice to the government – that they needed 'one final push'[14] was being carefully considered in the corridors of Whitehall.

SHAC were also being discussed in another of London's landmarks. After years of legal wrangling and unrelenting persistence, in late 2007 campaigners Simon Dally and Max Gaston convinced the High Court to soften some restrictions in HLS' injunction. For the first time in four years, SHAC were allowed to hold a protest with more than twenty-five people outside HLS itself.[15]

We seized the opportunity and immediately announced a national demonstration at the laboratory. Activists from across the UK rallied to the call. Dozens of local groups arranged minibuses and coaches to ensure as many activists as possible could bring SHAC's message back to HLS' doorstep.

The original injunction had made international headlines. *Sky News*, the BBC, and Channel 4 all arranged for journalists to attend the demonstration to interview activists and report on the next chapter in the HLS saga.

The protest began with 700 activists marching around Huntingdon town centre before moving on to the laboratory itself. The protest crowded the narrow confines of Woolley Road to bursting point. The Cambridgeshire countryside roared with passionate voices, megaphones, klaxons, drums, and air horns, but amidst speculation of interference by the Serious Organised Crime Agency (SOCA), not a single reporter showed up.

With the police noting down every word I said, I addressed the crowd:

> This campaign was never about just three people. This is a massive, unstoppable global movement that took on and defeated some of the largest and most powerful companies in the world.
>
> I stand here today with a message for the police, for the government, and for Huntingdon Life Sciences. My message is this: you can kick down my door every day of the week. You can drag me out of bed and ransack my house whenever you like. But I will be back here time and again with the same message. Huntingdon Life Sciences are going to close.

Campaigners across the globe echoed my passion. Sixty activists protested outside the Eurotox conference in Amsterdam. The delegates, who included many of HLS' customers and competitors, attempted to escape in boats to attend a lavish meal. However, as their boats docked, they found the protestors waiting to greet them.

In the first days of 2008, activists in Chile secured a major victory with their own SHAC-inspired campaign. After two years of activism, the Coalición por los Derechos Animales (CDA) closed the Universidad Catolica's primate research laboratory. The Chilean Air Force flew eighty-eight monkeys to Monkey World in the UK. The monkeys had been imprisoned in solitary confinement for up to twenty years.[16]

Days later, the ALF in Britain carried out a rescue operation at Highgate Rabbits in Lincolnshire. They had identified the previously unknown farm from a research paper and discovered the breeder was a major supplier to HLS and other labs. An anonymous ALF communiqué described the raid:

> A ventilation fan was forcibly removed to evade the alarm systems on the doors. Inside, rabbits were lined in barren cages breathing in the stench of shit and urea, waiting to be tortured to death in animal testing labs. But tonight, the activists had a more compassionate fate for them. They loaded a total of 129 rabbits in friendship groups into bags and whisked them immediately to safety. Never will they have to know or experience an experimental facility or university lab. Some of the rabbits were visibly excited when they reached their new lives, playing in the straw and munching carrots happily.[17]

27

SHAC the RIPA: 2008

The activists have made it pretty clear that they have a long-term strategy; the end of all animal research in this company, and the end of all animal research in this country.[18]

— Brian Cass, HLS' managing director

SHAC's use of encryption frustrated the police. With no evidence that any of the SHAC defendants were connected to crime, the entire case hinged on them finding something – *anything* – on one of the dozens of computers they had seized. However, SHAC stored sensitive documents such as donor lists, legal communications, and whistle-blower information on encrypted drives on computers using PGP software.

As part of the 'War on Terror', Tony Blair's government had considered laws to force terrorism suspects to hand over their encryption passwords. With lawyers, journalists, and politicians all relying upon similar encryption, the wider ramifications of such invasive powers shelved the laws for several years.[19] Despite being too controversial for terrorism cases, when it came to SHAC, the government left nothing off the table. Within five months of the raids, Regulation of Investigatory Powers Act (RIPA) laws were pushed through Parliament, and the Crown Prosecution Service (CPS) served the first-ever Section 49 notices on all SHAC arrestees.[20]

The notices demanded people hand over their passwords whether they had been charged or not. However, a secure encryption password is over thirty-two characters long, and tends to be hard to guess and easy to forget. Lynn Sawyer explained to the *Guardian* that she had never accessed the PGP files on her computer, as she didn't even understand how the program worked. If she had been able to, as someone not even charged with a crime, she failed to see why she should be obligated to open her life to the police:

> In a so-called democracy I am being threatened with prison simply because I cannot access encrypted files on my computer.
>
> The police are my enemy; I know that they have given information about me to Huntingdon Life Sciences (as well as hospitalising me). Would I really want them to see and then pass around private communications with my solicitors, which could be used against me at a later date in the civil courts? Medical records, embarrassing poetry which was never meant to be read by anyone else, soppy love letters or personal financial transactions?[21]

It emerged that Lynn had no legal obligation to hand over her passwords anyway. In the confusion and excitement of new legislation, the Crown Prosecution Service (CPS) had delivered the Section 49 notices, rather than the police, making them invalid. By the time the police eventually served their own notice, too much time had passed and they dropped the matter.

The passwords were required because the May 2007 raids took place in the early hours, before people had woken up, turned on their computers, and opened encrypted volumes. In January 2008, the police circumvented this problem.

It was mid-morning, and I was helping design a new website for SHAC North America. Three years after a judge had ordered the end of SHAC USA, Camille from Win Animal Rights in New York was preparing a rebrand.

Suddenly, our front door exploded off its hinges. I barely had time to pull the plug out of the computer before a riot cop in full armour flung me from my chair and ground my face into the carpet.

Police led Nicci and me from our home in handcuffs and threw us into the back of a police van in full view of our neighbours as a *BBC News* team filmed. Once again, the police meticulously tore our home to pieces and loaded everything into a fleet of vehicles. Strangely, they barely touched the room our housemate occupied at the time; all they took from her room was the eMac I recovered from the SHAC office in 2007.

This time, police raided two houses and arrested the most prominent spokespeople for SHAC. The 'evidence' they presented to us in interview was that we had phoned the police to arrange peaceful protests, attended those protests, answered the SHAC phone line, given press interviews, and responded to emails and letters.

The police immediately requested our encryption passwords, but our solicitor informed them that they had once again made a technical error, and they withdrew their demand. Two homicide detectives were pulled off a murder investigation to interview Nicci and myself over thirty-one hours. Each time our solicitor requested our immediate release through lack of evidence, they promised something important that never materialised. I later saw one of the interviewing detectives during a court hearing. He told me the whole thing had been a bizarre experience for him, and that the evidence was the most tenuous he'd ever seen.

Eventually we were allowed to go home, under strict conditions preventing us from protesting against HLS. Sarah Whitehead, Nicci Tapping, and I were charged with conspiracy to blackmail. We were the first defendants added to 'Trial Two'. Nicole Vosper, Jason 'JJ' Mullen, and Alfie Fitzpatrick were added later.

We spent a further two years awaiting trial. While we waited, I continued my involvement behind the scenes: researching, maintaining the website, producing the newsletter, and organising campaign merchandise, but I couldn't arrange or attend demonstrations. Even though a barrister regularly approved it, the police attempted to take down the campaign website by intimidating the domain host. As we transferred it to a more resilient server, I rebuilt the website, making it more contemporary and user friendly.

At the same time, the campaign bank account was frozen. We switched providers, only for the same thing to happen again. With neither a warrant nor judicial oversight, the Serious Organised Crime Agency (SOCA) had notified all banks not to provide SHAC with an account.[22] It seemed, however, that HSBC missed the notification, as they offered their banking services without issue.

Weeks after the second set of police raids, Nicci and I received some good news: the Navy was scrapping deep-diving tests due to our SHAC-inspired pressure campaign. They released all the goats which remained at the Qinetiq testing facility to a sanctuary. Amidst the stress of the raids, we were buoyed by the knowledge that we had not only kept SHAC alive, but through SARC we had also secured the freedom of thirty-two goats and saved many hundreds more by ending the cruel and pointless military experiments.[23]

Our focus on HLS' shareholders was so successful that we quickly wiped out the modest gains their share price had made following the initial police raids. We switched our attention back to their customers, hosting a national protest for World Day for Laboratory Animals outside Novartis in Sussex.[24] The march around Horsham and subsequent protest at the company's primate research facility was an anathema for Novartis, who had been promised all protests would end a year before.

In Barcelona, a city renowned for its revolutionary spirit, the Spanish national march against Novartis took a more direct tack. Hundreds of campaigners thronged the streets with banners, placards, and flares, while others broke windows and daubed slogans on walls.

During a protest outside Novartis' global headquarters in Switzerland, an older lady accepted a leaflet from the protestors; what she read enraged her so much that she kicked over a bike belonging to a Novartis employee, gave the activists a thumbs up and ambled off. The police watched on in shock. In France, a giant rabbit invaded a Novartis conference and informed delegates about the company's connections with HLS, before security chased them out of the building.

With a surge of protest against the company, a global week of action was called against Novartis. Protests erupted across four continents.

In South Africa campaigners reported:

The demo was well received by the public. While distributing 170 pamphlets to the other residents in the office park, every single person we spoke to was definitely on our side, horrified by the idea that animal testing is funded by a company in their midst, and they ended by wishing us luck.

SHAC Italia followed suit:

We screamed and chanted against all the workers coming out. We will never forget the images of agonising monkeys on their cage floors, and we will never forget that these experiments were paid for by Novartis.[25]

With global activism pressuring Novartis across the world, I knew one thing for certain would force them to renounce HLS. The 1997 undercover exposé decimated HLS' revenue as their customers rushed to distance themselves from the scandal. Another covert investigation would surely push them over the edge.

I contacted an undercover reporter. She had never been named publicly for her work, and she was eager to get inside the laboratory, despite risking up to two years in prison under the Animals in Scientific Procedures Act.[26]

I met her regularly in neutral locations, communicating on a safe 'burner' phone which I never turned on within twenty miles of my home. I helped her set up a new life in Huntingdon, where she lived under the pretence of separating from her husband. Over six months, she joined the local rowing team and got a job working at the Peterborough Greyhound Stadium. From there it was just a matter of applying for positions at the area's most prolific – and desperate – recruiter for low-skilled jobs: HLS.

Her first interview was a great success. The interviewer commented as much as he rounded up. A few days later, she found a tracking device on her car. HLS were desperate for staff, but they were also paranoid. For a company with 'nothing to hide', they went to incredible lengths to keep it hidden.

After a few weeks of being monitored, HLS called her in for a second interview. Her background checked out, there were no perceivable security issues, and she left confident she had the job. But then communication stopped. HLS never phoned her back and refused to answer her calls. Something had spooked them, and they blacklisted her.

It was heart breaking. Had our plan worked, we could have revealed to the world what was happening inside not just HLS, but all animal testing laboratories. HLS would surely have closed, and we would have been armed with fresh evidence to force further change. We tried to find other investigators, but none of them came as close to getting inside the laboratory.

As my plan collapsed, the state was developing perhaps their most bizarre strategy.

The year before, animal liberation campaigners launched a blog called *NETCU Watch*,[27] reporting sightings of the secretive police agency. With the National Extremism Tactical Coordination Unit (NETCU) exempt from Freedom of Information Act (FoIA) requests, or any public scrutiny, the blog shone a light on an otherwise unaccountable police unit.

A blunt comment on *NETCU Watch* from a user called Max: 'What a load of useless tossers'[28] would have been easy to dismiss, but 'Max' wasn't just another internet troll. The post originated from an internal government proxy, gateway-303. energis.gsi.gov.uk, which NETCU used to access the internet.[29]

In early 2008, a new blog appeared in response to *NETCU Watch*, called *SHAC Watch*.[30] The blog's primary purpose was to insult campaigners, while also trying to divide them. When they began posting personal information about SHAC activists, web hosts WordPress took the site offline, noting that it was updated from an 'unusual' IP address.

Migrating to a new host, *SHAC Watch* continued to spread misinformation. Posts also began appearing on radical news forum *Indymedia*, either signed 'SHAC Watch' or copy-and-pasted to both sites almost simultaneously.

Indymedia refused to record the IP addresses of its visitors or contributors. However, the admin team were suspicious, and programmed the site to flag specific IPs if they posted or commented. Virtually all the suspicious posts originated from government computers.

In an intensive campaign between 2008 and 2011, the posts took a variety of approaches and targeted a wide range of activists, disproportionately focusing on SHAC. Most posts were simply insulting or abusive. Others showed a more nuanced approach to dividing and deterring the movement:

> The SHAC campaign has caused considerable damage to HLS, but it is still running. Compare the effects against the impact of police action on the campaigns and individuals and you have to question if the [animal rights] route is the one to follow.[31]

As well as dissuading other campaigns from imitating the targeted effectiveness of SHAC, the police were also eager to encourage actions that could lead to easy arrests. Commenting on a planned Greenpeace protest against a coal-fired power station, they declared:

> Let's not all stand around like lemmings – lets shut the place! Bring ladders and wire cutters. If there are enough of us, we can shut it![32]

After several years of internal conflict over whether to admit that they had logged IP addresses – albeit ones exclusively used by the British state – *Indymedia* exposed the posts, marking the beginning of the end for the website. With police weaponising their site, *Indymedia* commented:

> The comments build a bewildering picture of a campaign of disparagement, incitement, and support, together with wry asides and outright attempts at demoralisation. A few really stand out as obvious incitement to illegality while some are so bizarre that we can't work out if they are part of a sinister master plan to bring down the whole activist scene – or just

the ramblings of bored coppers with faces full of doughnuts and nothing better to do.[33]

Activists weren't the only ones under attack. The same IP addresses also edited pages on Wikipedia, including that of Jean Charles de Menezes, an innocent man shot dead in error by a police marksman following the 2004 suicide bombings in London. The crass amendment police added to his Wikipedia page read:

There has been some public backlash against Menezes, with British tabloid newspaper in particular protesting that he has received more publicity than any of the fifty-two people who died in the bombings. 'Anti-war' groups who champion Menezes' case, ignore the fate of the victims of the bombings, other than to 'understand' why the attacks occurred due to the UK's role in Iraq.[34]

In the USA, activists protested regularly on the doorsteps of NYSE Euronext executives. When it emerged that one of those executives was running to be governor of North Carolina, they made parodies of his campaign flyers and handed them to people outside his campaign offices, securing interviews with the media to publicly highlight his links to HLS.[35]

Suddenly, and with little warning, an unanticipated problem hit HLS as they found themselves embroiled in a global crisis. The US housing bubble had burst, sending house prices crashing and causing an international recession. By the summer of 2008, investment banks were collapsing or being bailed out in government schemes.[36] Families across the world were struggling, and businesses were forced to tighten their belts. Companies such as HLS, who relied upon external contracts, were hit hard.

Combined with pressure from SHAC, HLS' share price tumbled by 75 per cent over the first months of the recession, and their third quarter results confirmed they were struggling. Their debt stood at $70 million. They'd only managed to repay $200,000.[37] With a little over two years left to clear the balance, their prospects looked bleak.

*　*　*

The FBI had brought about the SHAC 7 case using CoIntelPro tactics, which they had refined to devastating effect against the Black Panther Party during the 1960s. These tactics had been successfully replicated in Canada and the UK. The British police who led the SHAC investigation believed they had the blueprint to ending not just SHAC, but all animal liberation globally.

By May 2008, the Austrian animal liberation movement had achieved a spate of victories. This included a ban on battery cages for hens, and the end of wild animals in circuses. However, a string of broken windows belonging to fur retailer Kleider Bauer drew the attention of the Austrian authorities. With no leads on who was behind the attacks, the British officers behind the SHAC prosecutions advised their Austrian counterparts that for most animal liberation activists, lawful campaigning was 'just the tip of the iceberg'.[38]

On 21 May, Austrian police raided twenty-three homes and offices connected to activists who had attended protests against Kleider Bauer. With no reason to believe any of them were connected to the broken windows, they remanded ten activists into prison without charge. Seven of the campaigners began a hunger strike, demanding they be charged or released. After sixteen days without food, Martin Balluch collapsed. As he fell to the floor, he muttered, 'I simply cannot believe this can happen in Austria.' He was taken to hospital on a stretcher.[39]

Eventually, police charged the activists with being members of a 'criminal organisation' under Section 278a of the Austrian Criminal Code. After 105 days in prison, they were released, pending trial. Martin Balluch gave observers a dire warning:

> The moment the politicians can portray you as terrorists and are believed, they have won this battle, no matter what.[40]

As their trial began, 300 people, including a nun, a priest, and a Member of Parliament, submitted signed confessions to the public prosecutor. They admitted that they too had taken part in social justice campaigns, aware that unknown persons had broken the law for the same cause.

Towards the end of their trial, the defendants uncovered evidence of a police spy working in their midst. Her intelligence reports, which prosecutors had attempted to hide, proved the innocence of the activists on trial. They were all found not guilty.[41] Section 278a of the Austrian Criminal Code was amended so it could never again be used against social justice campaigners.[42]

Meanwhile, three of the British SHAC defendants pleaded guilty.[43] The charge of blackmail required that an unwarranted demand had been made, with menaces. The prosecution claimed someone called 'Paul' had telephoned companies connected to HLS and demanded they stop working with the laboratory. If they didn't, Paul would publish their company details on the SHAC website. He finished with a thinly veiled threat that direct action could follow. The unwarranted demand was 'Stop dealing with HLS', and the menaces were 'Or else ...'

Gregg and Natasha were the first to plead. When they made this decision, they believed Adrian Radford was a close friend suffering from a terminal illness. The voice of 'Paul' belonged to Adrian. On a visit to Natasha in prison, she informed me that she was willing to act as a 'lightning rod' to protect others.

Shortly afterwards, Dan Amos followed their lead and entered a guilty plea. His support group released a statement explaining that the amount of circumstantial evidence being presented would overwhelm and sway a jury. They conveyed his reluctance to attend a trial every day for six months.[44] Under British law, suspects usually have one third of their sentence removed if they plead guilty at the earliest possibility. Because of his decision, Dan was eventually released from prison two years earlier than he would have been had he attended trial and been found guilty.

A few weeks after Dan pleaded guilty – and for the third time in a year – the police smashed down our front door.

This time it was for a specific incident, though the action wasn't actually criminal and didn't involve us. Two young activists had hung a banner from a bridge near to a Novartis-owned facility. Their banner was outside the injunction's exclusion zone, and they stayed with it to make sure it was safe. The police attended, took their details, and left. Later, however, another officer decided that the red spray paint used on the banner looked like red spray paint that had been used to write 'Puppy killers' on a branch of one of HLS' shareholders, Barclays Bank.

The two activists were visiting our house for a few days, so the police took the opportunity to snoop around our property once more. As they rifled through our possessions, officers repeatedly insisted that they were only interested in the other two and that it had nothing to do with us. However, they didn't search any other address connected to the two activists, not even their own home.[45]

28

Trials and Tribulations: 2008

The prosecution of these activists was political and an attack on the individual's right to voice their anger and dissent against corporate greed.[46]

– Corporate Watch

When the Serious Organised Crime Agency (SOCA) was announced in 2004, Tony Blair had sent them a clear dog whistle, declaring that if a criminal case was 'big enough', they should not 'take the normal burden'.[47]

Since 1780, the normal burden in a British criminal trial demands a suspect's guilt be proven 'beyond a reasonable doubt'.[48] SOCA's task was to convince juries to convict when doubt remained. According to Seema Parikh, Managing Partner for MPR Solicitors:

SOCA is well known for having larger budgets and resources to investigate and prosecute their cases.

A conspiracy charge can assist the prosecution in convicting some conspirators at the expense of others. Those individuals with very minor roles, often not knowing the full details of the conspiracy, or having no knowledge of the conspiracy at all, are accused of being professional criminals. This can often lead to undeserving long custodial sentences if convicted after a trial. Or, worse still, pressure being put on them to plead guilty at an earlier stage in the proceedings.[49]

The prosecution's biggest challenge was proving a lawful campaign group was a blackmail conspiracy. Despite their best intentions, Gregg, Natasha, and Dan's guilty pleas had – from a legal perspective – achieved this. Rather than shielding others, they had inadvertently agreed that a conspiracy existed.

As a result, Heather Nicholson, Dan Wadham, Gerrah Selby, Gavin Medd-Hall, and Trevor Holmes stood trial in Winchester Crown Court, accused of attending protests, and to varying degrees coordinating the day-to-day functioning of a protest campaign. There was no specific evidence which would convince a jury that any of them were connected to a blackmail conspiracy, so SOCA took a different approach.

Using a tactic known as infoxication, they overwhelmed the jury with emotional testimonies and a mountain of information they could never reasonably be expected to analyse. Neuroscientist Dr Anders Sandberg from the University of Oxford explains:

> Memory research unequivocally suggests that juries tend to be both forgetful and suffer from information overload. Worse, human memory has various biases that may affect jury decisions (e.g., something causing an emotional reaction is easier to recall than something neutral) and these can be exploited.[50]

With the trial scheduled to last for up to six months, any potential juror with a job was allowed to excuse themselves. The same applied for childcare commitments, health care issues, or holiday plans. As a result, the jury for this highly complex court case, involving computer forensics, questions of human rights, and an intricate web of alleged conspiracy, consisted of the only twelve people who could be found in the

Winchester area with absolutely no life plans or commitments for a specific six-month period.

SOCA's plan to emotionally pummel the jury began immediately, as the prosecution unleashed a conveyor belt of witness testimonies. Some witnesses had received criminal damage attacks to their property by the ALF. Most had seen lawful protests outside their companies. Several had received letters, emails, and phone calls from unknown members of the public which were overwhelmingly polite, but occasionally threatening or abusive. Some companies had received no form of attack or protest activity at all but were allowed to explain in detail the actions police had warned them could happen.

Since 2001, a barrister had routinely approved the *SHAC Newsletter* and website. The prosecution refused to acknowledge that every newsletter carried at least one disclaimer, giving advice such as:

> Be polite and informative at all times, these people may be animal lovers too, and many of them are very supportive of our aims once they are given the info on HLS.[51]

> These companies are listed here for the purpose of polite communications and protests only. SHAC does not encourage illegal actions of any kind against these companies. Remember people power works, so please call, email, fax or hold some demonstrations at these offices. A lot of these people will be sympathetic and probably really shocked to hear about HLS and what sort of company they are.[52]

The fact that SHAC – and those on trial – had neither encouraged nor carried out any of the acts described in court made little difference. From behind screens, witnesses sobbed as they recounted their stories. The defence asked that the screens be removed as they added unnecessary theatrics to the prosecution's performance; the witnesses' identities were already known to anyone who wanted to know. Justice Butterfield denied their request.

Gerrah struggled to understand why she was on trial, and not the people who had carried out the alleged criminality:

The day our trial started, my legal team warned me about our judge. When their colleagues asked them who was trying our case, they all responded in the same way: by sucking air through their teeth and grimacing.

Most of the actions brought up in court occurred long before I was involved in SHAC, while I was still at high school and living in a different country. ALF actions were repeatedly brought before the jury, not SHAC actions, but it appeared that the two were purposefully conflated to poison the jury against anyone who believed in the concept of animal liberation.

Our barristers didn't know how to respond. They didn't even cross-examine any of the witnesses, as their testimony didn't relate to us or anything we had done.

While we started the trial confident in a jury seeing through the prosecution's lies and misconstrued evidence, we grew concerned when our barristers noticed that the senior police officer was winking at the jury foreman.

The prosecution presented peaceful protests and polite phone calls as sinister works of extremism, comparable to and indistinguishable from the direct action and criminal damage carried out by the ALF and others. Of the criminal acts described in the courtroom, not even one was attributed to any of the defendants. The prosecution relied upon a broader 'climate of fear' that furthered SHAC's – entirely lawful – aims.

The prosecution ignored the police's role in creating the climate of fear. Specialist police units such as NETCU relied upon supplementary funding from consultancy work. To maintain this revenue stream, they dramatically played up the threat to corporate clients.[53] The father of one animal liberation activist, who worked as a pharmaceutical reseller, was shown a video by the police. The video included arson attacks and a compilation of the most aggressive protest footage they could find from around the world. Officers told the company's employees that the things in the video would all happen to them if they were ever subjected to an animal rights campaign. They were advised not to engage in discussions with campaigners, to always look over their shoulders, and to prevent their children from joining any protest groups.

After two months of emotionally charged witness testimonies, the prosecution had failed to connect the defendants to the events being described. To drag them into the conspiracy, they required more. Stretching the evidence to fit their designs, prosecutors insisted that SHAC held quarterly planning meetings, which were the nexus of a sinister conspiracy of direct action against HLS.[54]

Gerrah was accused of attending one such meeting:

I had been invited to attend a Sunday BBQ and turned up with vegan brownies. It seemed like a joke when the prosecution began to label this barbecue hosted by Natasha and Gregg as a conspiracy meeting. It was so far removed from the truth, but the prosecution took the idea and ran with it.

Of course, we chatted about the SHAC campaign, and animal rights in general, but it was a social BBQ with friends, not a planning meeting, and nobody discussed anything criminal. The police had microphones hidden around the house, which proved this, but they chose not to focus on that detail.

It didn't seem to matter that not all the defendants had attended the barbecue, nor that there were other people (including children) present who hadn't been arrested or charged.

None of the evidence presented implicated Gerrah in anything more than attending protests and a barbecue. Her legal team applied to have her case dismissed, but the judge, Mr Justice Butterfield, refused.

The prosecution case for Trial One ended, and the focus shifted to the defence. Heather took the stand:

Giving evidence in court is exhausting. I was in the dock for three days, answering questions asked by my lawyer, having to go into great depth about the most banal things: why I had attended a BBQ with my friends, why I had telephoned the police to arrange lawful protests, why I had gone to the garden shed to collect placards and leaflets. It all just felt so absurd. The jury must have wondered why I was even there, and I was waiting for the judge to cancel the whole thing at any moment.

Despite being under surveillance for months, I was never seen going out at night, posting letters, or doing anything even vaguely criminal. In over a thousand pages of transcripts from microphones hidden in our houses, it was clear that I had never discussed blackmail or anything else illegal.

I finished the first day feeling really positive. I was certain the jury must surely see through this charade. But the next day, everything changed.

As I was preparing to face cross-examination, the prosecuting QC suddenly declared that they had some fresh evidence. It was a document they claimed they had just found on a computer, which apparently listed targets for ALF actions. It was a document I had never seen before in my life.

What I do know is that the police seized our computers two and a half years before, and yet conveniently found this document three months into our trial, just as everything was going our way and the prosecution could see their case crumbling.

I don't know where that document came from, or who put it there, but I do know it had nothing to do with me.

In later media interviews, police spy Adrian Radford admitted involvement in the 'target list'.[55] This led to the defendants speculating whether the prosecution withheld it for so long because they were aware of, and were protecting, its real creator. No similar document was found on any SHAC computers seized in police raids prior to Adrian Radford's deployment in the campaign.

Following the sudden revelation of undisclosed evidence, defence solicitor Steven Bird noted to his clients that there were 'dark forces at work'.

The target list mentioned three nicknames: 'Pony', 'Kidda', and 'Mumsy'. It remains unclear who attributed those nicknames, but the name Pony appeared on a separate text document which mentioned that Dan and Pony 'didn't want to do any more at the moment'. The prosecution deduced that this must refer to Dan Wadham and, with nothing else to corroborate their claim, insisted that it referred to his involvement in criminal damage attacks.

Dan firmly denied the allegation. He described how he had spent weeks sitting in bushes outside HLS to keep track of which companies came and went from the site to identify protest targets. It was a lawful endeavour, but hiding for hours at a time on the edge of HLS' injunction zone was physically draining and carried risks of the police arresting first and asking questions later. This was what he had decided to take a break from.

Overnight, Gavin Med-Hall – who was registered blind – faced the insinuation that he must have been involved in researching the target list. There was no evidence on his computer, nor anywhere else, to support this theory, but it suited the false narrative of him being SHAC's 'computer expert'.

On the face of it, the document did nothing to change the case against Gerrah and Trevor. They remained confident that the actions of others should not negate their right to protest against HLS. Nor did the document make SHAC itself, and its thousands of supporters, a criminal conspiracy.

As the trial came to a close, the jury were sent out to deliberate. After four days they failed to reach a verdict, but they had to make a decision as Christmas was just days away. The foreman of the jury returned to the courtroom to ask the judge whether words and phrases shouted on protests were enough on their own to serve as proof of involvement in a blackmail conspiracy. With little consideration, and despite the protests in question being approved, observed, and licensed by the police, Justice Butterfield agreed that they were.

On the final day of court before Christmas, the jury delivered their verdict. One juror refused to appear, and the media widely implied that he was scared for his safety.[56] In reality, he was feeling guilty for what was about to happen. Following the trial, he contacted the SHAC campaign to find out how he could get involved.

Trevor was acquitted and released from court a free man. However, Gerrah was convicted by ten out of twelve jurors and sentenced to four years in prison for taking part in lawful protests and attending a barbecue with her friends while she was a teenager.

Dan Wadham was convicted by eleven of the twelve jury members and received five years. For occasionally helping to research companies for legitimate protest, Gavin was convicted and sentenced to eight years. Dan Amos, who had earlier pleaded guilty believing he wouldn't receive a fair trial, received four years, and both Gregg and Natasha received nine. Heather, who had co-founded a campaign that she still maintains was lawful, and who was not directly connected to any of the criminal actions, received an eleven-year prison sentence.

As he handed down sentences totalling fifty years, Justice Butterfield called for a change in the law: he wanted to allow activists convicted of blackmail to be detained indefinitely.[57] On the behest of the police he gave anti-social behaviour orders (ASBOs) to each of the defendants. For most, these prohibited taking part in any lawful protest against HLS or any company connected to them for between five and ten years. Gregg, Natasha, and Heather were banned from any anti-vivisection campaigning for the rest of their lives.[58] If any doubt remained that the trial was aimed at silencing protest, rather than preventing criminal damage, the gagging orders made this clear.

As she stood beside her friends to receive her four-year sentence, Gerrah was heartbroken:

I did my best to maintain a passive expression while the sentence was read out, aware that the eyes of the media were on me, aware that any reaction would be reported on and plastered across the front pages of papers across the country. Don't cry. Be brave. When I was led down to the cells, I burst into tears. Again. Why must I cry? Even today, I wish that I could have been braver, stronger, more resilient. I hate that I cried when I should have been angry. I hate that I was crying because I got sentenced to four years while my kind, sensitive, and amazing friends had received sentences of up to eleven years. I hated that I was crying when the animals had never even received a trial; they'd simply been sentenced to die inside HLS. Compared to them, I was fortunate.

Following the convictions, the police's media drive went into effect. They passed press releases to every major news outlet, including photos and descriptions of the most shocking actions the ALF and other unknown individuals had taken against HLS since 2001. They made no attempt to clarify that the defendants were linked to none of them. As a result, when it came to explaining the convictions, the *Evening Standard* could only go as far as:

> Medd-Hall, from Croydon, was a computer and research expert who uncovered the links that firms had with HLS. Wadham, of Bromley, regularly attended demonstrations against the firms and HLS. Selby, from Chiswick, was also a regular activist at protests in Britain and Europe.[59]

Corporate Watch, whose journalists were the only media outlet to attend the full trial, gave a more in-depth summary:

> The prosecution essentially argued that SHAC operated legally but gave tacit support to direct action. In some cases, particularly where activists had not been involved in SHAC for long and could not be painted as organisers, the prosecution argued that words they had said on demonstrations, ranging from threats to articulate speeches about the need to end vivisection, were evidence of 'conspiracy to blackmail'.[60]

Having been remanded following the raids in 2007, Gregg, Natasha, and Heather had already been in prison for nearly three years. The others, including Gerrah, now experienced British jails for themselves:

Nothing can prepare you for imprisonment. The first night, when you're separated from your co-defendants and sent to a high-security prison all by yourself. The second night, when you're scared to take a shower because you fear you might be assaulted so you keep your underwear on. The third night, when you start to tick off the first days of the next four years of your life. When you're in prison, you wish your life away. Another day, another week, another month, another year. You try to put on a brave face. 'I'm fine!' you lie, pretending you haven't been affected by your incarceration, pretending it's not slowly tearing you apart, pretending you don't dream of another life, one where this is not happening, one where you are not locked away from everything and everyone you hold dear.

What made it even harder was knowing that we had been silenced by the state, our activism conflated with terrorism, so few people cared when we were sentenced to years in prison for our non-violent activism. I wanted to scream about the injustice as loudly as I could, but at the same time, I was afraid of the consequences. My words had been used to jail me; if I told the truth, I risked putting other people off speaking up for animals. My other option was to lie and pretend I had done something criminal. I chose to stay silent, too hurt and confused to know how to articulate my words into easy-to-digest soundbites for a public that had believed all the lies they'd been told about us.

A warning had been sent to the animal liberation movement in the most striking and heavy-handed manner. The question was, would the movement listen?

29

Baker Bailout: 2009

Huntingdon have shown the rest of UK plc how not to do it.[61]

– Investors' Chronicle

With seven British SHAC activists sentenced to a total of fifty years in prison, HLS went on the PR offensive. They used the convictions as proof that protests were an unfortunate speck in their rear-view mirror. Speaking to the *Telegraph*, HLS' CEO Andrew Baker declared:

We intend to return to Britain in the near future. We are an English company – we shouldn't be based in America.

We are in the middle of trying to get an English bank account and an English loan. We currently have a $60 million loan in the US and about $30 million in cash. But we are borrowing from foreign lenders. We are paying an interest rate of more than ten per cent and being treated as if we were a bankrupt company when, in fact, we are highly profitable. This is grossly unfair.[62]

While still trying to sound hopeful, the triumphalism of Brian Cass' statements following the 2007 police raids had been dampened. There had been a brief lull in activism, but by the time the SHAC defendants were sentenced in January 2009 the campaign was back in full swing. HLS' dreams of an English bank account and loan remained a pipe dream.

The year 2008 had seen over 700 SHAC protests across six continents,[63] with major shareholders, including Barclays Bank, Wells Fargo, and the Bank of New York Mellon joining the boycott of HLS. Following the sentencing, hundreds of SHAC activists attended a national protest in the City of London. The impact of SHAC was so ingrained in the national consciousness that the band Blur used a photo from this protest on the cover of their *Midlife* album, alongside other iconic images of the early twenty-first century.

In the first weeks of 2009, HLS once more found themselves on a cliff edge.

The lenders who replaced Stephens Inc. had driven a hard bargain. HLS were a high-risk investment, and having sold most of their assets, they had little left to bargain with. Their lenders had confidentiality clauses, which allowed them to recall the loan should their identity be revealed, as well as an extortionate 15 per cent interest rate,[64] far higher than the 10 per cent Andrew Baker publicly admitted. Every year HLS had to pay around $10 million in interest alone.

It was too much for the struggling laboratory. In January 2009, they could not manage even the basic interest repayments and defaulted on their loan.[65]

In July, HLS published a report revealing their desperate situation. 'Plymouth Report: Project Atlantic' was sent to HLS' shareholders, with every effort made to stop it reaching SHAC.[66]

The USA's financial regulator, the SEC, had agreed an unprecedented deal with HLS which allowed the Plymouth Report to refer to HLS by the pseudonym 'Atlantic'. However, they were unaware of SHAC North America's informant within the SEC, who leaked the report to the campaign.

The Plymouth Report outlined HLS' last-ditch attempt to remain solvent. They had contacted fifty companies to gauge interest in a buyout. Four of those companies, including HLS' own CEO Andrew Baker, put in first round proposals. Concerns over SHAC and an over-valuation of the company caused all but Andrew Baker to retract their offers. With no other options, the laboratory's remaining shareholders were handed an ultimatum: sell their shares to Andrew Baker and allow the company to become private, or let HLS close and receive nothing. They were given a few months to decide.

Buried in the Plymouth Report were two names which had eluded SHAC for seven years. Nicci Tapping was one of those who uncovered them:

When Stephens Inc. sold their loan, HLS borrowed nearly $100 million from 'a consortium of US lenders'. We never found those lenders, but the Plymouth Report revealed the loan was sold again to 'Anchor Sub Funding' and 'Progress Funding' in 2006. HLS owed Anchor $30 million, and Progress $40 million. The report stated that if SHAC identified these lenders, they could recall the loan immediately. Potentially, all we needed to do was send them an email from SHAC and it would all be over!

Unfortunately, we soon realised that neither of these companies actually existed. We worked tirelessly with WAR in New York, checking through old SEC filings, trawling websites and all the paperwork we could get our hands on.

Days later, we found evidence that Anchor had been set up in 2006 by a company called BDO in Luxembourg.

BDO's website promised they would be 'as innovative and entrepreneurial as our clients'.[67] By setting up the shell company Anchor Sub Funding in Luxembourg, they left virtually no paper trail. All investigations led straight back to the gatekeepers at BDO, rather than the actual lender, but that was

all SHAC needed. Campaigners held thirteen peaceful protests against BDO in quick succession across the UK, Ireland,
Sweden, and New York.

In Luxembourg, the Animal Rights Militia (ARM) took
matters into their own hands. They set fire to vehicles belonging to the two BDO employees who had created Anchor Sub
Funding. Ten days later, BDO closed Anchor,[68] and contacted
SHAC to leak the name of the company who had employed
them: the Fortress Investment Group.

On the first weekend of action against Fortress, business-
men turned up at protests in both New York and London.
They handed protestors notes on headed paper stating that
Fortress had sold its financial interest in HLS. The notes were
unsigned, and the men who delivered them refused to offer
any further comment. When Fortress were asked for clarification, they refused to respond. HLS' share price didn't flutter,
and there was no indication that a move as significant as
losing their lenders had occurred. While protests were paused
for just over a week to be certain, they swiftly resumed across
North America and Europe.

Amidst this backdrop, Nicole Vosper, one of my co-defendants in Trial Two, pleaded guilty, causing me to consider my
own position.

I had been on bail for over two years, repeatedly and violently arrested in my own home, and constantly barraged with
fresh 'evidence'. The evidence consisted of everything that the
police could scrape from the long-abandoned depths of my
computers' hard drives; boxes of emails dug from my spam
folder which had never been read, advertising Viagra, or
informing me I had won a fictitious lottery.

I knew I was innocent. I have never blackmailed anybody.
But I was certain the same was true for many, if not all, of
those in Trial One. Receiving a third off a potential sentence

for a guilty plea was tempting; a common feeling for those facing trial;[69] 40 per cent of cases referred to the Court of Appeal as potential miscarriages of justice involve defendants who pleaded guilty.[70]

When Nicole pleaded guilty, I offered to do the same, on one condition: they had to drop the blackmail charges against my partner, Nicci. I hoped at least one of us could go back to some kind of normality. The prosecution refused my offer.

As we prepared for trial, Adrian Radford outed himself as a spy working for the police.[71] In an interview for *The Times*, he explained how he had infiltrated SHAC and then formed his own ALF cell. He had led protests and criminal actions, all directed by the police. He was also interviewed for Dutch national television, where he expanded on his claims:

The whole coordinated approach to infiltrating the Animal Liberation Front was done at a very strategic level with a very large team of people behind it. It wasn't just me on my own as a spy, it was an enormous group of people. Every-thing was planned out and very succinctly developed, so we knew exactly what we were doing and where we're going to be doing it.[72]

The interviews were intended to garner interest for a forthcoming biography, written by *The Times* journalist Nick Fielding, who had been in contact throughout Adri-an's deployment. The book, *Target: ALF* was completed, but remains unpublished.[73]

For those awaiting trial, the revelations presented a glimmer of hope. Adrian had admitted accessing and researching the 'target' list from Trial One which lay at the heart of the con-victions. We hoped there would now be an opportunity to investigate his actions as an agent provocateur directed by the police.

We requested full disclosure relating to Adrian's role in SHAC. The CPS firmly rebuffed our requests. Remarkably, we were told that we had no power to compel him to be a witness or use his interviews as evidence.

* * *

In mainland Europe, the attack on the BDO employees' cars, claimed by the Animal Rights Militia (ARM), marked the start of a rising militancy.

According to former NETCU officer Gordon Mills, the imprisonment of SHAC's main coordinators had little impact on the severity of actions by unaffiliated groups such as the ALF and ARM.[74]

In April 2009, activists doused vehicles belonging to six German employees of Bayer and Novartis with paint stripper. The ALF and the previously unknown Militant Forces Against HLS (MFAH) claimed the attack.[75] A month later, the MFAH struck again in Germany, setting fire to a car belonging to a vivisector at HLS' customer Sanofi Aventis. French activists carried out the next MFAH action, damaging several cars belonging to NYSE Euronext directors before burning one of the vehicles. That same month, a Novartis sports complex on the Franco-Swiss border was set on fire, cars were vandalised in Belgium, and more vehicles were torched in Luxembourg and Germany.

As the MFAH spread across Europe, an animal rights activist called Vicky stood trial in the UK. In stark contrast to the militancy on the continent, her alleged crime was walking around the property of HLS' rabbit supplier Highgate Farm. In Britain, a trespassing offence would not normally be criminal, but under Section 145 of SOCPA it potentially carried a heavy custodial sentence. It was enough to convince Vicky's three companions to cut their losses and plead guilty.[76]

Vicky stood her ground; to 'interfere with the contractual relationships of an animal research organisation' there had to be evidence of lost income. The prosecution alleged this was a reconnaissance trip for an unspecified action planned for an unspecified future date. Vicky claimed a different story. She had been, as discreetly as possible, looking for evidence of cruelty. Had she not been caught on CCTV, farm owner Geoffrey Douglas would never have known she was there. The judge agreed and halted the case, directing the jury to acquit Vicky on the spot.

Speaking to the press afterwards, Vicky told gathered reporters:

> I think the legislation is prejudiced against animal rights people, so me being found not guilty is a small and significant victory. I am very happy. I am pleased with the outcome, and it was the right outcome.[77]

During the case, Geoffrey Douglas admitted that following the ALF rescue in 2008, he had cancelled his contracts with animal research companies and planned to close his business. However, something changed his mind:

> Special Branch and a number of other people came round. They convinced me things were not as I thought they were, and they would try to help me stay in business.[78]

Amongst those 'other people' were representatives from HLS, who installed a £60,000 state-of-the-art security system at the farm.[79] HLS and the police were not prepared to allow Highgate to close.

With Mr Douglas so close to throwing in the towel, SHAC started a focused campaign against Highgate. In July, activists established a protest camp. They were planning a week of protests to convince Geoffrey Douglas to reconsider his position. Chris Potter, a camp organiser, told the media:

We are here to peacefully protest and are trying to keep it non-confrontational.

We're here just to be here, to act as a gentle reminder to the farmer that it's an unacceptable way to make a living and to let local people know we're here.[80]

The Chief Inspector of Lincolnshire Police visited the camp and left without complaint, while local officers came and went in good spirits. Residents put up supportive posters in the nearby town and drove past the camp honking their horns. The sun was shining literally and metaphorically on the campers.

Mr Douglas brusquely told the press:

We are very much animal orientated, and most of our animals go on to develop vaccines for animals.[81]

His claims were on shaky ground due to video footage ALF recorded inside his breeding sheds. The evidence showed row after row of rabbits forced into cramped, dirty metal cages. During the protest camp, a dead rabbit with a noose around its neck was flung towards the campers from the direction of the farm, doing little to help Douglas' position.

SHAC supplied research papers to the press, revealing that HLS used Douglas' rabbits to test an artificial sweetener called

Advantame. During the experiments, female rabbits were impregnated before having tubes forced down their throats. Extreme doses of the sweetener were administered via the tubes to slowly poison them:

One [female rabbit] showed hunched and unsteady posture, hypoactivity, low muscle tone, weight loss, and reduced food consumption, and was killed on day seventeen. The colon and rectum contained a 'dark amorphous material with soft granular material'.

One [female rabbit] exhibited collapsed posture, loss of coordination and locomotion, vocalisation and respiratory difficulties, and was sacrificed on day twenty-seven. The internal surfaces of the kidneys were stained green, with punctate foci also observed on both kidneys.

A control [rabbit] was killed on day seventeen shortly after dosing due to 'convulsive-like signs, vocalisation and respiratory distress'. No other abnormalities were observed. Green, purple or pink staining of the cage tray paper was observed for the majority of treated [rabbits], with green/purple/blue or pink urine.[82]

Once these observations had been made, the remaining rabbits were killed, before all were dissected and inspected for living foetuses.[83]

When the press confronted Mr Douglas about these experiments, his bluster faltered:

I don't know anything about it to tell you the truth. I don't know what the rabbits were used for. The testing of artificial sweeteners is a legal requirement. They are a part of life.[84]

A part of life they may be, but the tests were not a legal requirement.

After a week, the camp voluntarily dispersed. But this was the beginning of a larger campaign. Activists began planning for a national protest at the farm under the banner of 'Operation Liberation'. On the day of the protest, police met campers with roadblocks, drones, Section 14 notices banning people from approaching the farm, and an army of police evidence gatherers. As a result, no one present dared take the opportunity to rescue more rabbits from Highgate. It did, however, spawn a new group, called Close Highgate Farm, who held regular protests at the facility in the years that followed.

Meanwhile, the MFAH attracted international attention when they set fire to a hunting lodge high in the Austrian Alps. The lodge belonged to Novartis' CEO Daniel Vasella.[85] Days before, MFAH activists had entered Vasella's family cemetery and added two crosses bearing the names of Novartis' CEO and his wife. They poured paint over the graves, and in a sinister escalation stole an urn of ashes, which they offered to return if Novartis ceased all business with HLS.[86]

*   *   *

Charged with blackmail, and under strict bail conditions preventing us protesting against HLS, Nicci and I had taken a backseat with SHAC. We continued to store and distribute campaign materials such as leaflets, petitions, and posters, but no longer organised or attended SHAC protests.

Nonetheless, in the early morning of 11 November, I heard a noise from our roof terrace. I looked outside to see a police officer in riot gear, surrounded by several of his colleagues, trying to cut through our patio doors. The door exploded in a maelstrom of glass and noise as police officers charged into our house screaming indecipherable words of warning. They arrested us for 'conspiracy to cause criminal damage'.[87]

As they ransacked our home, Chris Potter answered a knock on his own door less than a mile away. A man dressed in a Royal Mail delivery uniform and carrying a cardboard box greeted him with 'Package for Potter'. Chris confirmed that was him and found himself pinned against his own front door as a dozen riot police bundled out of an unmarked van and stormed past him.

The evidence that prompted the raids was a single tin of spray paint Chris had left in a communal cupboard in our house when it was searched the year before. The can bore Chris' fingerprints and came from the same batch as one used to paint slogans onto the side of a Barclays' bank. Shoes belonging to Chris and his partner Maria showed traces of the same paint, and CCTV recorded Chris' car pulling up outside a bank before two figures got out to apply the spray paint.

Officers hauled us directly from the police station to the magistrates' court, where the prosecution attempted to have Nicci and I remanded immediately to prison. Facing a complete lack of evidence, the magistrates refused. Instead, they released us under house arrest with an electronic tag and curfew. We were ordered not to:

> Participate in, assist travel arrangements, facilitate, or organise in any way any animal rights related activity, stall, website, protest or demonstration.

SHAC, however, refused to be silenced, and HLS' prospects continued to fade.

In December 2009, the Baker deal became reality. Using his investment firm FHP Realty, HLS' CEO borrowed roughly $200 million from a variety of lenders. He set up a string of private shell companies, through which he funnelled the money. The final shell company, Lion Holdings, purchased all of HLS' shares and merged with the laboratory. As a result, the money was never in the hands of a public company, and the lenders never needed to be named in SEC filings, or anywhere else. Only Andrew Baker and the investors themselves knew their identity.[88]

For the first time in over twenty years, HLS were a private company without shareholders. Their dreams of listing on the New York Stock Exchange were dashed once and for all.

30

A Sting in the Tale: 2009–11

The world of political activism is watching this campaign, because SHAC is doing something that has never been done before.[89]

– HLS

In the first month of 2010, SHAC activists held thirty-nine protests in eight countries, across four continents.[90] Despite the best efforts of the British government, the police, the pharmaceutical industry, multinational financial institutions, and private investigators, the threat of HLS' closure loomed large. The loss of a financial lender, or one large customer, would spell their doom.

With SHAC's founders in prison and others on stringent bail conditions and unable to organise, police acquired a search warrant for the company hosting SHAC's postal address. Finding Debbie Vincent's name on the account, they made neutralising her their prime objective.

*   *   *

Prior to the police raids in 2007, Novartis had been one of HLS' key customers. A network of informants within courier and freight companies confirmed this. Yet, in 2009, Novartis told the *Financial Times* that they no longer dealt with HLS,[91] and after the police action, many of those informants refused to work with SHAC.

To clear the matter up, SHAC dispatched a letter to Novartis:

You claimed in recent media articles that you have not used HLS in recent years. If this is indeed the case, we would like to request that you make a statement to the SHAC campaign stating that you are no longer using HLS and are not going to be using HLS again in the future. If you would prefer, we can privately accept such a statement and ask groups both in the UK and globally to cease demonstrations against you in a discreet manner; we will not publish your statement as any kind of campaign victory.

Finally, we feel it would be highly beneficial to have a meeting with representatives from yourselves and SHAC. We are happy to send members of the SHAC campaign to meet with you at your Switzerland headquarters where we can discuss these matters in a more efficient and personal manner.[92]

Novartis' head of security, Andrew Jackson, received the letter and promptly informed the British police. Although the letter was polite and reasonable, the police planned an elaborate sting. A meeting was arranged between Debbie and Max Gaston from SHAC, and Andrew Jackson and James Adams from Novartis. Covert audio recordings later revealed that 'James Adams' was a little more than he seemed:

I am a serving law enforcement officer who, for the purposes of this operation, will be known as James. Today is the 10th of March 2010 and the time is 8:17 in the morning. I have just activated this recording device which will be used during a meeting between myself, a representative of Novartis and two people who will also be attending the meeting who I understand are Debbie and Max. I am now going to switch this device off until it is required again.[93]

Unknown to Debbie and Max, the proposed meeting room in a London hotel was selected and hired by SO15, the Metropolitan Police's Counter Terrorism Command. Their officers were covertly distributed throughout the hotel, and they searched Debbie and Max as they entered, posing as Novartis security.[94]

Novartis had only proposed the meeting to instigate the return of CEO Daniel Vasella's missing urn. Asking two almost random activists in a completely different country whether they could 'sort it out' was an exercise in futility. James Adam's recording device captured Debbie attempting to explain:

The fact is, what you do, many thousands of people oppose.

The way democracy is, these sorts of meetings are very rare. Usually, we can't go and talk to the people who make decisions. We can't go and talk to heads of state, or government officials about policy. We're just normal, everyday members of the public so the only thing people can do is try petitions, try lobbying their MP, they try all sorts of other methods. And of course, that leads to frustration because things don't change … companies like yours have to realise that you've got to take comment from grassroots campaigns. If you don't, if you just ignore us, then you can see the escalation, and that's totally beyond our control.

We can't give you any guarantees, we've got absolutely no idea who did it, it's countries away from where we are. I actually answered the phone when the media phoned about it and that was the first time I'd heard anything about it.[95]

Another meeting was arranged, following an almost identical format. Pushed four times to give information about the urn, Debbie and Max explained they knew no more about it than anyone else in the room. Debbie was clear: they only had the power to stop SHAC protests, and not ALF or MFAH activists. She also expressed a concern:

We have no idea who is involved, as we have said before, or even what country they are from. The reason they did that allegedly is to do with your links to HLS. So, then it logically follows that once you have made a statement about HLS, they don't need to keep hold of them.

This is a very sensitive issue. We have seen in the past that law enforcement are grasping at straws, and us having this meeting, if it was found out … all the actual facts get lost. So, it would be claimed that me and Max were blackmailing you.[96]

After a further meeting, the police arranged for 'James Adams' to bump into Debbie on the London Underground. Debbie continued to explain that she didn't support the MFAH action, that she had played no part in it, and that she had no way of liaising with those who had. SHAC had only contacted Novartis to ask them whether they still dealt with HLS or not.

* * *

In August 2010, Dan Amos was the first person from Trial One released from prison, under strict conditions not to talk to other activists, use the internet, or take part in any animal liberation campaigning. Dan left prison as Trial Two was about to begin. With Sarah Whitehead and Nicole Vosper having pleaded guilty to blackmail, four of us remained, preparing to face the court.

Alfie Fitzpatrick had been involved in SHAC for only a few months. He had gone on lawful protests in Paris which were arranged with the police and attended by a lawyer.

When Jason 'JJ' Mullen was charged, the police believed he was an ALF activist code-named Kidda, a 'male from North London'. However, further scrutiny of JJ's activity proved beyond doubt that he could not have been Kidda, causing panic in the CPS.

Nicci and I were charged because we helped coordinate SHAC following the 2007 police raids. Despite the prosecution's sweeping claims, there was no legal issue with the newsletters we designed and distributed. Neither was anything wrong with the protests we organised, nor the barrister approved website or email lists. I had also attended lawful protests in Paris and forwarded two anonymously received emails to the American website Bite Back, which served as a news clearing house for animal liberation actions. All four of us had attended the barbecue, vilified by the prosecution in Trial One.

Despite the weak case, Alfie had seen his partner, Gerrah, sentenced on similarly ethereal evidence. He decided he couldn't go through it again:

I had followed every day of Gerrah's trial, which was incredibly draining and stressful, and when she was found guilty for something I knew she hadn't done, it just got worse.

I decided during one of our court appearances that I just didn't want to do it again. I had lost all faith in our legal system. I told my barrister that I wanted to plead guilty to a lesser offence, either a public order offence, or at worst SOCPA. I asked him to check with everyone else's barristers, which he was positive about, as he thought they might go for a group plea that ended the trial.

The prosecution agreed to accept a guilty plea for SOCPA. My barrister told me everyone else was working on plea deals, too. I figured I was unlikely to get a high sentence, so I accepted the deal.

The SOCPA legislation is entirely absurd. Like so many other ridiculous laws, I'm convinced that one day it will be struck off the statute book. I am happy to be guilty of the so-called 'crime' of interfering with the contractual relationships of an animal research facility. We have a moral duty to ignore unjust laws.

While JJ wasn't 'Kidda', he had attended similar protests to Gerrah, who had been convicted. French authorities raised no issues with his behaviour, but that hadn't made a difference in Trial One. Despite Section 145 SOCPA not applying to protests outside the UK, JJ cut his losses and accepted the same offer as Alfie.

Nicci and I faced Trial Two alone. The jury were sworn in and we stood in the dock waiting for the case to begin when prosecuting QC, Michael Bowes, approached our legal team. As chief prosecutor for the Financial Services Authority, he was responsible for an unrelated fraud case which was far more important to his career than a second SHAC trial. Realising that we wouldn't be pressured into pleading guilty to blackmail, he relented and offered us a deal. If I admitted to blackmail, then Nicci could plead to Section 145 SOCPA, reducing her maximum possible sentence from fourteen years to three.

We accepted the deal. We had done nothing in furtherance of a criminal conspiracy, but had no faith in receiving a fair trial.

On 21 October 2010, we all lined up in Winchester Crown Court to be sentenced. For blackmail, Sarah received six years, I was sentenced to four, and Nicole was handed three and a half. For Section 145 SOCPA, JJ was given three years, Nicci fifteen months, and Alfie a suspended sentence.

* * *

Taking their injunction back to the High Court, Novartis requested a ban on vivisection being referred to as murder or torture, and the prohibition of activists wearing rabbit costumes. Their demands were refused. Demonstrations against them continued in Liverpool, Sussex, London, and Hampshire, as well as across the USA, Chile, Sweden, France, and Norway.[97]

In London, HLS lender Fortress removed all signage from their offices in the hope that they could hide in plain sight. The plan failed. Regular demonstrations continued, causing Fortress to eventually replace their signs. At an investment conference in Baltimore, protestors attached a huge banner denouncing Fortress to helium balloons and suspended it from the ceiling.[98]

In Russia, SHAC activists carried out protests and anti-HLS street theatre in St Petersburg, Krasnodar, Saratov, and Moscow. Under cover of darkness, a separate group of over a dozen people attacked Novartis' Moscow offices with paint, stones, and smoke bombs.[99]

In Mexico, activists went even further. A homemade bomb was discovered outside Novartis' offices in Guadalajara. It was the second live device to be found at the facility, and activists followed it by placing a hoax bomb near Novartis in Mexico City.[100]

With SHAC's coordinators all in prison or under intense surveillance, the individuals and groups taking unlawful direct action remained largely unaffected by the clampdown. The MFAH continued their aggressive campaign, torching vehicles connected to Fortress in Germany and France. In the most militant action in the UK for several years, they also struck against Highgate rabbit farm, setting fire to their delivery vans on two separate occasions.

Peaceful actions by the anti-Highgate protest group, which had sprung from the SHAC national demonstration, continued with regularity. In August 2010, they erected a second protest camp outside the farm, but the police moved them on, claiming it contravened laws against protesting outside a home. The following day, campaigners tried again, pitching camp further down the road. Police promptly arrested two protestors and threatened the rest with the same if they did not move. On the third day, the camp was moved to the local town, where protestors dressed in rabbit costumes handed out leaflets to the local community and conducted interviews with the media. The two arrested activists were released without charge.

In Israel, another HLS animal supplier faced problems. Mazor Farm caught wild macaque monkeys in Mauritius, shipped them to their facility in Israel, and bred them for experimentation. Inspired by SHAC, activists launched 365 Days to Close Mazor Farm. Israeli activist Yael Gabay recalls:

In lots of ways the SHAC campaign influenced our campaign. Particularly, the idea to pressure El Al Airlines at all of their branches around the world, and not limiting ourselves to the firm itself, came from SHAC.

El Al were the only airline willing to export the primates out of Israel, so the optimistically named 365 Days to Close Mazor Farm launched a campaign against them, reigniting Gateway to Hell in Israel, the UK, and across the world. After several months of pressure, EL Al cut all ties with the vivisection industry.[101] It would take another four years of campaigning before the government closed the farm and declared:

> Israel will no longer be a country from which monkeys are exported for experimentation. This is a great achievement of the Environmental Protection Ministry, and we must give credit to all of the organisations that led the struggle and whose voice was heard. Together, we brought relief to the monkeys.[102]

A total of 650 wild-caught monkeys were taken to the safety of the Ben Shemen monkey sanctuary. Unfortunately, the Israeli government reneged on its promise to fund the care of the remaining 1,250, and it took many more years before the rest left captivity.[103]

As El Al distanced themselves from the vivisection industry, the BUAV launched an investigation into wild monkeys illegally trapped in the jungles of Laos and Cambodia. The monkeys were kept in bags before being moved to factory farms. On the farms, babies were taken from their mothers at six months old before being shipped to China and Vietnam, and then on to the UK for experimentation.[104] When pressed by MPs on whether there should be an inquiry, the British government responded, 'We have received no evidence to suggest one is needed.'[105]

Primate Products Inc. (PPI) transported some of the primates held in China to HLS. The Animal Liberation Investigation Unit (ALIU) acquired a stash of photos demonstrating horrific abuse. The photos, taken by PPI's own veterinary staff, depicted monkeys with injuries to their heads and bodies. The owner of PPI, Don Bradford, told journalists that despite wounds which exposed large sections of skull, the pictures portrayed 'completely healed, healthy, beautiful animals'.[106]

The US Department of Agriculture announced an investigation, and several research establishments distanced themselves from PPI. HLS continued to use them. Five years later PETA would expose PPI again, prompting the US Department of Agriculture to cite them for over twenty-five violations of federal animal welfare regulations.[107]

In Italy, Morini Farm finally threw in the towel after an intense seven-year fight.[108] Virtually every activist involved in the campaign had been banned from the area around the puppy farm, and protests had all but stopped two years before. Nevertheless, the economic damage they had inflicted was irreparable, and the financial incentive of turning the land into houses proved too tempting. Campaigners worked tirelessly to ensure every single animal inside was rescued, finding suitable homes for thousands of rats, mice, hamsters, and 283 beagles. Without pausing for breath, Claudio and the other organisers moved straight on to their next target, Green Hill:

> Green Hill were Italy's only other beagle breeder, and they had been very lucky. With all our attention on Morini, a lot of their customers had switched to Green Hill.
>
> We knew we had to do something, but after the SHAC arrests in the UK, it was time for us to stop and reflect on how we worked. Several activists from across Europe discussed what we should do with SHAC, and we decided we couldn't keep going on as we had. It wasn't sustainable. Eventually the government would just stop us, so we had to win public support.

We started the Green Hill campaign after someone leaked us inside information. They worked in the offices and hadn't been aware of what the company did. When they found out, they told us that Green Hill wanted to double their capacity – from 2,500 dogs to 5,000. Some of the dogs would be kept in pens buried under the ground, and it would have made them the biggest beagle breeder in Europe. We launched a campaign to stop them from getting planning permission to expand, and we called a national demonstration. The city council immediately announced they would never allow Green Hill to expand, and so we won before we even held our first protest.

With such an easy victory, the campaign switched to closing the existing farm. Concentrating on public relations, they became an effective campaigning machine. Mainland Europe saw its largest-ever anti-vivisection protest, with 10,000 people marching against Green Hill through the streets of Rome,[109] and thousands of others gathered at events around the country.

SHAC activists in the UK relaunched Beagle Day and toured facilities owned by HLS and their key supporters. With megaphones, placards, and flyers, the protestors reminded those supporting HLS of the countless animals dying inside their laboratories.

* * *

In the early hours of 10 December 2010, Debbie Vincent was rudely awoken yet again:

I was volunteering at an animal sanctuary when the police raided us at 8 am. With their lights and sirens on, they rushed me by unmarked car from Croydon all the way into Belgravia station. Other officers spent nearly twelve hours searching and removing property from the small building I lived in.

They had arrested me for an entirely fabricated allegation of fraud, and after five interviews, during which I remained silent, they released me on bail. Two years later the charges would be dropped, but the police had not finished with me yet.

The same could be said for Nicci and me. In January 2011, we returned to court to face criminal damage charges with Maria Neal and Chris Potter. As Chris and Maria pleaded guilty, I was confident the CPS would drop the case against Nicci and me, as we had done nothing more than let the couple stay in our home. However, Judge Cutler had other ideas.

The CPS requested the jury be told of my recent blackmail conviction. They admitted that without that, they had no case against me. Nothing suggested that I had carried out, organised, or even knew about the criminal damage. They argued that because I had pleaded guilty to a similar crime, I must also be guilty of this one.

Remarkably, Judge Cutler agreed to their request and put me in an impossible position. No matter how convincing my defence was, it would always be tainted with suspicion. Nicci was days from being released from prison, so I agreed to a deal. I pleaded guilty to criminal damage on the condition that they drop the case against her and allowed her to go home. In another inexplicable move, Judge Cutler added a year to my prison sentence, while Chris and Maria each walked out of court with suspended sentences.

31
Endgame: 2011–18

[HLS] is a chaotic, stressful hell-hole. Do not work here.[110]
– HLS' toxicology study director

In March 2011, the ALF liberated dozens of trout in two rescue operations at HLS' supplier Brown Well Fisheries in Yorkshire.[111] As the fish swam to freedom, Nicci was released from HMP Bronzefield 200 miles further south. She was the third activist to be released from Trials One and Two. As with Gerrah Selby, Dan Amos, and everyone who came after, she was subjected to a raft of restrictions aimed to 'frustrate political activity'.[112] These conditions forbade her from contacting her co-defendants, using the internet, and taking part in any protest, meeting, or website in support of animal welfare. She was ordered to sleep at her mother's house every night and given a five-year ASBO, which prevented any campaigning at all against HLS.

With activists like myself and Gerrah sentenced to years in jail, Nicci's comparatively brief sentence of fifteen months visibly frustrated the senior police officers who attended court. Following her release, they put a plan into action to extend her prison time:

I was at my mum's house baking vegan cakes for a local dental surgery's staff meeting. Two police officers knocked on the door, and arrested me for breaking my licence conditions. I asked what I had done wrong, but they claimed not to know.

When I arrived at prison, the officers said I knew what I had done and implied I was being difficult. I was told I would receive paperwork explaining my recall within five days. You only have fourteen days to appeal a recall, so time was ticking. After five days, it became clear I was being unlawfully denied access to my 'recall dossier'. After ten days, my lawyer threatened to take the prison governor to court, and I was briefly allowed to see the document under strict supervision. It was another two days before they gave my lawyer a copy.

The document claimed that 'Jon Lord' from Kent Police had received intelligence that I was living at my dad's house instead of my mum's. Kent Police later denied any knowledge of Jon Lord. The document claimed that Nick Brown from Dorset Police investigated and confirmed the claim. I later spoke to Nick Brown, who adamantly denied this. I've never solved who 'Jon Lord' really was, nor who fabricated Nick Brown's statement.

I was also accused of 'continuing animal rights activities unabated', breaking my ASBO, being badly behaved, and not taking my licence conditions seriously. All those accusations were lies, and I've never been given any clarification or specifics.

My solicitor, Louisa Kirk, wrote an amazing appeal document to submit to the parole board. She interviewed witnesses and went through every claim, providing extensive evidence to prove them false.

Incredibly, I lost the appeal, and I wasn't allowed to know why. Louisa phoned the parole board, who looked at the decision and immediately cancelled it, admitted something looked 'unusual'. We appealed again but lost because my defence documents 'went missing'. Again, the decision was cancelled. I lost my third appeal because the parole board claimed the allegations made by the police were 'unusually vague and lacking information', 'did not provide any details', and they were therefore unable to determine what I was accused of. Somehow this convinced them I couldn't be released.

Before I could appeal again, my licence period came to an end, and they were forced to free me.

In Britain, there is a process that even the most serious offenders follow to aid rehabilitation and assimilation back into society. This often includes ending their sentence in an 'open' prison, and day release to reconnect with family and pursue employment.[113] With the *Observer* reporting that the home secretary went 'squinty-eyed about these types of cases',[114] pressure was applied to ensure SHAC campaigners were not treated like normal prisoners.

Before his release in 2010, Dan Amos was taken to HMP Ford open prison, but was immediately shipped back to a higher category institution, with a guard muttering, 'This isn't for you.' Home Office representatives visited the governor of another prison to inform him that if a SHAC prisoner were afforded any 'perks' he would lose his job. The perks they referred to were open prison and day release; the accepted norms of rehabilitation.

When Gregg arranged an inter-prison visit with his wife Natasha, the police fed the story to the *Telegraph*, who ran the headline '£110 taxi bill for animal right's thug's visit to wife in prison'.[115] In another story, Natasha was lambasted because she was allowed to wear non-leather boots and have access to ethical cosmetics. A police 'source' declared, 'She's living the good life as happy as Larry on the prison farm growing organic veg in her plastic boots.'[116] In reality, having had her entire life taken away, being separated from her husband, and spending four and a half years in prison, followed by another four and a half on severe licence conditions was about as far from as 'happy as Larry' as Natasha could be.

The police informed the media that Heather had befriended notorious child murderer Rose West.[117] Heather was sickened by the idea that she would associate with such a person and explained this to *Wales Online*.[118] For telling her truth, Heather was called before the prison governor and threatened with severe sanctions.

Despite the Liberal Democrats' justice spokesperson decrying the politicisation of the probation service as 'a grotesque abuse of power',[119] most of the SHAC prisoners were told at the last minute that they would be released to bail hostels rather than their own homes. In the case of Gregg and Natasha, a married couple, this meant separate hostels, many miles apart. They were allowed out of the hostel for a few hours a day, under strict conditions, and were banned from using the internet or contacting other activists. Gerrah recalls her release:

> My original probation officer had advocated for me to receive a non-custodial sentence, as I 'literally wouldn't hurt a fly'. However, I had a new probation officer assigned while in prison. Without even meeting me, on advice from the police, he decided that forcing me to live in a halfway house with women suffering from severe mental health and addiction issues was necessary for my rehabilitation. I was listed as MAPPA level 3, which is the highest level of multi-agency supervision that any prisoner can receive. I was forbidden from going to London during the royal wedding and was visited by anti-terrorism officers in the run-up to the London 2012 Olympics. I'm not a violent person, and I

was involved in non-violent protests. Yet apparently, I now ranked alongside the most violent and dangerous offenders in the country, because the police had insisted that my teenage activism was a threat to national security. It felt like a sick joke, funny if it weren't so damaging.

For two more years, I learned to have no hopes or dreams because I knew I would not be allowed to follow them. The threat of losing my freedom again loomed constantly, and I was petrified that the slightest misunderstanding would put me back behind bars. I was banned from using a computer, a smartphone, or the internet, and from working for any organisation involved in human rights, animal rights, animal welfare, or the environment. My probation officer refused to let me intern with a charity which offers legal advice to people on death row, and they banned me from accepting a film mentorship from the Koestler Trust.

For Heather, five and a half years in high-security prisons followed by a sudden release to a bail hostel took a toll:

At the beginning of my sentence, every day I thought, 'I don't belong here. I need to be out there, looking up at the sky.'

After a little while, I began to accept it. 'This is my world. I don't want to go out there. I don't belong out there.' So, when it came to my release, I had a nervous breakdown. I didn't want to go. I couldn't imagine life outside of prison.

The reason they have open prisons is to prepare you for your release. Without that, it's just a horrific situation. You could be a child murderer, or a sex offender, or anything else, but if you behave, then you go to open prison to get you ready for the outside world. If you're an animal rights activist, however: no chance.

With activists from Trial One and Trial Two trickling out of prison, several of us appealed to the Director of Public Prosecutions, Sir Keir Starmer, to review our case. By not disclosing the existence of Adrian Radford, whose testimony could have acquitted many of us, we had been subjected to a grievous abuse of process. Starmer's response was blunt:

> It is well established practice that the police and prosecution will neither confirm nor deny the existence of a Covert Human Intelligence Source, past or present. The mere fact that a person claims in public to have been tasked by an investigative agency to act as a CHIS is insufficient reason to deviate from that practice.[120]

Keir Starmer knew SHAC was a lawful organisation. In fact, he was one of the barristers SHAC instructed for advice to ensure that was the case. Nonetheless, Starmer had no intention of looking into the matter himself. He relied upon the word of his old friend, and the CPS' Domestic Extremism Co-ordinator, Nick Paul.[121] The pair had co-founded the Doughty Street legal practice and had worked together as far back as the 1980s as editors on *Socialist Lawyer*.[122]

Environmental activists later accused Starmer and Paul of conspiring to cover up a similar case. The campaigners were arrested during a planned incursion of the Ratcliffe-on-Soar power station, but their trial collapsed when one of the organisers was exposed as an undercover police officer. Starmer should have disclosed that fact immediately, but instead stayed silent.[123]

Keir Starmer went on to become leader of the Labour Party, using his position to stop MPs voting against a controversial bill which allows undercover operatives to commit serious criminality, including rape and murder, without repercussions.[124]

* * *

Debbie remained unaware that her meetings with Novartis were police entrapment, so when Fortress asked to meet with SHAC, she agreed. These meetings were genuine, and Fortress agreed on an amicable arrangement. They supplied a signed statement and SEC filings to show that they had cut ties with HLS,[125] refused to sign the loan over to another company, and applied to the High Court to cancel their injunction.[126]

Once again, HLS scrambled to find a new lender, securing an undisclosed agreement with US Bank.

Photos taken by activists at HLS' New Jersey laboratory showed buildings falling into disrepair.[127] On industry recruitment pages, negative comments from ex-employees piled up, such as this from a former toxicology study director:

The company is very inefficient, takes a long time to conduct a study and as a result has poor profit margins. It is very clearly slowly bleeding to death.

[HLS] is a chaotic, stressful hell-hole. Do not work here.[128]

To secure HLS' future, their CEO Andrew Baker conceived another scheme. Under the False Claims Act, US citizens are encouraged to file lawsuits against corporations they believe have defrauded the federal government. If the prosecution is successful, the whistle-blower receives a portion of any money recovered.[129]

Before joining HLS, Baker and two other executives held top positions at a competitor called Unilab. They brazenly filed a lawsuit against Unilab, claiming $1 billion in damages for offences which took place under their own management. If successful, the scheme promised Andrew Baker a $150 million pay-out – enough to save HLS. However, to bring the claim HLS' attorney Mark Bibi unlawfully disclosed confidential information, and the judge dismissed the lawsuit.¹³⁰

SHAC delivered a further blow by uncovering experiments recently conducted inside HLS. In one test, HLS exposed sixteen rhesus monkeys to a toxic PCB coolant which had been banned in the UK since 1981. In another, they fed hundreds of rats a herbal supplement made by MegaNatural, before gassing them and examining their organs. Other products tested on rabbits and rats included food preservatives, soybean fibre, food additives, unleaded petrol, and Botox. Amongst the studies was a surprisingly frank admission:

> These studies show the rat is a very poor model for humans and toxicity in the rat cannot be extrapolated to humans.[131]

This strongly contradicted HLS' public claims. During a disruption at Imperial College London's science fair in February 2012, an activist posing as a student filmed an HLS' representative claiming that 'one mouse can save 100 lives'.[132] The phoney student filming asked if that meant HLS had already saved the entire population of earth, based on the number of rodents they tested on. The peaceful disruption barely lasted five minutes before security ejected protestors.

Protests continued across the USA too. In Los Angeles, sixty protestors gathered outside houses belonging to executives from HLS' shareholders and customers. In New Jersey, another crowd voiced their horror against the New Jersey Association for Biomedical Research's 'Enrichment Extravaganza', which focused on how to 'deal with' laboratory animals. When SHAC called a week of action against top HLS' customer AstraZeneca, activists in seven US states carried out protests.

Canada and Chile also saw demonstrations, as well as countries across Europe. In the centre of Bilboa, thirty-four activists in white paper suits stood in a line, holding laptops playing undercover footage from inside the laboratory. French and Greek campaigners took to the streets outside Astra-Zeneca offices, while black-clad Dutch protestors roared their anger through megaphones. In London, campaigners rushed into the Drug Transporters' conference, disrupting a speech by an AstraZeneca representative. Protestors including Debbie super-glued their hands together and marched through the reception area of the company's flagship London offices. When security eventually evicted them, the protestors formed a barrier across the entrance.

In Loughborough, activists including Jon White set up a protest camp outside HLS' supplier Harlan, to protest their breeding of dogs, rabbits, and other animals for laboratories:

We positioned the camp near the entrance, so we regularly came face to face with Harlan's staff. The protest lasted for several days, and the police raised no complaints at the time. However, two of us were later arrested under the SOCPA legislation.

The charges related to two incidents. One night, a bull and a group of cows chased us across a nearby field, and we were forced to scale Harlan's perimeter fence to escape. This was entirely true, but unsurprisingly the police did not believe us at all. Nonetheless, that charge was later dropped.

The second SOCPA charge concerned frequent argu-ments with Harlan's staff as we confronted them head-on during the protest. The case went all the way to Crown Court before we reluctantly pleaded guilty. It felt like all we had done was loudly protest, but the environment around anti-vivisection campaigning had changed.

By 2012, the British government considered any form of protest against vivisection an act of extremism, which had to be quashed. As a result of SOCPA, shouting during a protest was now treated as a serious crime. While Jon received a suspended sentence, his co-defendant, Luke Steele, received eighteen months in prison. The pair were handed ASBOs, preventing them from owning or using a megaphone for three years. Professor Roger Morris, head of bioscience at King's College, made it clear why protests against animal suppliers were particularly feared:

We are now down to our last three major breeders in the UK. We can manage with that, but if we lose another, we will be in a very uncomfortable situation.[133]

This situation became reality in Italy, during the most significant animal liberation protest of this period. Following an ALF raid at HLS' beagle supplier Green Hill, which saw five dogs liberated, another more brazen rescue took place. The Green Hill campaign had become so successful that satellite groups sprung up with the same aims. One group organised a march against the facility for World Day for Animals in Laboratories, which they publicised before the Green Hill campaign had announced their own protest. In the confusion of two identical events, Green Hill organisers saw an opportunity. They arranged a march within the march, diverting activists towards the back of the facility and cutting open the fences.

Dozens of activists entered the compound and made their way into breeding units. They freed thirty puppies and passed them back over the barbed wire into the waiting hands of other campaigners. Twenty-two dogs were smuggled to freedom, but for several campaigners, this was their first brush with the reality of animal liberation. Several older campaigners boarded their coach home, still carrying dogs, while younger activists posed for selfies with rescued animals, unaware that they were hot property and needed to be gone. As social media feeds filled with photos of the dogs inside, and far away from the farm, police arrested thirteen campaigners and seized eight dogs. Their photos and internet posts had put themselves and their canine companions at risk, but their live streams of the protest had gone viral. People across the world watched a dramatic and inspirational act of animal liberation unfold live on their phone screens.[134]

Green Hill campaign founder Claudio had seen two possibilities for the daring plan:

> One was that the dogs would be liberated, and the protest would get a lot of publicity and inspire people. The other was that people would get beaten and arrested by the police, and no dogs would get rescued. But we thought that maybe the second option was even better, as millions of people supported our campaign across Italy. If the police attacked us – like they had at Morini – there would have been outrage. We had won the public's support.
>
> Whatever happened, we were certain more people would join the campaign.
>
> Because of the public's support, when the protest happened, the police knew they couldn't charge in and beat or arrest us. They were almost helpful in the liberation. There were all these new activists who were just walking around the farm, laughing, chatting, smoking. The police just let it happen, until eventually they said, 'Now it's enough, please leave.'

The twenty-two dogs who made it to safety were never recovered and were free to live out their lives as beloved family members.

Green Hill attempted to sue the campaigners who had been arrested, but animal rights group Legambiente counter-sued, using evidence of cruelty taken during the rescue. The judges overseeing the case visited the farm. Upon seeing the state of the facility, they ordered police to seize all the dogs, and handed 2,700 beagles to animal rights groups for rehoming.[135] Three Green Hill employees were convicted and sentenced to prison for cruelty,[136] and despite trying to prove that they could turn their business around, Green Hill officially closed a few years later. While the dogs were free, it took a further eight years before all the activists were finally acquitted.[137]

In Sweden, more laboratory beagles were making headlines. In a forest an hour outside of Malmö, in a supposedly secret facility, AstraZeneca bred dogs for their laboratories. The secrecy had evaporated during several ALF liberations over the years, and the site was well known to animal liberation activists. The company announced a billion-euro cost-cutting drive, involving 7,300 job losses, and declared that they were going to stop breeding their own dogs and start buying them from third-party suppliers.[138] Daniel from Djurrättsalliansen (Animal Rights Alliance) seized the moment:

> I contacted a worker at the breeding unit. They told me the plan was to kill 400 dogs before the public found out or sell them to another laboratory such as HLS.
>
> We started the campaign 'Let the Astra-Dogs Live' and made sure it went out in the international media. Animal lovers all over the world joined the campaign, and we organised demonstrations at the site, even though it was in the middle of the winter with really deep snow. We targeted

all companies involved with them and contacted every possible airport that the dogs could be flown from. We had homes ready for every dog.

I convinced employees from the breeding facility to smuggle some of the dogs to safety, but most of them were flown out of the country by Aeronova. People chained their necks to the gates of the breeding site and tried to block the lorries from leaving. When they got past us, we protested at the airport right up until we could see the dogs being loaded onto aeroplanes. Activists begged for their freedom using megaphones, but the company was only interested in money, so the dogs left Sweden. We learnt they were being flown to Manchester and organised with our British friends to be ready at the airport to meet them.

When British campaigners discovered the dogs were going to be experimented on at an AstraZeneca facility in Chester, they blockaded the laboratory. It was to no avail. The police moved protestors aside and escorted the dogs into the next phase of their tragic lives. This inspired Victoria Fraser, an activist on her first protest, to launch a new group called Unite to Care. The group campaign for the rehoming of laboratory beagles following experimentation.[139]

*   *   *

By 2012, a small core of regular activists kept SHAC alive in the UK. While hundreds joined them on larger protests, a handful of groups scattered across the country protested almost daily against companies connected to HLS.

Removing Debbie and the persistent group of activists she protested with remained the police's priority.

An officer from the National Domestic Extremism Unit (NDEU, formerly NETCU) stumbled upon a YouTube video from the peaceful disruption of the Imperial College London's science fair. Although no complaints were made at the time, police tracked down and arrested two activists, accusing them of breaching HLS' injunction. The campaigners were brought before the Old Bailey, only to be ushered out shortly afterwards when a breach of process by the police caused the case to collapse.

The police had a contingency in place, having already arrested one of those activists, Lorna Potter, along with several other campaigners on a raft of SOCPA charges. Alexis Raven Báthory was arrested alongside her:

> We realised the police were following us to a protest in Milton Keynes. They pulled us over and immediately arrested Debbie on a spurious traffic offence. None of the rest of us could drive, so a police officer got in our car and started driving us away. I immediately clocked that we were being driven to a police station and shouted, 'We're getting nicked, everyone out.'
>
> We threw ourselves out of the moving car. If we were getting arrested, it was going to be on our terms. As we tried to run, several of us were quickly rounded up and caught, but we were determined not to make it easy for them. We went limp and made them drag us to police vehicles.

For the arrested activists, this was the beginning of a lengthy legal ordeal. Lorna recalls:

> Three of us were arrested under SOCPA for a protest we had held two months before, with a fourth person arrested a few weeks later.

We were placed on bail with conditions preventing us from campaigning against HLS or going within a mile of any animal rights protest in Buckinghamshire, Berkshire, and Oxfordshire. We were instructed 'not to gather at any company listed as a target, past or present, on the SHAC website'. This effectively barred us from standing outside our own high-street banks or being in a car as it was refuelled. Our solicitors successfully fought to have 'past' targets removed from the wording, as no one was able to list them all.

Over the next eight months we were re-bailed repeatedly until January 2013, when the four of us, along with two others, woke up during the night to the sound of police battering down the doors of our houses to arrest us yet again. They now accused us of twenty-five breaches of SOCPA legislation between October 2011 to June 2012.

The police weren't messing around. In an excessive show of force, at least one sleeping activist was woken with a gun pointing at their face. Emma Phipps recalls being added to the charge, completing the 'SOCPA 7':

There were around twenty-seven incidents listed as reasons for our arrests and prosecution, none of them involving violence, most not even involving trespass. One incident involved us turning up to a business address for a protest, only to find that the company was run by a guy from his home, so we immediately left.

Two of the incidents involved criminal damage against companies connected to HLS, which none of us were accused of doing. They were included simply because they had happened during the period we were under investigation. As the people who committed the criminal damage offences were never identified, it was clear you were more likely to be prosecuted for peaceful protests than if you hid your identity and caused damage to property in the dead of night.

Because SOCPA criminalised trespass against companies connected to animal testing, we were forced to agree to a plea deal with the Crown Prosecution Service (CPS). Prior to sentencing, the CPS showed footage of our behaviour to the judge, who repeatedly yawned through videos of us holding placards and handing out leaflets while accidentally being a couple of metres inside a private car park. Even footage of us chanting and handing out leaflets inside office buildings didn't seem to wake him up.

After two years on bail, during which we were barred from protesting against HLS, we were given suspended prison sentences, large cost orders and fines. It was a great relief to avoid prison, but the threat was not over. The suspended sentences hung over us for a further two years, with the risk of immediate imprisonment if we were arrested for anything else.

The SHAC campaign lost some of its last remaining regular protestors, and in the UK daily protests dropped to one or two a month. Across the world, without influence from the UK, protests against HLS began to dwindle. The last SHAC Newsletter was released in mid-2012, and with it the final cry for help for the animals imprisoned within the laboratory. However, even as it prepared its final gasp, the SHAC campaign continued to prove its efficacy, as HLS was forced to shed 6 per cent of its workforce to remain solvent.[140]

With the SOCPA 7 banned from protesting, and SHAC struggling to survive, the police might have finished there.

They were, however, keen to wrap up one final, and significant, matter.

During the height of the MFAH attacks across Europe, police had pulled over an activist named Sven van Hasselt during a random patrol in Luxembourg. The stop happened near the house of someone connected to Fortress, and as the police let Sven on his way, a car parked outside that house caught fire. A year later police arrested him on suspicion of arson while he crossed the border by train into Germany, but dropped the case due to lack of evidence.

While the authorities in mainland Europe showed little interest in prosecuting Sven, he was the only potential lead British police had into who was behind MFAH actions. If planned in the UK, blackmail is one of the few offences British police can prosecute when carried out abroad.[141] Sven, however, was a Dutch national, and while his partner was British, she had lived with him in the Netherlands for several years.

The police found a convenient bridge in Debbie. The call register on her phone logged hundreds of messages and calls to people across the global animal rights community. By picking out a handful of calls to Sven's partner Tasha, the police tenuously linked Debbie in the UK to Tasha in the Netherlands. From there it was just one small step to Sven. It was enough to see Debbie charged for conspiracy to blackmail.

Sven and Tasha were being prosecuted in the Netherlands for an attempted liberation at a fur farm and could not leave the country. As a result, in 2014, Debbie stood trial alone.

Aside from several friendly phone calls to Tasha, the crux of Debbie's case were the meetings with Novartis in which she clearly denied any knowledge of, or connection to, the ALF or MFAH. Despite the meetings taking place four years prior, the prosecution only admitted two weeks before trial that Novartis' 'Special Projects Manager' James Adams was really a police officer. Novartis' head of security, Andrew Jackson, was even encouraged to write a false witness statement, implying James Adams was his employee.[142]

Launching a bid to have the case dismissed, James Woods QC was scathing:

> This is not just a case of tacit investigation, but a case where an undercover police officer has instigated contact with the defendant in order to seek to entrap her into crossing the line into participation in a criminal conspiracy.[143]

Despite significant breach of disclosure rules, and the suppression of information which all but proved Debbie's innocence, the trial continued.

Desperate to prove there was more to the case, the prosecution pointed to Debbie possessing a copy of *Animal Farm*. A threatening email claimed by the MFAH was signed 'George Orwell', which they insisted proved her connection. The author's name was the default signature for the mail provider, which was not mentioned until the prosecution's computer expert was cross-examined.

Having witnessed the extent of the prosecution's case, James Woods QC attempted again to have the trial dismissed:

> There is no evidence that Debbie Vincent was a party to a conspiracy to blackmail.
>
> She has neither threatened damage nor been a party to such a threat. The undercover material makes this clear.

The request was once more denied. Despite the incredibly weak case, the prosecution had proven in Trial One that enough emotional testimony could compel a jury to convict. Unfortunately for Debbie, she was the only person on trial, and swayed by graphic details of crimes she played no part in, the jury convicted her, and she was sentenced to six years in prison. The twelve weeks before her sentencing was the only period between 2000 and 2020 without an anti-HLS activist in prison.

With the last stalwart of SHAC removed, the campaign made a tough decision:

SHAC has been the biggest and most effective grassroots animal rights campaign the world has ever seen. Since we started, thousands of people across the globe have taken up the fight to close down Europe's largest animal testing laboratory, HLS.

We've all played our part in this revolutionary campaign. Through determination, anger, and ground breaking new tactics, we've decimated the finances and reputation of the massive multinational corporation HLS.

Right now, HLS is over $100 million in debt, is struggling to win or keep customers, has steadily decreasing year end profits and is at serious risk of bankruptcy. The only reason they've survived this long is because of the UK government.

Since 2007 dozens of activists have been arrested, with some receiving lengthy prison sentences. Campaigners have also been given extreme bail and licence conditions to silence them from speaking out against animal testing and isolate them from the animal rights movement.

With the onslaught of government repression against animal rights activists in the UK, it's time to reassess our methods, obstacles, and opponent's weaknesses, to build up our solidarity network for activists and to start healing the effects of repression.

Although we're announcing the closure of the SHAC campaign, it will always be an important part of our history and a reminder of the ingenuity and power of the animal rights movement.[144]

It would be another four years before Sven and Tasha were extradited to face the British courts. With SHAC and the mythos surrounding it resigned to the past, there was no one left to deter. Tasha and Sven pleaded guilty to blackmail, and in the last act of the British state – who had spent tens of millions in crushing the campaign – Tasha received a suspended sentence and Sven was imprisoned for five years.

As the dust settled, Gordon Mills, a retired officer from the specialist NETCU police unit, observed:

The post-2004 era witnessed a new age of animal rights activity and associated extremism; however, it also witnessed a new era in policing protest that will continue to have huge ramifications for our democracy.[145]

32

Epilogue: 2014–22

After trying to silence and suppress SHAC through every possible channel, the British state had decisively brought its iron boot down on the campaign. In handing out prison sentences of over eighty years to anyone who dared coordinate or speak on behalf of SHAC, they forced the campaign out of existence.

However, with its last breath, SHAC had one final move to play. HLS outlasted SHAC through sheer determination, unprecedented governmental support, and creative accounting, but was it sustainable? Believing the financial damage was irreparable, SHAC publicly announced its cessation. They hoped HLS would take the opportunity to quietly close, without appearing to have conceded defeat.

In a literal sense, the tactic worked. To evade financial ruin, in September 2015 the laboratory merged with animal breeder and feed supplier Harlan to rebrand as Envigo.[1] The following year, the process began to officially dissolve Huntingdon Life Sciences.[2] The merger failed, and three years later the part of Envigo which had been HLS was sold to their rival Covance and later rebranded LabCorp.[3]

Against all odds, SHAC forced HLS out of business, but it was a hollow victory. On paper, HLS is no more. But Lab-Corp's laboratories remain open, and animals continue to be exploited and killed in their tens of thousands.

Governments on either side of the Atlantic framed their extreme reaction to SHAC as an inevitable response to the ALF. However, in many cases, those sent to prison had no role in militant tactics. The efficacy of the campaign, and its potential impact on big business and the economy, rather than the criminality of its supporters, dictated the state's behaviour. History repeats in a pattern all radical activists should take note of.

In 2011, during the twilight of SHAC, the FBI replicated their repressive tactics against the Occupy Wall Street movement.[4] Amidst mass surveillance and smears of terrorism, over 2,600 anti-capitalist campaigners were arrested. Here, the police focused on cracking skulls and spraying CS gas rather than holding show trials.[5] Police were accused of breaching international law on multiple occasions,[6] but the short burst of extreme state violence was enough to suppress a movement.

A decade later, Britain's home secretary, Priti Patel, declared, 'I don't support protest',[7] before drafting a swathe of draconian new laws.[8] The Police, Crime, Sentencing and Courts Bill targeted Extinction Rebellion (XR) and Black Lives Matter (BLM) following a string of non-violent protests and publicity stunts. The Act, which became law in April 2022, dramatically increases police powers to clamp down on protests, effectively extending the SOCPA legislation that blighted SHAC to all social justice causes. While XR and BLM are comparable to SHAC, they were not supported by an equivalent to the ALF. Even without the spectre of militant allies, the net which snared SHAC now encircles them too. Counter-terrorism police have added organisations as mainstream as Greenpeace and PETA to watch lists distributed to schools and hospitals.[9]

During the bombing of Gaza in 2021, Richard Barnard, an activist from Palestine Action Network, carried out a rooftop occupation at the landlords of an arms factory. In a chilling repeat of history, he was charged with blackmail. The unwarranted demand was to stop arms sales to Israel, the menaces were the threat of further protest stunts.[10] The charge soon developed into an alleged conspiracy, with several of his colleagues added to the case.

As former NETCU officer Gordon Mills observed:

> The government, the police, and the targeted industries robustly responded [to SHAC] in a coordinated strategic approach to reduce animal rights crimes. However, the success of this initiative has had far-reaching implications for human rights and the ability of people to protest in a democratic society.[11]

The culture which allowed Adrian Radford to infiltrate and incriminate SHAC campaigners was highlighted in 2014, when Home Secretary Theresa May launched a government inquiry into spy cops. She was forced to act after evidence revealed that for decades, undercover police officers had formed intimate relationships and even fathered children with unwitting social justice activists. The inquiry uncovered documents detailing the significant role that police agent provocateurs have played in the Animal Liberation Front (ALF). They were instrumental in burning down department stores selling fur,[12] drafting an anti-McDonald's leaflet which led to the infamous McLibel trial,[13] raiding fur farms,[14] and liberating animals from facilities including Wickham Laboratories.[15] At the time of publication, five of those imprisoned for SHAC activism are named victims in the miscarriage of justice category of the inquiry. Attempts to appeal our convictions, and secure justice, continue.

Questions surrounding Lord Sainsbury's donation and subsequent rise to power resurfaced as a fresh 'cash for honours' scandal broke in late 2021. The ruling Conservative Party were exposed offering donors' seats in the House of Lords, with a former Conservative chair claiming, 'Once you pay your £3m, you get your peerage.'[16] Seats were granted despite concerns from MI5 and the House of Lords Appointment Commission.[17] MPs called on the Metropolitan Police to investigate but they chose not to, refusing to explain their decision.[18]

Many prominent SHAC activists now hold leading roles in organisations including Stop the Cull, the Save Movement, Essere Animali, SPA Canada, Freedom for Animals, the Beagle Freedom Project, Djurrättsalliansen, and others. Their influence permeates the international animal liberation movement. However, for many of those caught in the final wave of repression, the psychological damage will last a lifetime. Violently dragged into a state conspiracy they were never prepared for, some were so traumatised by what they endured they left the UK and mainland USA permanently.

The campaign against HLS, and the response it provoked, left deep scars in the British anti-vivisection movement. However, in 2018 local campaigners resumed protests against the facility once known as HLS, under the banner of 'Stop Animal Cruelty Huntingdon' (SACH). In January 2021, ALF activists liberated eighty fire salamanders in the first raid on a British laboratory supplier in a decade.[19] Months later a second raid followed, targeting a breeder who activists claim was connected to the vivisection industry. They rescued and rehomed over 400 guinea pigs.[20]

In June 2021, campaigners released footage gathered using hidden cameras over the course of a year. The recordings showed hundreds of beagle puppies being forced into crates at MBR Acres in Cambridgeshire – formerly known as Harlan Interfauna. The dogs were sent to animal testing laboratories, and the *Daily Mirror* ran a two-page feature exposing the 'factory farm'.[21]

Echoing 1997, the harrowing report led to activists erecting a long-term protest camp, dubbed Camp Beagle, outside of MBR Acres,[22] attracting hundreds of protestors to the site.[23] For forty days and forty nights, they put the facility under siege, preventing dogs being shipped to laboratories. As a result of the footage and protest camp, Home Secretary Priti Patel announced a review, tasking officials with finding ways to end animal testing in the UK once and for all.[24] Just like New Labour's 1997 promise of a Royal Commission, the review failed to materialise.[25] After three months of protest, MBR followed HLS' lead and applied for an injunction to have Camp Beagle removed. This time, however, the attempt failed, and the camp was allowed to remain,[26] attracting wide support which saw pop star Will Young breach the injunction and chain himself to the gates.[27] Campers insisted that they would remain in place until MBR closed, and in June 2022 released new footage from inside the facility, revealing dogs in severe distress, without bedding or any form of enrichment.[28]

In the USA, a facility born out of HLS' failed 2015 merger was exposed by PETA. Throughout 2021, Envigo's beagle breeding facility in Virginia was infiltrated by an investigator who recorded staff using high-pressure hoses on puppies, injecting euthanasia drugs directly into their hearts, leaving them to fall into drains and die, and starving pregnant mothers.[29] The exposé prompted federal agents to seize nearly 450 dogs[30] and in June 2022, with legal proceedings ongoing, Envigo announced they were permanently closing the site, along with three others;[31] 4,000 dogs were removed from the facility and adopted by loving families, including Prince Harry and Meghan Markle,[32] who voiced their support for an end to animal research.[33]

In June 2022, as Camp Beagle neared its twelfth month of continuous protest, twenty-five activists connected to Animal Rebellion snuck past their tents and climbed inside MBR Acres.[34] Live streaming their protest, they showed the world the reality of life for dogs inside the UK's largest commercial puppy farm. As they were arrested and removed, they revealed it to be a factory farm, as intensive, filthy, and cruel as any other. The following morning, under the noses of scores of police officers, several of the activists returned. In the most dramatic anti-vivisection protest on UK soil in well over a decade, they brazenly liberated five beagle puppies. As MBR's security looked on helpless, the dogs were spirited away into the morning light and given the chance to live free from abuse in loving homes.[35] The police hunted in vain for the missing puppies, even searching the home of Camp Beagle's 101-year-old patron, Ron Green.[36] As they did so, three activists handed themselves in, taking full responsibility and demanding a trial by jury.[37] In order to prove their guilt, the focus would be on their motives rather than their actions. The ethics, efficacy, and legitimacy of animal research faced public scrutiny in a way never before seen. In the age of social media, an industry which thrives in shadows faced its archaic dogma being thrust into the cultural zeitgeist. It wasn't a risk they were willing to take. Just two weeks after the rescue, the Crown Prosecution Service dropped all charges. Despite three confessions, CCTV from multiple angles, eyewitnesses, and photos of the five missing dogs, they claimed there was 'insufficient evidence' to pursue the case. Days before Christmas, Animal Rebellion returned, rescuing and rehoming eighteen dogs before handing themselves in to the police voluntarily. Two further dogs, Love and Libby, were seized by police during the action and, despite international outrage, were returned to MBR Acres.[38]

As history repeats, and from the shadow of SHAC, a new era is dawning. The grassroots anti-vivisection movement is poised for a resurgence and is determined to finish what its predecessors started. The power and the passion of the anti-

HLS campaigns was not created in a vacuum. While state-led extremism may silence dissent for a time, until a government is brave enough to hold a science-led review of the industry, it seems inevitable that activists will emerge to force that change.

You've read our history. The future is yours.

Photographs

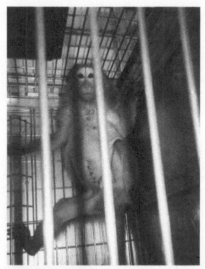

Figure 1   1997: A macaque is photographed inside Huntingdon Life Sciences in New Jersey by an undercover investigator. The monkey's identifier is crudely tattooed onto their chest, and rough stitching and heavy bruising are clearly visible on the abdomen and stomach.

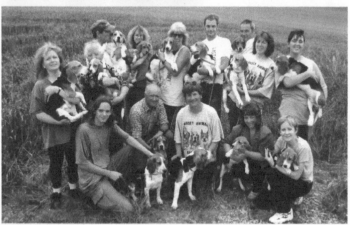

Figure 2   July 1997: Consort campaigners cradle rescued beagles destined for laboratory experiments. Heather Nicholson and Liz Stewart are standing at the right end of the back row, having secured the dogs' freedom.

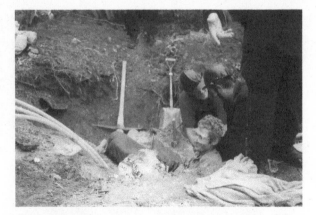

Figure 3 September 1997: Amid the eviction of Camp Rena, bailiffs struggle to unchain Gamal, anchored to a safe at the entrance to an underground tunnel. HDSC activist Greta is barricaded inside the tunnel beneath him.

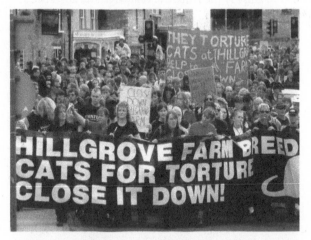

Figure 4 6 September 1998: Over 2,000 campaigners march through Witney, united against the animal research breeder, Hill Grove Cat Farm.

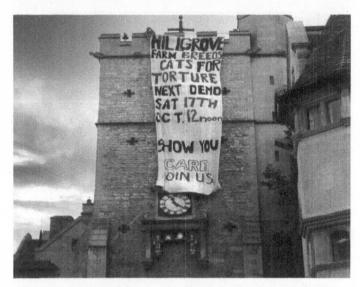

Figure 5　1998: Activists scale Oxford's Carfax Tower, unfurling a banner to amplify the Hillgrove campaign and advertise an upcoming protest.

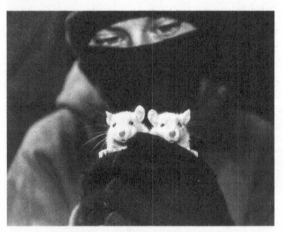

Figure 6　Early 2000: An ALF activist holds two of 400 rats, freed from HLS supplier Tuck and Son in Essex by underground campaigners.

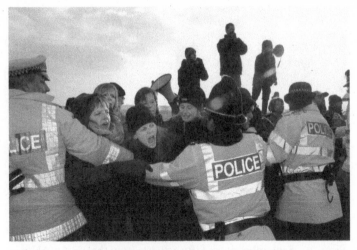

Figure 7   2000: Protestors express their anguish and fury towards HLS' employees, confronting them as they depart from work.

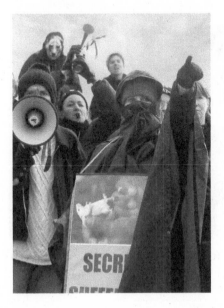

Figure 8   2000: Activists congregate at the gates of Huntingdon Life Sciences, berating staff as they exit, during a daily protest.

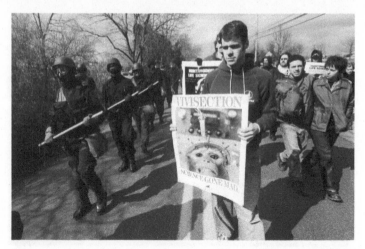

Figure 9   September 2000: Fifty activists from the nascent SHAC USA march towards HLS' New Jersey laboratory in the campaign's first significant North American protest.

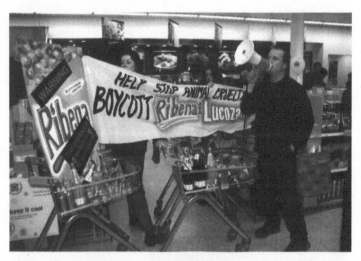

Figure 10   Activists fill a trolley with GlaxoSmithKline products in a Liverpool supermarket, highlighting the HLS connection while obstructing the checkout.

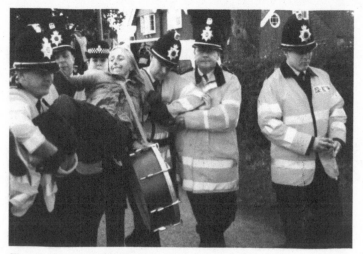

Figure 11   2001: SHAC campaigner Sarah Gisborne is seized and removed by police during a home demonstration.

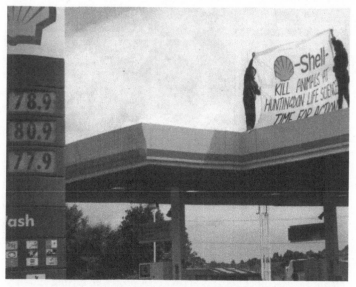

Figure 12   2001: Activists occupy a Shell petrol station canopy for the first time, a protest action that would soon echo across the UK.

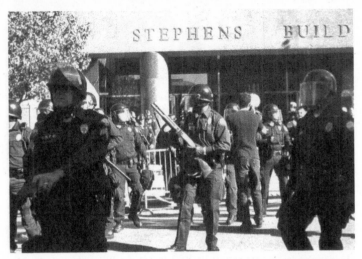

Figure 13 October 2001: Police prepare to riot outside of Stephens Inc.'s imposing headquarters in Little Rock, Arkansas. Local hospitals are braced to receive the victims of their tear gas.

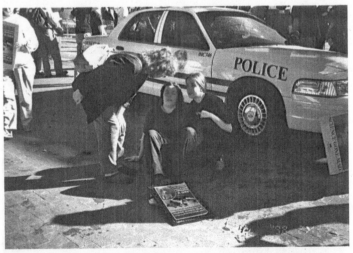

Figure 14 October 2001: A SHAC USA protester, reeling and in shock, post tear gas assault outside Stephens Inc. in Little Rock, Arkansas. (Photo: Brenda Shoss)

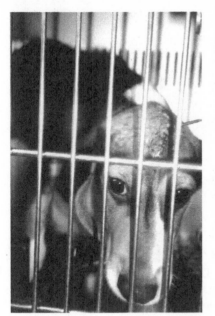

Figure 15 2002: A beagle puppy with an electrode stitched into their brain peers out of a cage inside a Japanese laboratory during Dawn Hurst's fact-finding investigation for SHAC. (Photo: Dawn Hurst)

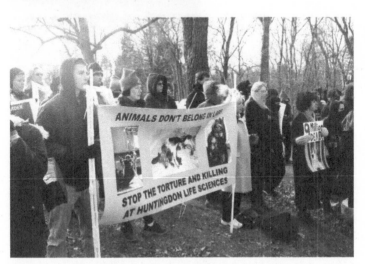

Figure 16 December 2002: Marking HLS' 50th anniversary, campaigners find themselves corralled away from the laboratory by New Jersey police.

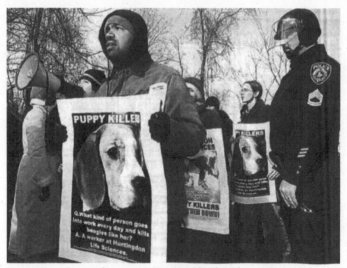

Figure 17   December 2002: During HLS' 50th anniversary protests, any activist straying from the police cordon faces immediate arrest and detention.

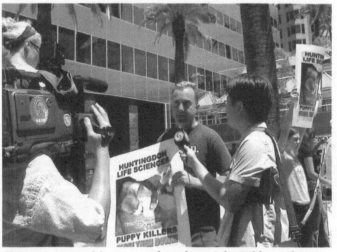

Figure 18   2002: Musician and producer John Feldman draws media attention as he protests against HLS's customer Sumitomo in California.

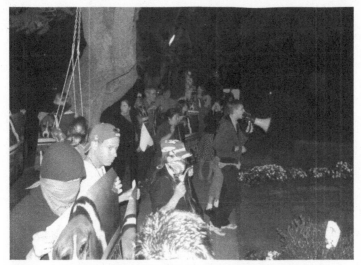

Figure 19 2005: After a full day of protest, SHAC USA campaigners press on into the night, holding home demonstrations outside an HLS financier's residence in Los Angeles.

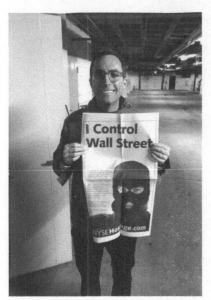

Figure 20 Following his release from prison, SHAC USA founder Kevin Jonas jokingly displays the dramatic newspaper ad funded by right-wing lobbyists the Center for Consumer Freedom. (Photo: Aaron Zellhoefer)

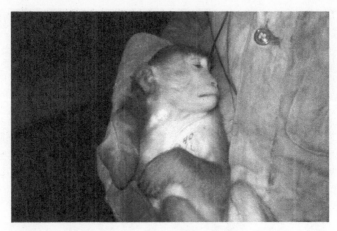

Figure 21   December 2006: A young primate is liberated from laboratory supplier Harlan in Italy by the ALF, before being spirited to a sanctuary to live out their natural life in safety.

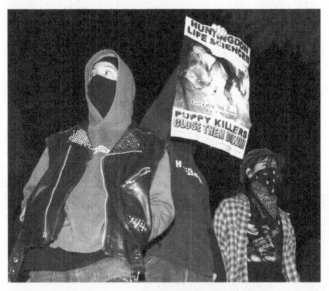

Figure 22   September 2006: Outside the home of Sumitomo's Canadian Vice President in Montreal, SHAC Canada protestors brandish SHAC's distinctive yellow poster.

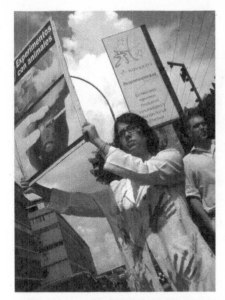

Figure 23　2007: In South America, a SHAC Venezuela activist wearing a blood-stained lab coat joins a protest against HLS customer Novartis.

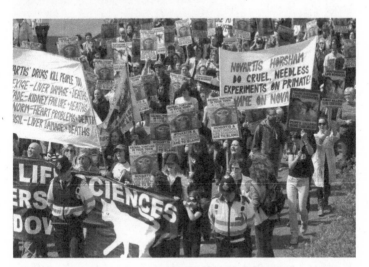

Figure 24　April 2008: A sea of SHAC placards fill the streets of Horsham during World Day for Animals in Laboratories outside of Novartis' UK primate facility.

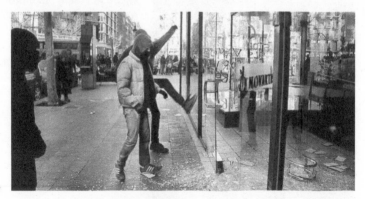

Figure 25 April 2008: Catalan activists attack a Novartis office during a march in support of World Day for Animals in Laboratories in Barcelona.

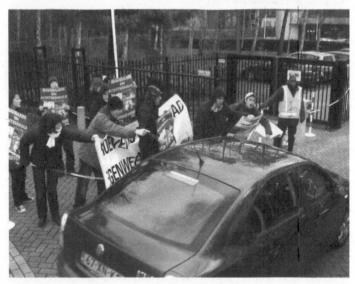

Figure 26 2008: Protestors from SHAC Belgium greet the staff of GlaxoSmithKline as they arrive for work.

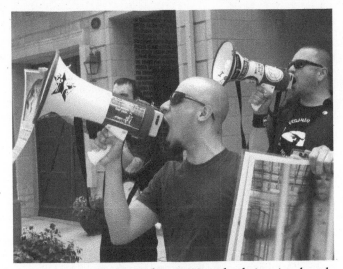

Figure 27   2008: Activists from WAR make their voices heard, holding a noisy protest outside a GlaxoSmithKline director's home on the USA's East Coast.

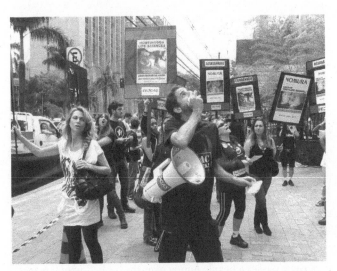

Figure 28   April 2010: SHAC Brasilia protest outside of HLS financiers Fortress' parent company Nomura in San Paulo.

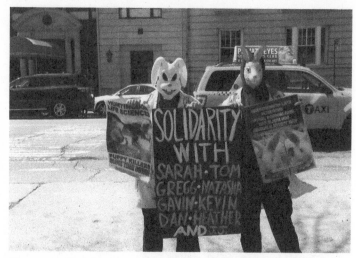

Figure 29 October 2010: As the second tranche of SHAC UK protestors are sent to prison, WAR hold a solidarity protest in New York.

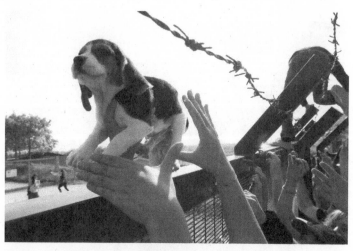

Figure 30 April 2012: World Day for Animals in Laboratories. An Italian activist passes a beagle puppy over the barbed wire fence of Green Hill's laboratory breeder, a spontaneous act of liberation that sets off a chain of events culminating in the farm's closure.

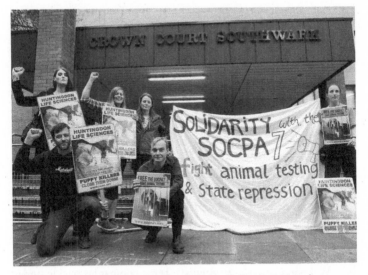

Figure 31 2012: In the final days of SHAC, the 'SOCPA 7' defendants stand defiant and united outside the courtroom during their trial.

Notes

The websites were last accessed on 5 October 2023.

PART I

1. Williams, A. (1997, 19 August). Lives ruined by animal terror-ists. *Independent*.
2. (2003). SHAC attack! Targeting companies animal rights style. *Do or Die, 10*.
3. (2003). Beagles saved and international trade in lab animals exposed. *Animal Defender*.
4. Boggan, S. (2006, 1 June). Money talks. *Guardian*.
5. (1994, 5 October). Livestock flights plan. *The Times*.
6. Wolmar, C. (1994, 20 August). Ferry companies buckle under public pressure over livestock. *Independent*.
7. Franklin, A. (2001). *Nature and Social Theory*. SAGE Publications.
8. (1996, 2 March). Exporter convicted. *The Times*.
9. Eccleston, B. (2021, 1 February). Jill Phipps: 26 years since campaigner died at Coventry Airport. *Coventry Telegraph*.
10. Cowell, A. (1996, 2 April). Britain asks Europe to pay most of cost of killing cows. *New York Times*.
11. Watson, S.M. (1998, 20 August). Dog 12 month oral (dietary) toxicity study. *AgrEvo Ltd*.
12. Mann, K. (2007, May). *From Dusk 'til Dawn*. Puppy Pincher Press.
13. Ibid.
14. Walsh, G. (2004, 1 August). Blair promised animal tests ban. *The Times*.
15. (2012, 24 July). The history of the NAVS. www.navs.org.uk.
16. (2005, May). Martin Balluch. *Bite Back, 10*, p. 14.
17. Ibid.

18. Ricks, M. (1997, 4 May). Animal rights protesters sue over police CS gas and baton attack. *Independent*.

19. Mann, *From Dusk 'til Dawn*.

20. Masood, E. (1997, 30 October). UK tightens regime for animal research. *Nature*.

21. (1997, 12 November). £15,000 to save the doomed beagles. *Eva*.

22. Lauchlan, I. (1997, 5 October). Save our beagles. *Sunday Mirror*.

23. Boggan, Money talks.

24. Ffrench, A. (1998, 8 September). Cat farm demos will 'fade away'. *Oxford Mail*.

25. Spark, K. (1998). Horror of Hillgrove Farm. *Oxford Courier*, p. 1.

26. Southworth, J. (1999, 4 January). He breeds cats for animal experiments … *Daily Mail*.

27. (1997, October). *Hillgrove Campaign Newsletter, 1*.

28. (1998, February). *Hillgrove Campaign Newsletter, 3*.

29. Horne, D. (1997, 29 October). Protestor injured in cat demo. *Oxford Mail*.

30. Ibid.

31. (1997, October). *Hillgrove Campaign Newsletter, 1*.

32. Spark, K. (1997, 17 October). Countess joins battle to shut down cat farm. *Oxford Journal*, p. 1.

33. Binns, J. (2008, November). Gulf War illness and the health of Gulf War veterans: scientific findings and recommendations. *Research Advisory Committee on Gulf War Veterans' Illnesses*, p. 128.

34. Horne, D. (1997). Cat protesters hit by pesticide. *Witney Gazette*.

35. Ibid.

36. Horne, D. (1997, 18 October). Manager spat at a protestor. *Oxford Mail*.

37. Hillier, J. (1998, 25 March). Brick attacks on cat worker and protestor. *Witney Gazette*.

38. Askwith, R. (1998, 5 September). Showdown on the farm. *Independent*.

39. Malle, A. (2002). *A Cat in Hell's Chance*. Slingshot Publications, p. 76.

40. (1998, 22 January). The force. *BBC Two*.

41. Spark, K. (1997). Hell Grove farm. *Oxford Courier.*
42. Williams, Lives ruined by animal terrorists.
43. (1999). *Hillgrove Campaign Newsletter, 11.*
44. Askwith, Showdown on the farm.
45. Horne, D. (1997, 14 July). Police turn 'blind eye' at cat farm. *Oxford Mail.*
46. (1998, March). *Hillgrove Campaign Newsletter, 4.*
47. (1998, 13 March). PC faces 'framing' claim. *Western Daily Press.*
48. (1998, 19 March). Trio cleared of cat farm burglary. *Western Daily Press.*
49. Askwith, Showdown on the farm.
50. Ibid.
51. Ffrench, A. (1998, 30 January). Police form new force to tackle cat farm demos. *Oxford Times.*
52. Ffrench, A. (1998, 20 April). The battle of Hillgrove. *Oxford Mail.*
53. (1998, 19 April). Mob of 1,000 storms cat experiment facility. *Sunday Express.*
54. Ffrench, The battle of Hillgrove.
55. (1998, 26 August). Case summary. *CPS.*
56. McGee, D. (1998, 19 April). Thousands battle with police at breeding farm. *Sunday Mirror.*
57. Ibid.
58. Askwith, Showdown on the farm.
59. Malle, *A Cat in Hell's Chance*, p. 76.
60. Brown, K. (1998, 28 July). Witness statement. *Thames Valley Police.*
61. Askwith, Showdown on the farm.
62. (1998, 8 June). I smuggled cat to safety. *Oxford Mail.*
63. Alford, D. (1998, 2 June). What's going on at Mr Brown's cat farm? *The Mirror.*
64. (1999, 4 January). *Daily Mail.*
65. Askwith, Showdown on the farm.
66. Brown, S. (1998, 17 July). Traffic chaos as demo switches to Oxford. *Oxford Times.*
67. (1998, 9 December). Torture of cats and kittens. *Early Day Motions.*

68. Hewison, F. (1998). A grilling over cat farm tactics. *South Oxfordshire Courier.*

69. (1998, October). *Hillgrove Campaign Newsletter, 9.*

70. (1998, 5 September). *Independent.*

71. (1999). *Hillgrove Campaign Newsletter, 10.*

72. Southworth, He breeds cats for animal experiments …

73. (1999). *Hillgrove Campaign Newsletter, 10.*

74. Perthen, A. (1999, 3 January). Straw security alert after threat by kitten protesters. *Sunday People.*

75. Malle, *A Cat in Hell's Chance*, p. 76.

76. Reid, T. (1999, 14 August). Besieged cat farmer quits. *The Times.*

77. Jankiewicz, A. (1999, 14 August). Cattery closure delights protesters. *Independent.*

78. (1999). *Hillgrove Campaign Newsletter.* Victory Newsletter.

PART II

1. Cliffe, C. (2000, 1 March). Dog days in Huntingdon: lessons from a corporate crisis. *Scrip Reports.*

2. Jones, D. (1989, 20 November). Inside Britain's beagle labs. *Today.*

3. (1989, 21 November). Shame shops to end this. *Today.*

4. Kite, S. (1990). Secret suffering. *BUAV.*

5. (2002, January). Attempted arson of HLS coach company. *ALFSG*, p. 19.

6. Broughton, Z. (1997, 26 March). Where blood runs cold. *Guardian.*

7. Ibid.

8. (1997, 26 March). Countryside Undercover: it's a dog's life. *Channel 4.*

9. Gimson, A. (2001, 20 Januaryo). Petrol bombs and threats are out of order. *Telegraph.*

10. Johnston, P. (1997, 25 July). Drug-test animal lab faces closure. *Telegraph.*

11. Daly, M. (1997, 8–14 December). Lords stop animal testers using animal-stalking law. *Big Issue.*

12. Pavitt, A. (1998, 21 January). The big questions answered. *Hunts Post.*

13. (1997, 4 July). Animal rights protestors wipe out HLS profits. *Cambridge Evening News.*

14. Rokke, M. (1997). The diary of Michele Rokke. *SHAC.*

15. Kolata, G. (1998, 16 April). New Jersey lab is fined over care of animals. *New York Times.*

16. (1998, January). PETA, Huntingdon settle lawsuit. *The Animals' Agenda, 18(1)*, p. 16.

17. Johnston, L. (1997, 15 June). Beagles' legs to be broken in drugs test. *Observer.*

18. (1997, 16 June). Basinger pleads to save puppies. *Independent.*

19. (1997, 3 July). Actress-animal rights activist Kim Basinger arrived at a research laboratory. *United Press International*

20. Johnson, L. (1997, 21 September). Shelters try to find homes for 40 beagles. *LA Times.*

21. Cliffe, Dog days in Huntingdon, p. 5.

22. (1998, January). Protest charges dropped. *Hunts Post.*

23. King, D. (1997, 22 September). Protestors on lab roof. *Huntingdon and St Ives Evening News.*

24. (1997, 24 September). Lab protestors to 'evade' eviction. *Huntingdon & St Ives Evening News.*

25. (1997, 1 October). Bailiffs clear animal protestors. *Independent.*

26. (2002). Buried alive. *SHAC USA Newsletter, 2(4).*

27. Morpeth, G. (1997, 1 October). Demo dig-in. *Cambridge News.*

28. (1997, 30 September). New camp for animal rights demo. *Cambridge Evening News.*

29. (2002). Buried alive. *SHAC USA Newsletter, 2(4).*

30. Pavitt, Protestors dig in at HLS.

31. (1997, 7 October). Cash to clear protestors 'well spent'. *Cambridge Evening News.*

32. Kirk, J. (1997, 22 October). Lab goes to court over harassment. *Town Crier.*

33. Daly, M. (1997, 8–14 December). Lords stop animal testers using anti-stalking law. *The Big Issue.*

34. (1998, 3 September). Drug research firm wins shares lifeline. *Cambridge Evening News.*

35. (1998, August). *HDSC Newsletter.*

36. (1998, June). *HDSC Newsletter*.

37. Cliffe, Dog days in Huntingdon, p. 5.

38. Ryle, S. (1998, July). Leading pharmaceutical companies are still shunning controversial drug research group. *Independent*.

39. (1999, 14 May). Deed of variation between Ciba Geigy and Huntingdon Life Sciences Ltd. *SEC*.

40. Ibid.

41. (1998, August). *HDSC Newsletter*.

42. (1998, 13 January). Insurance firm target of protest. *Cambridge Evening News*.

43. (2007, 25 July). The fall of the ethical bank. *Marketing Week*.

44. Bloom, J. (2002, 7 January). HLS tale includes a lesson for all CEOs. *PR Week*.

45. Taylor, P. (1998, July). Lab's future is in the balance. *Wilmslow Express*.

46. (1999, 12 July). Agreement for the sale of freehold property known as Stamford Lodge, Altrincham Road Wilmslow. *SEC*.

47. (1998, 31 December). Annual report. *Huntingdon Life Sciences Group Plc*.

48. Green, D. (1997, 11 April). Militancy fears over dog laboratory plans. *East Anglia Daily Times*.

49. Brown, N. (1997, 12 December). Joy as laboratory plans thrown out. *Diss Express*.

50. Lennard, D. (1998, 14 September). Protestors vow to go on until the tests stop. *East Anglia Daily Times*.

51. (1998, 7 January). Coach for HLS staff damaged. *Hunts Post*.

52. (1998, June). AGM scandal. *HDSC Newsletter*.

53. (1998, 7 August). Deed of variation between Huntingdon Life Sciences Limited as the Company and Huntingdon Life Sciences Group plc and Christopher Cliffe as the director. *SEC*.

54. German, C. (1998, 11 August). Pounds 20m rescue bid for Huntingdon. *Independent*.

55. Ibid.

56. (1998, 29 April). *White Coat Revolution*. York Press.

57. (2000). New UK govt/industry task force to deal with concerns over UK-based pharma. *Pharma Letter*.

58. (2000, 15 April). Task-force to strengthen industry. *Pharmaceutical Journal*.

59. (2002). *SHAC Newsletter, 16.*
60. Jones, D. (1999, 29 June). Horror of the beagle factory. *Daily Mail.*
61. Ibid.
62. Prescott, M. (1999, 12 December). Scientific experiments on dogs to be banned. *The Times.*
63. (2000, 30 August). Animal rights extremists targeted. *BBC News.*

PART III

1. Doward, J. (2004, 11 April). Sex and violence allegations split animal rights campaign. *Guardian.*
2. Mondics, C. (2002, 11 August). Animal-rights campaign targets N.J. firm, workers. *Baltimore Sun.*
3. Feltham, C. Huntingdon is hit by fund's sell-off at 1p. *Daily Mail.*
4. Boggan, S. (2006, 1 June). Money talks. *Guardian.*
5. (1999, 3 December). Braintree: animal protests outside bank. *Daily Gazette.*
6. (1999). *SHAC Newsletter, 1.*
7. (1999). *SHAC Newsletter, 2.*
8. Boggan, Money talks.
9. (2000). *SHAC Newsletter, 3.*
10. Wilson, G. (2000, 24 January). Labour's animal dilemma. *Daily Mail.*
11. Naik, G. (2001, 27 April. Rights group goes to scary extremes to close down a UK lab. *Wall Street Journal.*
12. (2000, 14 February). Animal rights activists target investors to dump Huntingdon research lab stock. *CNN News.*
13. (2000). *SHAC Newsletter, 4.*
14. Ibid.
15. Vidal, J. (2000, 12 April). This time it's personal. *Guardian.*
16. Ibid.
17. Boggan, Money talks.
18. Braid, M. (2000, 22 July). The siege of Huntingdon. *Independent.*
19. (2000, 30 March). Huntingdon Life Sciences Group Plc 10-K – annual report. *SEC.*

20. (2000, 5 May). Huntingdon Life Sciences Group Plc 10-Q – quarterly report. *SEC.*

21. Doward, Sex and violence allegations split animal rights campaign.

22. Calvesbert, A. (2000, 17 August). Dawn swoop by police in Vale. *Evesham Journal*, p. 1.

23. Boggan, Money talks.

24. (1999, 29 April). Royal Commission of vivisection, EDM 598. *UK Parliament.*

25. (2000, March). Budget 2000. *HM Treasury.*

26. (2001, March). Final report. *Pharmaceutical Industry Competitiveness Task Force.*

27. (2020). Worldwide animal research statistics. *Speaking of Research.*

28. McKerron, I. (2001, 14 January). Bank pulls plug on UK's biggest animal testing laboratory. *Mail on Sunday.*

29. (2000, January). *SHAC Newsletter, 2.*

30. Johnston, P. (2000, 31 August). Animal activists may face new laws. *Telegraph.*

31. Toynbee, P. (2001, 17 January). Running scared. *Guardian.*

32. Lyons, D. (2000). Diaries of despair. *Uncaged Campaigns.*

33. Davies, D. (2000, 27 September). Police consider charges after leak. *Hunts Post.*

34. Johnston, L. (2000, 28 September). Animal lab shuts down after we reveal horrors. *Express.*

35. (2000, 9 September). Demo-hit biotech company to quit city. *Cambridge Evening News.*

36. http://web.archive.org/web/20010418010616fw/http:/www.freespeech.org/sharelist/SHACTEMP/archives/000921a.html.

37. Logan, C. (2000, 12 March). Victory for the Mail on Sunday as baboon farm is shut down. *Mail on Sunday.*

38. (2000). *SHAC Newsletter, 8.*

39. (2000). *SHAC Newsletter, 7.*

40. (2000, 11 June). Animal firm seeks overseas cash. *This Is Money.*

41. (2001, June). Financial houses scared off by vivisectionist threats. *Nature.*

42. (2001, 8 January). Lab firm seeks debt extension. *BBC News.*

43. Braid, The siege of Huntingdon.

44. (2000, December). Who slipped up in 2000? *Investors Chronicle.*
45. (2000, 15 August). Huntingdon announces refinancing. HLS press release.
46. Nathan, S. (2000, 21 August). Day of protests. *Cambridge Evening News.*
47. (2000). *Shares Magazine.*
48. Shrimsley, R. (2001, 17 January). Ministers in bid to save HLS. *Financial Times.*
49. Alleyne, R. (2001, 20 January). Scientists defend animal tests. *Telegraph.*
50. Ibid.
51. Firn, D. (2001, 18 January). 'Forgotten' workers try to remember why they support animal experiments. *Financial Times.*
52. Harrison, D. (2001, 21 January). Minister set up deal to save animal lab. *Telegraph.*
53. http://web.archive.org/web/20210318000901/http://www.lobbywatch.org/profile1.asp?PrId=116.
54. Ibid.
55. Williams, M. (2002, July). Funding of research facts re: Sainsbury. *Margaret Williams.*
56. (2001, 22 January). Animal lab saved. *New Scientist.*
57. Walsh, D. (2001, 21 January). City stands firm over HLS. *The Times.*
58. White, M. (2001, 13 March). Straw attacks banks that dumped protest firm. *Guardian.*
59. McKerron, Bank pulls plug on UK's biggest animal testing laboratory.
60. (2000, 25 September). Loan facility letter between Andrew H. Baker and Huntingdon Life Sciences Group plc. *SEC.*
61. Treanor, J. (2001, 22 January). Testing at animal lab may grow under US backers. *Guardian.*
62. Murray-West, R. (2001, 16 January). Don't give in to animal lab activists, warns minister. *Telegraph.*
63. Pears, C. (2001, 22 January). Business as usual at HLS. *Cambridge Evening News.*
64. Cox, S. (2004, 18 November). How animal rights took on the world. *BBC Radio 4.*

65. McKenzie, S. (1999, 7 April). Animal Liberation Front takes credit for destruction. *Minnesota Daily.*
66. Suchan, C. (2019). *The Animal People.* Bird Street Productions.
67. Woodward, W. (1999, 5 November). On campus, animal rights vs. animal research. *Washington Post.*
68. Kettle, M. (1999, 6 April). Animal activists vandalise US labs. *Guardian.*
69. (1999). ALF raids Minnesota Laboratory. *No Compromise, 13,* p. 27.
70. Thomas, D. (2002, 11 November). Animal rights advocates and university researchers clash. *Minnesota Daily.*
71. Suchan, *The Animal People.*
72. Ibid.
73. Mondics, Animal-rights campaign targets N.J. firm, workers.
74. (2000). *SHAC Newsletter, 7.*
75. Suchan, *The Animal People.*
76. Best, S. (2006, June). Rethinking revolution. *The International Journal of Inclusive Democracy, 3.*
77. (2002). *SHAC USA Newsletter, 2(4).*
78. Meeks, F. (2012, 3 November). The king of Little Rock. *Barrons.*
79. Satchell, M. (2002, 8 April). Animal-rights activists are close to destroying a major drug-testing firm. *US News.*
80. Ith, I. (2002, 11 July). Smoke bombs halt workday at offices. *Seattle Times.*
81. (2001). *SHAC Newsletter, 10.*
82. (2003, May). Prisoners in the struggle. *Earth First!*
83. Suchan, *The Animal People.*
84. (2003, July). SHAC attack. *Do or Die, 10,* p. 102.
85. Alleyne, Scientists defend animal tests.
86. (2001). *SHAC Newsletter, 6.*
87. (2001, 22 January. Animal rights group to target Glaxo-SmithKline. *New Scientist.*
88. Taylor, B. (2001, 12 February). Animal rights mob of 1,000 on rampage. *Daily Mail.*
89. (2001). *SHAC Newsletter, 10.*
90. Lewis, P. (2020, 28 October). Secrets and lies: untangling the UK 'spy cops' scandal. *Guardian.*

91. (2001, 12 March). Animal experimentation (intimidation of staff). *UK Parliament.*

92. Corney, Z. (2001), Animal activists storm Novartis. *Grimsby Telegraph.*

93. (2001). *SHAC Newsletter, 11.*

94. Naik, Rights group goes to scary extremes to close down a UK lab company.

95. (2001). *SHAC Newsletter, 13.*

96. (2002). Breaking into hell. *Bite Back, 1(1),* p. 8.

97. Llanos, M. (2003, 5 December). New activism: up close and personal. *NBC News.*

98. (1991, 9 February). A tribute to Mike Hill. *North West Hunt Sabs.*

99. Mann, *From Dusk 'til Dawn.*

100. Babbington, A. (2000, 3 September). Hunt kennels raided in hunt sabs' revenge attack. *Independent.*

101. (2001, 5 September). Case dropped against huntsman. *BBC News.*

102. (2013, 27 January). It's official - Crown Prosecution Service say it is OK to try to kill hunt saboteurs. *HSA.*

103. Taylor, B. (2001, 24 February). Defiance of the animal testing chief attacked on his doorstep. *Daily Mail.*

104. Peachey, P. (2001, 24 February). Animal test lab director beaten by masked gang. *Independent.*

105. Alleyne, R. (2001, 24 February). He got off lightly, says militant who began 'liberation struggle'. *Telegraph.*

106. Taylor, Defiance of the animal testing chief attacked on his doorstep.

107. Steele, J. (2001, 24 February). Pro-animal violence 'is work of 100 extremists'. *Telegraph.*

108. Horne, D. (1999, 4 December). Revealed: £4.8m cat farm fight bill. *Oxford Mail.*

109. Bennett, R. (2001, 25 February). Director's privacy law follows attack. *Financial Times.*

110. (2001). Time for action II. *SHAC.*

111. (2002, July 28). How Cass bought Huntingdon back to life. *Telegraph.*

112. Gerard, J. (2001, January 21). A human being at bay from the animal rights mob. *The Sunday Times.*

113. Steele, J. (2001, 24 February). Pro-animal violence 'is work of 100 extremists'. *Telegraph.*

114. (2001). Pharmaceutical Industry Competitive Task Force Final Report. *PICTF.*

115. Mansell, I. (2004, 9 September). Drugs giants' threat on animal terrorism. *The Times.*

116. Pilling, D. (2001, 29 March). Easier licensing for animal tests. *Financial Times.*

117. Jenkin (2001, 4 April). Criminal Justice and Police Bill. *UK Parliament.*

118. (2001). Animal Experimentation. *UK Parliament.*

119. Dyer, C. (2001, 7 May). Justice bill 'endangers press freedom'. *Guardian.*

120. (2001). Criminal Justice and Police Bill. *UK Parliament.*

121. (2001). *SHAC Newsletter, 12.*

122. http://web.archive.org/web/20010830043016/http://www.shacusa.net/news/04-26-01c.html.

123. (2001). Activists 'lock-on' in the City. *SHAC Newsletter, 12,* p. 4.

124. (2001, 2 July). Bank of England agrees to bail out animal testing company. *Independent.*

125. Clark, A. (2001, 2 July). Bank of last resort. *Guardian.*

126. Huband, M. (2003, 30 May). Activists pose big threat, bosses warned. *Financial Times.*

127. Alleyne, Scientists defined animal tests.

128. Bright, M. (2001, 21 January). Inside the labs where lives hang heavy in the balance. *Observer.*

129. (2009, 9 June). Shell settles Nigeria deaths case. *BBC News.*

130. Laville, S. (2020, 23 June). Shell faces UK supreme court case over Niger delta pollution. *Guardian.*

131. (2004, 19 October). 2-methyl-2-butene. *UNEP Publications.*

132. (2001). *SHAC Newsletter, 12.*

133. Montagu-Smith, N. (2001, 16 July). Huntingdon protesters target Shell. *Telegraph.*

134. (2001, 7 September). Refinery at standstill. *Daily Post.*

135. Hamilton, M. (2001, 5 Augus). Sweetener slaughter. *Sunday Mirror.*

136. (2001). Jobs from hell. *ITV.*
137. (2001). *SHAC Newsletter, 11.*
138. Laville, S. (2007, 22 February). Police crack down on animal rights fundraising stalls. *Guardian.*
139. (2001). *SHAC Newsletter, 14.*
140. Malkani, G. (2001, 29 March). Shareholders take stock at a testing time. *Financial Times.*
141. Ibid.
142. (2001). *SHAC Newsletter, 13.*
143. Potter, W. (2011). *Green Is the New Red.* City Lights Publishers, p. 96.
144. (2001, 8 June). Huntingdon postpones shareholder meet. *Reuters.*
145. (2001, 2 September). Protesters call for HLS AGM. *Independent Commodity Intelligence Services.*
146. Judd, T. (2001, 30 August). Laboratory protesters threaten to sue Hewitt. *Independent.*
147. (2001, 9 November). HLS did not hold AGM court told. *Cambridge News.*
148. Wehner, P. (2001, 20 April). Offensive action. *New Scientist.*
149. (2002). HLS fails in multi-million-dollar lawsuit. *SHAC USA Newsletter, 2(3),* p. 6.
150. (2006, 27 November). Animal extremist law bolstered. *Washington Times.*
151. (2001). *SHAC Newsletter, 12.*
152. (2001). Sicherheitsmaßnahmen. *Kölner Stadt-Anzeiger.*
153. Moss, A. (1961). Valiant crusade: the history of the RSPCA. *Cassell*, pp. 20–2.
154. Mason, P. (1997). The brown dog affair. *Two Sevens.*
155. (2014). League Against Cruel Sports 1924–2014: celebrating 90 years of protecting wildlife. *League Against Cruel Sports.*
156. (2003). HSA history Part 1. *Howl, 79.*
157. The Animal Liberation primer. *Anonymous.*
158. (2001, July). Huntingdon Life Sciences – die kampagne gegen das folterlaboratorium. *Voice, 26.*
159. (2001). *SHAC Newsletter, 13.*
160. (2001). *SHAC Newsletter, 14.*

161. McGhie, T. (2001, 22 April). Treasury plan to shield animal lab. *Financial Mail.*

162. Young, E. (2002, 10 January). Animal research company loses backer. *New Scientist.*

163. Mansell, P. (2009, 4 March). CEO Baker puts in offer for Life Sciences Research. *Pharma Times.*

164. (2001). *SHAC Newsletter, 15.*

165. (2001, 24 December). Animal lab firm to abandon London. *BBC News.*

166. Clark, A. (2001, 10 October). Huntingdon Life Sciences to list in US. *Guardian.*

167. http://web.archive.org/web/20020305063928fw_/http://www.shac.net/archives/011207b.html.

PART IV

1. Cox, S. (2004, 18 November). Battle for influence: animal rights. *BBC Radio 4.*

2. Sayle, A. (2000, 5 September). Those who cut up animals deserve a bit of harassment. *Independent.*

3. (2000, 22 June). The siege of Huntingdon. *Independent.*

4. (2001, 29 January). UK scientists call for legal protection from animal rights activists. *Cordis.*

5. Grimston, J. (2004, 8 February). Rise of suburban terrorist has British scientists on the run. *Sunday Times.*

6. (2002, 16 January). Engagements. *UK Parliament.*

7. (2002, 3 October). Cops clamp down on protest. *The Comet.*

8. Bush, G. (2001, 11 September). Address to the Nation.

9. Smith, A. (2001, 15 October). Cops, docs plan for animal rights protest. *Arkansas Business.*

10. (2001, 18 September). Public assembly permit. *City of Little Rock.*

11. Suchan, C. (2019). *The Animal People.* Bird Street Productions.

12. Shoss, B. (2001). Inside/out: diary of madness. *Kinship Circle.*

13. Suchan, *The Animal People.*

14. Smith, A. (2001, 30 October). Police make arrests at Stephens protest. *Arkansas Business.*

15. Shoss, Inside/out: diary of madness.

16. Bennetto, J. (2001, 15 November). Animal rights trio jailed for inciting lab harassment. *Independent.*

17. (2001, 15 November). Hate campaign leaders jailed. *Cambridge Evening News.*

18. Fresco, A. (2001, 15 November). Animal rights activists jailed for harassment. *The Times.*

19. (2001, 15 November). HLS/police fail with their show trial. SHAC press release.

20. Hall, S. (2001, 6 November). Animal activists mourn their martyr. *Guardian.*

21. Best, S. (2004). *Terrorists or Freedom Fighters?* Lantern Books, p. 91.

22. Foggo, D. (2001, 2 December). Animal welfare thugs funded via US charity. *Telegraph.*

23. (2002, 20 October). SHAC's attack goes multinational. *Telegraph.*

24. (2002). *SHAC Newsletter, 15.*

25. (2002). *SHAC Newsletter, 16.*

26. (2011, 6 October). Planning application, Littlemore House. *East Area Planning Committee.*

27. (2003, 28 May). Brand bij Yamanouchi. *Sleutelstad.*

28. Adetunji, L. (2005, 7 September). Huntingdon forced to postpone NYSE listing. *Financial Times.*

29. Market place rules. *SEC.*

30. (2002, May). *SHAC Newsletter, 17.*

31. Barry, D. (2002, 4 February). Forum in New York protests. *New York Times.*

32. (2009, 6 January). USA v Darius Fulmer. *US Court of Appeals for the Third Circuit.*

33. (2002, 10 May). Life Sciences Research: schedule 14a. *SEC.*

34. (2001, 14 October). *Financial Times.*

35. Young, E. (2002, 10 January). Animal research company loses backer. *New Scientist.*

36. (2002, 20 September). SHAC threatens terrorist style attack. *The Intelligence Report.*

37. Moran, N. (2002, 16 January). Protesters force Stephens group to sell position in Huntingdon. *BioWorld.*

38. Suchan, *The Animal People.*

39. Wootliff, B. (2001, 21 January1). Police alert the City over animal protests. *Telegraph.*

40. Veysey, S. (2002, 12 May). HLS activists take protest to Marsh. *Business Insurance.*

41. (2013). Common causes of large losses in the global power industry. *Marsh.*

42. (2002). Marsh under pressure. *SHAC Newsletter, 16*, p. 6.

43. (2002, 29 April). Protesters tear down fence. *Eastern Daily Press.*

44. (2002, May). *SHAC Newsletter, 17.*

45. (2016, 1 November). How a theory of crime and policing was born, and went terribly wrong. *NPR.*

46. Gross, M. (2003, 11 July). Rikers Island inmates seek different menu behind bars. *Forward.*

47. Suchan, *The Animal People.*

48. Peachey, P. (2002, 9 July). Activists find new targets in fight against animal tests. *Independent.*

49. (2004, July). Animal welfare – human Rights: protecting people from animal rights extremists. *Home Office.*

50. Ith, I. (2002, 11 July). Smoke bombs halt workday at offices. *Seattle Times.*

51. Peachey, Activists find new targets in fight against animal tests.

52. (2002). *SHAC Newsletter, 18.*

53. (2004, 5 February). The honours system. *UK Parliament.*

54. Milner, M. (2002, 15 June). CBE for animal test boss Cass. *Guardian.*

55. (2002, 19 August). Carla sends back OBE. *The Argus.*

56. (2002). *SHAC Newsletter, 19.*

57. (2002, 21 October). Protester's sentence is reduced. *Cambridge News.*

58. (2002). *SHAC Newsletter, 18.*

59. Kurosawa, T.M. (2008, 11 January). Alternatives to animal experimentation vs. animal right terrorism. *Pharmaceutical Society of Japan.*

60. Cyranoski, D. (2003, 10 July). UK shock tactics repel animal-rights activists in Japan. *Nature.*

61. (2002). *SHAC Newsletter, 19.*

62. (2002). *SHAC Newsletter, 17.*

63. Ibid.
64. (2002). *SHAC Newsletter, 19.*
65. Haythornthwaite, A. (2003, 1 April). Clients too hot to handle? *Accountancy Daily.*
66. State anti-SLAPP laws. *Public Participation Project.*
67. Castagnera, J. (2015, 15 March). Counter terrorism issues: case studies in the courtroom. *CRC Press.*
68. (2002). *SHAC Newsletter, 19.*
69. Ibid.
70. Ith, Smoke bombs halt workday at offices.
71. (2002). *SHAC Newsletter, 20.*
72. (2010). Blood & honour, Britain's far-right militants. *Centre for Social Cohesion.*
73. (1999, 29 July). *An Phoblacht: Republican News.*
74. (1999). *ALF Supporters Group Newsletter.*
75. (2004, 28 October). Campaigner claims firm trying to make her homeless. *Worcester News.*
76. (2002, 19 September). Lab link fury sparks crematorium protest. *Cambridge News.*
77. (2002). *SHAC Bewsletter, 19.*
78. (2004, 15 April). Playing terrorists. *Economist.*
79. Doughty, S. (2007, 17 September). Boss of animal researchers HLS attacks other companies for shunning his firm. *Daily Mail.*
80. http://web.archive.org/web/20031027173157/http://www.shac.net/ARCHIVES/2003/06/4b.html.
81. (2004). *SHAC Newsletter, 30.*
82. Hencke, D. (2002, 22 July). Pro-hunt militants target Labour MPs. *Guardian.*
83. Foggo, D. (2002, 17 November). Militant group declares 'war' on hunt ban. *Telegraph.*
84. Beckett, A. (2002, 30 August). We've been acting like the IRA. *Guardian.*
85. (2002, 8 September). Pro-hunt rebels plot 'air mayhem'. *The Times.*
86. Vallely, P. (2003, 5 September). Commandos of the country-side. *Independent.*
87. (2004, 15 September). Fox hunting activists disrupt debate on ban. *NBC News.*

88. (2002, 8 November). Rocket attack shocks father. *Western Gazette*.

89. Vallely, Commandos of the countryside.

90. Townsend, M. (2005, 20 February). Anti-hunt MPs to get 24-hour bodyguards. *Guardian*.

91. (2003, 9 July). Hunt saboteur filmed attack. *The Argus*.

92. Vallely, Commandos of the countryside.

93. (2002, 20 September) Arson strikes claim in hunt row. *Western Daily Press*.

94. (2001, 28 September). Reward to uncover activist's attackers. *Northern Echo*.

95. Vallely, Commandos of the countryside.

96. http://web.archive.org/web/20210321101944/https://www.ucpi.org.uk/core-participants-list.

97. Fogg, D. (2003, 16 February). Into battle at dawn with the Real CA. *Telegraph*.

98. Bennetto, J. (2004, 16 September). Rise of the countryside militants. *Independent*.

99. Barnett, A. (2002, 8 August). Tory MP embroiled in 'cash for question' row. *Observer*.

100. (2002, 25 August). Retraction. *Observer*.

101. https://web.archive.org/web/20201121111714/http://search.electoralcommission.org.uk.

102. (2002, 16 January). Engagements. *Hansard*.

103. (2002, 3 October). Cops clamp down on protest. *The Comet*.

104. (2003). 2003 – it's payback time. *SHAC USA Newsletter, 3(1)*, p. 17.

105. (2005). Talking tactics with the FBI. *Bite Back, 8*, p. 20.

106. Haythornwaite, Clients too hot to handle?

107. Murray-W. (2002, 18 December). Government turns insurer and banker for Huntingdon. *Telegraph*.

108. http://web.archive.org/web/20040902191805/http://www.shac.net/ARCHIVES/2002/12/18.html.

109. Grant, P. (2003, 27 February). SHAC attacks Big Four firm. *Accountancy Age*.

110. Chrisafis, A. (2003, 20 February). Auditors under fire over animal rights. *Guardian*.

111. http://web.archive.org/web/20040101064205/http://www.shac. net/ARCHIVES/2003/02/22.html.

112. Grant, P. (2003, 29 May). SHAC on trail of Huntingdon's next auditor. *Accountancy Age*.

113. Grant, P. (2005, 17 November). Huntingdon audit saga ends in secrecy. *Accountancy Age*.

114. (2002, 31 December). Report of the Animal Procedures Committee for 2002. *UK Parliament*, p. 10.

115. Ibid., p. 16.

116. (2003). *SHAC Newsletter, 22*.

117. Yates, J. (2003, 16 February). Two strategies, same goal in activism for animals. *Chicago Tribune*.

118. Doward, J. (2005, 3 April). FBI monitored British activists. *Guardian*.

119. (2005, 9 September). *BBC Radio 4*.

120. (2002, 25 July). Form 424B3 Life Sciences Research Inc. *SEC*.

121. (2003). *SHAC Newsletter, 22*.

122. Wilson, J. (2005, 20 May). FBI calls UK animal activists terrorists. *Guardian*.

123. Cass, B. (2004). *Police statement*.

124. (2003, 19 March). Animal experiments. *Hansard*.

125. (2002, 16 July). Animals in scientific procedures – report. *UK Parliament*.

126. Doward, FBI monitored British activists.

127. Lewis, J. (2005, 26 October). Investigating and preventing animal rights extremism. *FBI*.

128. (2003). Editorial. *SHAC USA Newsletter, 3(1.5)*, p. 2.

129. Elliot, V. (2003, 25 April). Japanese firms face animal protest violence. *The Times*.

130. (2003). *SHAC Newsletter, 25*.

131. (2003).*SHAC Newsletter, 23*.

132. (2003).*SHAC Newsletter, 25*.

133. (1995). Assessment of cardiac sensitization potential in dogs. *HRC*.

134. (2003). *SHAC Newsletter, 26*.

135. Doward, J. (2004, 11 April). Sex and violence allegations split animal rights campaign. *Guardian*.

136. (2003, 8 May). Note of the meeting of the Ministerial Industry Strategy Group. *Department of Health.*

137. (2003). USDA covers up for HLS. *SHAC USA Newsletter, 3(2),* p. 4.

138. Taylor, N. (2009, 24 September). Court orders USDA to disclose HLS investigation files. *Outsourcing Pharma.*

139. (2003). Time to pay for your crimes. *SHAC Newsletter, 23,* p. 2.

140. http://web.archive.org/web/20190326152925/http://direct action.info/news_dec19_03.htm.

141. (2003). *SHAC Newsletter, 24.*

142. http://web.archive.org/web/20190326153017/http://direct action.info/news_apr11_03.htm.

143. Huband, M. (2003, 20 May). Activists pose big threat, bosses warned. *Financial Times.*

144. (2019, 9 May). Tim Lawson-Cruttenden obituary. *The Times.*

145. (2007, 26 October). The solicitor protestors love to hate. *Inside Out.*

146. Woolcock, N. (2003, 27 August). Anti-stalker law used against animal activists. *Telegraph.*

147. Bowcott, O. (2003, 17 April). Exclusion zone bars animal tests protest. *Guardian.*

148. (2021, 1 March). www.linkedin.com/in/ken-smith-b5833182.

149. (2006, 10 May). GSK wins injunction against animal rights activists. *PharmaTimes.*

150. Woolcock, N. (2004, 26 May). Animal activists could be barred near labs. *The Times.*

151. (2003). Anti-Social Behaviour Bill. *Hansard.*

152. Monbiot, G. (2005, 4 October). Protesters are criminals. *Guardian.*

153. (2003). Animals in Scientific Procedures. *Hansard.*

154. Gibson, I. (2003, 19 March). *Animal Experiments.*

155. (2003, 20 November). Letter from Caroline Flint.

156. (2001, 27 April). Inter-agency liaison on animal rights demonstrations: Crown Prosection Servce prosecution policy. *CPS.*

157. Waya, T. (2020, 12 February). Freedom of Information Act 2000 (FOIA) Decision notice, Ref: FS50832982. Information Commissioner's Office.

158. (2004, 1 June). Briefing for the Attorney General from an AGO official.

159. (2004, 15 June). Letter from the Attorney General's Office to Caroline Flint MP.

160. (2004, July). Ministerial Committee on Animal Rights Activists.

161. (2004, 28 July). Script on animal rights extremism. *National Forum*.

162. (2004). ALF: the frontline 3. *Anon*.

163. (2007, 26 August). Application re allocation of case. *Portsmouth Crown Court*.

164. (2003). Diary of actions. *Bite Back*.

165. Ibid.

166. Fimrite, P. (2003, 5 December). $50,000 reward in Chiron probe/FBI seeking fresh tips on blast suspect. *SFGate*.

167. (2014, 12 March). FBI hunting Hawaii for most-wanted domestic terrorist. *USA Today*.

168. Finz, S. (2003, 10 October). FBI seeks suspect in East Bay bombings. *San Francisco Chronicle*.

169. (2003, October). SHAC USA press release.

170. (2003). *SHAC Newsletter, 27*.

171. Horsnell, M. (2003, 28 August). Sacked chauffeur betrayed drugs firm to protestors. *The Times*.

172. (2003, 8 September). Animal rights campaigners cleared. *BBC News*.

173. (2003). *SHAC Newsletter, 28*.

174. (2003, 4 June). CPS fuels crops HLS. www.shac.net.

175. Huband, Activists pose big threat, bosses warned.

176. (2003, 10 January). LSR press release.

177. (2003, 14 January). What a shambles. www.shac.net.

178. (2006, 22 May). USA v. SHAC USA, Inc. *US District Court NJ*.

179. (2003, 12 May). Registration of Transfer Agent Life Sciences Research Inc. *SEC*.

180. (2004, 19 March). LSR announces 2003 results. *LSR*.

181. (2003). *SHAC Newsletter, 27*.

182. (2002, 24 November). 'Terrorists' steal 128 beagles. *Associated Press*.

183. (2003, 27 November). Report to the first Secretary of State. Ref: APP/W0530/A/02/1090108.

184. (2003, 8 January). Animal rights group condemns Cambridge. *Guardian*.
185. (2003, 27 November). Report to the first Secretary of State.
186. Curtis, P. (2003, November). Cambridge wins approval for new animal research lab. *Guardian*.
187. (2002, 31 December). Report of the Animal Procedures Committee for 2002. *UK Parliament*, p. 17.

PART V

1. (2006, 19 May). Eco-warriors are 'US terror risk'. *BBC News*.
2. (2001). *SHAC Newsletter, 5*.
3. Henderson, M. (2004). Monkey lab is cancelled over terror fears. *The Times*.
4. (2003, 28 October). Note of the meeting of the Ministerial Industry Strategy Group. *Department of Health*.
5. (2004, 22 April). Note of the meeting of the Ministerial Industry Strategy Group. *Department of Health*.
6. Walsh, G. (2004, 8 February). Rise of suburban terrorist has British scientists on the run. *The Times*.
7. Pope, C. (2006, 21 September). Combating animal rights extremism in the UK. *Royal United Services Institute*.
8. Monbiot, G. (2009, 18 May). As the political consensus collapses, now all dissenters face suppression. *Guardian*.
9. Coburg, T. (2016, 14 October). Revealed: the insider evidence that shines a light on one of the biggest police scandals in British history. *The Canary*.
10. http://web.archive.org/web/20070314143728/http://www.netcu.org.uk/links.jsp.
11. (2021, 10 March). www.linkedin.com/in/steve-pearl-b734223.
12. Alderson, A. (2006, 14 May). Labour 'has allowed Britain to be bullied by animal rights terrorists'. *Telegraph*.
13. Murray-West, R. (2004, 31 January). Securicor to quit animal testing lab. *Telegraph*.
14. (2004, 26 April). Victims of Animal Rights Extremism Early Day Motion. *UK Parliament*.
15. Pinnock, S. (2004, 22 April). Animal activist victims unite. *The Scientist*.

16. Elliott, V. (2004, 29 July). Government inaction 'spurs extremists'. *The Times.*
17. (2004, 19 April). City stands still as protest hits. *Cambridge Evening News.*
18. Mozingo, J. (2006, 5 September). A thin line on animal rights. *Los Angeles Times.*
19. (2004, 3 September). Doctors don't trust animal experiments. *Europeans for Medical Progress.*
20. Ibid.
21. Ibid.
22. (2004). *SHAC Newsletter, 30.*
23. Best, S. (2009, 3 May). Who's afraid of Jerry Vlasak? *OpEdNews.*
24. Ibid.
25. MacLeod, D. (2005, 31 August). Britain uses hate law to ban animal rights campaigner. *Guardian.*
26. Smallwood, S. (2005, 9 September). Britain bans American professor who speaks on behalf of Animal Liberation Front. *The Chronicle of Higher Education.*
27. (2005, 7 August). *Dagens Nyheter.*
28. Schorn, D. (2005, 11 November). Interview with ALF cell member. *CBS News.*
29. Doward, J. (2005, 3 April). FBI monitored British activists. *Guardian.*
30. (2005). Talking tactics with the FBI. *Bite Back, 8*, p. 19.
31. (2013, 19 July). An infographic: Magic Lantern, a keystroke logging software developed by the FBI. *Daily Host News.*
32. Apuzzo, M. (2016, 13 April). F.B.I. used hacking software decade before iPhone fight. *New York Times.*
33. Lewis, J. (2005, 26 October). investigating and preventing animal rights extremism. *FBI.*
34. (1992, 8 April). Animal Enterprise Protection Act of 1992. *US Congress.*
35. Suchan, C. (2019). *The Animal People.* Bird Street Productions.
36. Ibid.
37. (2004). Letter from Attorney General.
38. (2004). Script on animal rights extremism. *UK Parliament.*
39. (2004). Animal rights extremists. *UK Parliament.*

40. Bowden, T. (2004, 17 July). Drug firms welcome prosecution of activists. *The Times.*

41. Pfeifer, S. (2004, 4 April). City fights back against SHAC attack. *Telegraph.*

42. (2004, 24 July). £25m bounty to combat animal rights terrorists. *The Times.*

43. Durodié, B. (2004, Autumn). Animal-rights terrorism and the demise of political debate. *World Defence Systems, 7(2).*

44. Woods, N. (2018, 19 March). Undercover officers need protection from Greenpeace? You're joking. *Guardian.*

45. Coles. (1996, March). Appendix A. *Special Demonstration Squad Tradecraft Manual.*

46. (2009, 1 March). Animal terrorist group foiled by informant dressed as a beagle. *The Times.*

47. (1998, 12 April). Outrage! in the Cathedral. *BBC News.*

48. Webb, T. (2011, 10 October). City speeds up squad to take on animal rights extremists. *Independent.*

49. Rodgers, S. (2001, 5 April). U.K. drug industry seeks legislation to fight animal-rights protesters. *Wall Street Journal.*

50. (2009). Interview with Adrian Radford. *NOS.*

51. (2004). *SHAC Newsletter, 32.*

52. Ibid.

53. Murray-West, R. (2004, 21 October). Animal test firm 'wants my home'. *Telegraph.*

54. (2004, 14 November). Fears as animal rights funds leap. *The Times.*

55. Jackson, N. (2006, 2 February). Oxford University: attacks mount in animal battle. *Independent.*

56. Cookson, C. (2005, 23 July). Targets of animal extremists to fight back. *Financial Times.*

57. (2005). *SHAC Newsletter, 35.*

58. Merrell, C. (2004, 1 December). Gas firm ends supply deal after staff threats. *The Times.*

59. (2005, 20 June). *Newsday.*

60. (2006). *SHAC Newsletter, 41.*

61. Graham, G. (2014, 22 January). Over 1,500 monkeys are imported into the UK for medical testing. *Telegraph.*

62. (2005, 3 March). Animal rights group target Heathrow. *BBC News.*

63. (2004, 6 December). City protest demo proves hoax. *Oxford Mail.*

64. Fielding, N. (2005, 27 February). Airports are new target of animal groups. *The Times.*

65. (2009). Interview With Adrian Radford. *NOS.*

66. http://web.archive.org/web/20190326152243/http://direct action.info/news_nov05b_04.htm.

67. (2004, November 23). Full text of 2004 Queen's Speech. *BBC News.*

68. Grimston, J. (2009, 1 March). Animal terrorist group foiled by informant dressed as a beagle. *The Times.*

69. (2009). Interview with Adrian Radford. *NOS.*

70. (2003) October 28). Note of the meeting of the Ministerial Industry Strategy Group. *Department of Health.*

71. Drayson. (2005, March 14). Serious Organised Crime and Police Bill. *UK Parliament.*

72. (2005). Serious Organised Crime and Police Act 2005. *UK Parliament.*

73. 2008. Memorandum submitted by the Research Defence Society. *UK Parliament.*

74. Clark, W. (2008, September). Memorandum submitted by Mrs Wendy V. R. Clark. *UK Parliament.*

75. Monbiot, G. (2004, 3 August). A threat to democracy. *Guardian.*

76. (2005, October 13). Animal rights activist wins a cut in prison sentence. *Surrey Live.*

77. Toomey, C. (2005, April 24). Fierce creatures. *The Times.*

78. (2013. August 19). David Miranda row: What is schedule 7? *BBC News.*

79. (2005). *The SHAC Newsletter, 39.*

80. (2005, September 20). British animal rights protestors arrested in Sweden. *The Local.*

81. (2005, September 8). *Daily Mail.*

82. (2005). *SHAC Newsletter, 37.*

83. (2005, September 9). *BBC Radio 4.*

84. (2005, November 14). Animal rights and wrongs. *Pharmafile.*

85. Inhofe, J. (2005, October 26). Eco-terrorism specifically examining SHAC. *US Congress.*

86. (2006) *SHAC Newsletter, 41.*

87. (2006). *SHAC Newsletter, 44.*

88. Scrivens, L. (2005, March 3). Animal rights group target Heathrow. *BBC News.*

89. (2005). *SHAC Newsletter, 35.*

90. (2007, March 7). Four years for animal rights terror plotter. *Daily Mail.*

91. Steele, J. (2007, March 7). Campaign ends in jail for animal extremists. *Telegraph.*

92. (1990, April 12). Freight company fined in beagles' deaths. *Associated Press.*

93. (2007, March 7). Three 'violent' activists jailed. *BBC News.*

94. Ibid.

95. (2007, March 7). Four years for animal rights terror plotter. *Daily Mail.*

96. (2005). *SHAC Newsletter, 37.*

97. (2005, September 9). *BBC Radio 4.*

98. (2005, 27 October). NYSE 'caved in' on lab firm float. *BBC News.*

99. (2005, November 3). LSR third quarter results. *LSR.*

100. (2002, January 31). Huntingdon buyer remains a mystery. *Arkansas Business.*

101. http://web.archive.org/web/20210319010246/https://www.inhofe.senate.gov/newsroom/press-releases/inhofe-named-most-conservative-senator.

102. Inhofe, J. (2012). The greatest hoax: how the global warming conspiracy threatens your future. *WND Books.*

103. McCarthy, T. (2017, June 1). The Republicans who urged Trump to pull out of Paris deal are big oil darlings. *Guardian.*

104. (2015, March 24). Senator Inhofe Throws Red Meat At Anti-LGBT Base. *Erie Gay News.*

105. (2002, December 31). Political Group Ratings on civil rights issues. *ACLU.*

106. Inhofe, J. (2005, October 26). Opening Statement. *US Senate Committee.*

107. http://web.archive.org/web/20210308191138/https://www.newamerica.org/in-depth/terrorism-in-america/what-threat-united-states-today.

108. Boruchin, S. (2006, November 17). Letter of acceptance, waiver and consent. *NASD*.

109. Asquith, M. (2010, October 8). Department of Enforcement vs. Legacy Trading Co. *Financial Industry Regulatory Authority*.

110. (2005). *SHAC Newsletter, 39*.

111. (2002, October 20). Shac's attack goes multinational. *Telegraph*.

112. (2005, October 26). Eco-terrorism specifically examining Stop Huntingdon Animal Cruelty (SHAC). *US Congress*.

113. Potter, W. (2011, 1 June). *Green Is the New Red*. City Lights Publishers.

114. Hitchins, T. (2006, June 19). *The SHAC 7*.

115. Suchan, *The Animal People*.

116. Ibid.

117. Duignan, B. (2010, September 13). Andy Stepanian, animal enterprise terrorist. *Advocacy for Animals*.

118. Strugar, M. (2007, October 29). US v. SHAC. *US Court of Appeals*.

119. (2006, October 15). Animal rights militants sentenced to federal prison. *AVMA*.

120. Katz, B. (2010, March 30). Locked up with militants, freed American talks. *Reuters*.

121. Duignan, Andy Stepanian, animal enterprise terrorist.

122. Thompson, A. (2009, October 14). US v. SHAC. *US Court of Appeals*.

123. Suchan, *The Animal People*.

124. Starostinetskaya, A. (2019, October 25). Joaquin Phoenix-backed animal rights film premieres in Texas. *Veg News*.

125. Brownell, C. (2018, July 31). Canada's richest places 2018. *MoneySense*.

126. Barry, M. (2006, 4 October). Westmount to keep close eye on animal rights protestors. *Westmount Examiner*.

127. Walby, K. (2011, March 10). Private eyes and public order: policing and surveillance in the suppression of animal rights activists in Canada. *Social Movement Studies*.

128. Ibid.

129. (2006, February 9). Ministerial Industry Strategy Group MISG 06(01). *Department of Health.*

130. (2003, December). *Journal of Life Sciences.*

131. Shalev, M. (2007, January). Animal Enterprise Terrorism Act becomes law. *Lab Animal.*

132. (2007). Guest editorial. *Close HLS, 2(1)*, p. 2.

133. (2006). *Close HLS, 1(1).*

134. Ibid.

135. (2006). *SHAC Newsletter, 39.*

136. (2007, January 19). NYSE still weighing Life Sciences listing. *Reuters.*

137. Eaglesham, J. (2013, 4 October). More than 5,000 stockbrokers from expelled firms still selling securities. *Wall Street Journal.*

138. (2006). *SHAC Newsletter, 41.*

139. Hayes, A. (2020, January 11). Gray Market. *Investopedia.*

140. (2006). *SHAC Newsletter, 44.*

141. (2005, May 4). What's a name? *USA Today.*

142. Lovitz, D. (2010). Muzzling a movement. *Lantern Books.*

143. (2006). *SHAC Newsletter, 41.*

144. Smith, W. (2006, 10 May). Animal liberationists threaten shareholders. *National Review.*

145. Murray-West, R. (2006, 9 May). Extremists target Glaxo shareholders. *Telegraph.*

146. Caldwell, C. (2006, May 13). Terror and the letter of the law. *Financial Times.*

147. (2012). A review of national police units which provide intelligence on criminality associated with protest. *HMIC.*

148. Walsh, F. (2006, 9 May). Animal rights activists tell drug firm's small investors to sell up or else. *Guardian.*

149. Woodward, W. (2006, 14 May). Blair backs secrecy laws to thwart animal activists. *Guardian.*

150. Murray-West, Extremists target Glaxo shareholders.

151. Edwards, R. (2008, May 13). 'British FBI' SOCA drops 130 cases against crime barons. *Telegraph.*

152. (2016). Appraisal Report. *Home Office.*

153. (2010, July 28). Culture secretary adds fuel to quango bonfire. *Channel 4 News.*

154. (2004, February 9). Blair unveils plan for 'British FBI'. *Guardian.*

155. Addley, E. (2006, August 18). Animal Liberation Front bomber faces jail after admitting arson bids. *Guardian.*

156. Addley, E. (2006, December 7). Animal Liberation Front bomber jailed for 12 years. *Guardian.*

157. (2006). Dr. Joe Harris. *SHAC Newsletter,* 45, p. 16.

158. Britten, N. (2006, September 21). Cancer researcher is jailed for sabotage. *Telegraph.*

159. (2005). Serious Organised Crime and Police Act 2005. *UK Parliament.*

160. (2005, December). Animals. *Channel 4.*

161. (2006). *SHAC Newsletter,* 42.

162. (2006). *SHAC Newsletter,* 43.

163. Hinks, G. (2005, October 30). Huntingdon accounts withheld until auditors can be hidden. *Independent.*

164. Laville, S. (2008, 23 December). From a Hampshire cottage, animal extremists plotted campaign of violence. *Guardian.*

165. (2006, February 9). Ministerial Industry Strategy Group MISG 06(01). *Department of Health.*

166. (2006, May 11). 12 years each for animal rights extremists. *Irish Examiner.*

167. Woolcock, N. (2006, 12 April). Guinea pig farm activists guilty. *The Times.*

168. (1968). Theft Act 1968. *UK Parliament.*

169. (2006, 11 May). 12 years each for animal rights extremists. *Irish Examiner.*

170. Tanner, B. (2008, 13 June). Animal rights activist jailed. *Hereford Times.*

171. (2016, 9 May). Flashback: 9 May 2006. *Red Black Green.*

172. (2009). State crackdown on anti-corporate dissent: the Animal Rights Movement. *Corporate Watch.*

173. Brown, J. (2011, 23 October). Judge who sentenced animal rights activist was fan of blood sports. *Independent.*

174. (2006, 14 May). PM criticised over animal testing. *BBC News.*

175. http://web.archive.org/web/20061213001914/http://the peoplespetition.org.uk.

176. (2006). *SHAC Newsletter,* 43.

177. (2006). *SHAC Newsletter,* 44.

178. (2007). *SHAC Newsletter,* 45.

179. http://web.archive.org/web/20190326153524/http://directaction.info/news_deco2_06.htm.

180. (2006, 5 October). Monkey factory-farms feed UK demand. *Politics.Co.Uk.*

181. (2006). *SHAC Newsletter, 43.*

182. Grant, P. (2004, 7 April). Mystery surrounds auditor of HLS. *Accountancy Age.*

183. Lee, E. (2005, 22 December). LSR to ccommence trading on NYSE Arca. *NJBIZ.*

184. (2006, 1 June). NYSE group and Euronext N.V. agree to a merger of equals. *Business Wire.*

185. (2007). *SHAC Newsletter, 45.*

186. Smit, M. (2007, 22 February). 21 'illegally' collected for animal rights terror. *This Is Local London.*

187. Laville, Police crack down on animal rights fundraising stalls.

188. O'Neill, B. (2006, 10 August). The truth about animal rights terrorism. *Spiked.*

189. Bibi, M. (2005, 26 October). Statement of Mark Bibi. *U.S. Senate Committee on Environment & Public Works.*

190. Laville, S. (2007, 2 May). Animal rights activists involved in bid to shut lab among 30 arrested in raids. *Guardian.*

191. Malone, A. (2010, 30 October). A terrorist called Mumsy: the retired nurse who was the mastermind behind a vicious and ruthless IRA-style gang of animal rights fanatics. *Daily Mail.*

192. Laville, Animal rights activists involved in bid to shut lab among 30 arrested in raids.

193. Fielding, N. (2005, 13 March). Vegan bodybuilder funds animal extremists. *The Sunday Times.*

194. Byers, D. (2007, 1 May). Police swoop on animal rights extremists in raids. *The Times.*

195. (2007, 3 May). Animal lib: nine charged. *Daily Mirror.*

196. Jack, A. (2008, 19 January). Arrests in animal rights inquiry. *Financial Times.*

197. (2007, 15 May). Seven in court over animal rights. *BBC News.*

198. Billy, J. (2007, 1 May). Statement of FBI Counterterrorism Division Assistant. *The FBI.*

199. Cookson, C. (2007, 9 May). FBI closely involved in UK animal rights arrests. *Financial Times.*

200. Alderson, A. (2007, 2 September). Animal testing protests have fizzled: lab boss. *Telegraph.*

PART VI

1. (2002, 4 December). True Spies 3, it could happen to you. *BBC Two.*
2. Jack, A. (2007, 16 September). Call to resist animal rights threats. *Financial Times.*
3. http://web.archive.org/web/20070710210921/http://www.shac.net.
4. (2009). Novartis Pharmaceuticals v. SHAC. *England and Wales High Court.*
5. http://web.archive.org/web/20210211070751/http://direct action.info/news_may07_07.htm.
6. (2007). *SHAC Newsletter, 46.*
7. Ibid.
8. (2007). Letter from Heather. *SHAC Newsletter, 47,* p. 15.
9. Mitchell, S. (2007, 4 May). Analysis: animal activists persist in U.S. *UPI.*
10. Beckford, M. (2007, 30 August). Animal rights group in Savlon poison claim. *The Telegraph.*
11. Hancock, L. (2016, 26 August). *Narratives of Identity in Social Movements, Conflicts and Change.* Emerald Group Publishing.
12. Batty, D. (2007, 30 August). Animal rights group 'has contaminated Savlon'. *Guardian.*
13. Alderson, A. (2007, 2 September). Animal testing protests have fizzled: lab boss. *Telegraph.*
14. Ibid.
15. (2007, 5 November). Animal rights protesters to gather on Saturday. *Hunts Post.*
16. (2008, 30 January). 88 capuchin monkeys saved from Chilean laboratory. *Guardian.*
17. http://web.archive.org/web/20210309100406/http://www.directaction.info/news_jan09_08.htm.
18. Murray-West, R. (2001, 16 January). Don't give in to animal lab activists, warns minister. *Telegraph.*

19. (2007, 1 March). The month: government delays introduction of RIPA part III legislation. *SC Media.*

20. Ward, M. (2007, 20 November). Campaigners hit by decryption law. *BBC News.*

21. Leyden, J. (2077, 14 November). Animal rights activist hit with RIPA key decrypt demand. *The Register.*

22. (2009, July). Extending our reach: a comprehensive approach to tackling serious organised crime. *Home Office.*

23. (2008, 6 February). UK navy to end goat experiments. *BBC News.*

24. (2008). *SHAC Newsletter, 48.*

25. (2008). *SHAC Newsletter, 49.*

26. (1986). Animals (Scientific Procedures) Act 1986. *UK Parliament.*

27. (2006, 21 September). Combating animal rights extremism in the UK. *RUSI.*

28. http://web.archive.org/web/20110811185817/http://arcops. wordpress.com/2007/09/03/cops-from-speak-march-1st-sept-2007.

29. (2005, 30 August). Code of connection for the GSi. *GSi Operations.*

30. http://web.archive.org/web/20170820134415/https:// shacwatch.wordpress.com.

31. https://www.indymedia.org.uk/en/2009/09/437487.html?c= all#c231935.

32. http://web.archive.org/web/20200119180848/https://sheffield. indymedia.org.uk/2011/01/472496.html.

33. Ibid.

34. Rawlinson, K. (2014, 7 August). Wikipedia edits made by government sought to minimise high-profile killings. *Guardian.*

35. (2008). *SHAC Newsletter, 48.*

36. Denning, S. (2011, 22 November). Lest we forget: why we had a financial crisis. *Forbes.*

37. (2008, 5 November). Form 10-Q Life Sciences Research Inc. *SEC.*

38. (2010, 2 March). Gesammelte Berichte der Tierschutz-causa. *Die grünen.*

39. Schonfeld, V. (2008, 5 June). Who's being caged? *Guardian.*

40. Ibid.
41. Potter, W. (2011, 2 May). Austrian animal rights activists acquitted of all charges. In *Green Is the New Red*. City Lights Publishers.
42. http://web.archive.org/web/20191203104641/https://vgt.at/en/work-repression.php.
43. Coghlan, A. (2009, 22 January). Brits jailed but animal rights activism rising in US. *New Scientist*.
44. http://web.archive.org/web/20170813070945/https://www.indymedia.org.uk/en/2008/08/405118.html.
45. Hampshire Police search log.
46. (2009). State crackdown on anti-corporate dissent. *Corporate Watch*.
47. Johnston, P. (2004, 10 February). Burden of proof could change to convict gangsters. *Telegraph*.
48. Smith, M. (2019, 3 October). How large can a 'reasonable doubt' be? *YouGov*.
49. http://web.archive.org/web/20200926052212/https://www.mprsolicitors.co.uk/site/blog/criminal-department-news/defending-largescale-conspiracies-and-organised-crime.
50. http://web.archive.org/web/20140814022023/http://blog.practicalethics.ox.ac.uk/2010/01/the-judge-is-out-on-juries.
51. (2005, December). *SHAC Newsletter, 38*.
52. (2004, July). *SHAC Newsletter, 31*.
53. (2001, 27 April). Protest Action: A Guidance Paper for Personal Safety. *Home Office*.
54. Laville, S. (2008, 23 December). From a Hampshire cottage, animal extremists plotted campaign of violence. *Guardian*.
55. (2009). Interview with Adrian Radford. *NOS*.
56. (2008, 23 December). Activists guilty of hate campaign. *BBC News*.
57. Yeoman, F. (2009, 22 January). Jail for animal rights extremists who waged six year blackmail campaign. *The Times*.
58. (2009). State crackdown on anti-corporate dissent. *Corporate Watch*.
59. Cheston, P. (2012, 13 April). Animal rights activists face 14 years jail for blackmail. *Evening Standard*.

60. (2009). State crackdown on anti-corporate dissent. *Corporate Watch.*

61. (2000, 16 December). The Golden Boot Awards – 2000. *Investors Chronicle*

62. Alderson, A. (2009, 17 January). Huntingdon Life Sciences to move back to UK. *Telegraph.*

63. (2008). *SHAC Newsletter, 50.*

64. (2009, 7 July). Project Atlantic. *Plymouth Partners LLC.*

65. Ibid.

66. Ibid.

67. www.bdo.co.uk.

68. (2014, June). *Militant Forces Against HLS (MFAH), Blackmail 3 & The SHAC Model.* Person(s) Unknown Publications.

69. Wright, O. (2016, 13 June). Court rule changes 'may drive innocent defendants into making guilty pleas'. *Guardian.*

70. Helm, R. (2019, September). Constrained waiver of trial rights? Incentives to plead guilty and the right to a fair trial. *Journal of Law and Society.*

71. Grimston, J. (2009, 1 March). Animal terrorist group foiled by informant dressed as a beagle. *The Times.*

72. (2009). Interview with Adrian Radford. *NOS.*

73. http://web.archive.org/web/20090715013651/http://adrian radford.com.

74. Mills, G. (2013, 1 April). The successes and failures of policing animal rights extremism in the UK 2004–2010. *International Journal of Police Science & Management.*

75. http://web.archive.org/web/20210224215218/http://www. directaction.info/news_apr07_09.htm.

76. (2009). Crackdown on anti-corporate dissent. *Corporate Watch.*

77. (2009, 8 May). Animal rights protester walks free. *Market Rasen Mail.*

78. (2009, 30 April). Rabbit breeder 'sick' after activist attack. *North West Evening Mail.*

79. Ibid.

80. Steed, M. (2009, 29 July). Protest camp at rabbit farm. *Market Rasen Mail.*

81. Ibid.

82. Fulcher, S.M. (2003). Study of effect on embryo-fetal toxicity in the rabbit by gavage administration. *Huntingdon Life Sciences.*

83. Ibid.

84. (2012, 31 March). Protest at Highgate Farm against breeding rabbits for research. *BBC News.*

85. http://web.archive.org/web/20190326153946/http://direct action.info/news_aug05_09.htm.

86. (2014, June). *Militant Forces Against HLS (MFAH), Blackmail 3 & The SHAC Model.*

87. (2009, 11 November). Two arrested in Evesham over animal rights extremism. *Evesham Journal.*

88. Bibi, M. (2009). Schedule 14a, Life Sciences Research Inc. *SEC.*

89. Beam, A. (2002, 25 April). Animal rights and wrongs. *Boston Globe.*

90. http://web.archive.org/web/20100307235848/http://www.shac.net.

91. Jack, A. (2009, 4 October). Novartis chief takes on animal activists. *Financial Times.*

92. Trial Evidence, The Queen v. Debbie Anne Vincent. *Winchester Crown Court.*

93. Trial Evidence, The Queen v. Debbie Anne Vincent, Exhibit No. James/200810/1800T. *Winchester Crown Court.*

94. Morris, S. (2014, 28 March). Animal rights campaigner convicted of Huntingdon Life Sciences conspiracy. *Guardian.*

95. Trial Evidence, The Queen v. Debbie Anne Vincent, Exhibit No. James/200810/1800T. *Winchester Crown Court.*

96. Trial Evidence, The Queen v. Debbie Anne Vincent, Exhibit No. James/030610/1013T. *Winchester Crown Court.*

97. (2010). *SHAC Newsletter, 54.*

98. (2010). *SHAC Newsletter, 55.*

99. http://web.archive.org/web/20190326154031/http://direct action.info/news_may02_10.htm.

100. http://web.archive.org/web/20200918164115/http://www.directaction.info/news2010.html.

101. Erlichman, E. (2010, 9 February). El Al says will stop transporting animals for experiments abroad. *Y Net.*

102. Udasin, S. (2015, 27 January). Last groups of Mazor Farm monkeys moved to Ben Shemen sanctuary. *Jerusalem Post.*

103. Lior, I. (2017, 13 April). Israel Finally transfers money to save monkeys on brink of starvation. *Haaretz*.

104. (2010, 23 February). BUAV exposes shocking role played by Laos in the international trade in primates for research. *PR Newswire*.

105. (2010). Wild monkeys send to British labs. *SHAC Newsletter*, 54, p. 2.

106. Swenson, K. (2013, 25 July). Smash HLS: post-PETA gorilla tactics. *Miami New Times*.

107. Mercado, M. (2015, 1 June). Inspection report: Primate Products Inc. *USDA*.

108. (2010, 9 June). L'allevamento 'Morini' chiude Il Comune compra i 'beagle'. *Il Resto del Carlino*.

109. Sanna, A. (2012, 16 June). Green Hill: oggi in 10.000 per il corteo a Roma. *Cronaca*.

110. https://www.glassdoor.co.uk/Reviews/Employee-Review-Envigo-RVW1042730.htm.

111. http://web.archive.org/web/20190319185614/www.directaction.info/news_mar18_11.htm.

112. (2011, January). Draft licence conditions, Gerrah Selby. *CPS*.

113. (2015, 7 September). Understanding Category D 'open' prisons: do they work. *Prison Phone*.

114. Doward, J. (2009, 27 December). Civil servants 'interfering with criminal justice system'. *Observer*.

115. Hope, C. (2009, 29 January). £110 taxi bill for animal right's thugs visit to wife in prison. *Telegraph*.

116. Kolirin, L. (2010, 13 January). Jail's 'vegan' boots for animal rights terrorist. *Express*.

117. Turner, R. (2009, 25 January). Jailed animal activist speaks from behind bars. *Wales on Sunday*.

118. Ibid.

119. Doward, Civil servants 'interfering with criminal justice system'.

120. (2013, 3 May). Letter from Keir Starmer.

121. (2009, January). Report of the Inspectorate of the Special Crime Division of CPS Headquarters. *HMcpsi*.

122. (1987, Autumn). Socialist Lawyer, 3. *Haldane Society of Socialist Lawyers*.

123. Evans, R. (2021, 4 February). Undercover policing inquiry: Keir Starmer urged to give evidence. *Guardian*.
124. Heffer, G. (2020, 16 October). Sir Keir Starmer hit by series of Labour resignations over Covert Human Intelligence Sources Bill. *Sky News*.
125. Mudd, D. (2011, 1 March). Form 10-K: Fortress Investment Group LLC. *SEC*.
126. (2011, 28 June). Application notice: HQ10X02725. *High Court*.
127. (2011). *SHAC Newsletter, 57*.
128. https://www.glassdoor.co.uk/Reviews/Envigo-Reviews-E1122651.htm.
129. http://web.archive.org/web/20210515000634/https://www.justice.gov/civil/false-claims-act.
130. Patterson, R. (2011, 5 April). Fair Laboratory Practices Associates v. Quest Diagnostics Inc. *US District Court Southern District of New York*.
131. Ford R.A. et al. (2001, February). The in vivo dermal absorption and metabolism of [4-14C] coumarin by rats and by human volunteers under simulated conditions of use in fragrances. *Food Chem Toxicol*.
132. (2012). *SHAC Newsletter, 58*, p. 2.
133. McKie, R. (2012, 29 July). Animal activists' terror tactics drive staff out of laboratories. *Guardian*.
134. (2012, 30 April). Il caso Green Hill. *Il Post*.
135. (2012, 23 July). Green Hill, via libera agli affidamenti Lav e Legambiente raccolgono adesioni. *La Repubblica Milano*.
136. Margottini, L. (2015, 26 January). Jail sentences for staff of Italian dog breeding facility. *Science*.
137. (2020, 5 March). Green Hill, assolti in appello gli animalisti che presero i beagle. *BS News*.
138. Clark, A. (2013, 7 January). Battle over future of lab test beagles. *The Times*.
139. Owen, P. (2013, 23 February). Help them: campaigners want beagles destined for AstraZeneca research centre to be rehomed. *Daily Mirror*.
140. (2012, 31 July). Huntingdon Life Sciences sheds research jobs in east. *BBC News*.
141. (2020, 2 September). Jurisdiction. *CPS*.

142. (2014, 9 February). The Queen v. Debbie Ann Vincent provisional skeleton argument on pre-trial issues and request for disclosure pursuant to Section 8 CPIA. *Winchester Crown Court*.

143. Ibid.

144. http://web.archive.org/web/20210224082125/https://earthfirst journal.org/newswire/2014/08/12/shac-ends-we-made-history-the-future-is-ours.

145. Mills, The successes and failures of policing animal rights extremism in the UK 2004–2010. *Science & Management*.

EPILOGUE

1. Garde, D. (2015, 25 June). Huntingdon Life Sciences and Harlan Laboratories to become Envigo. *Fierce Biotech*.

2. (2016, 16 November). Application to strike the company off the register. *Companies House*.

3. Adams, B. (2019, 25 April). LabCorp spends $485M as its CRO unit snaps up Envigo's nonclinical business. *Fierce Biotech*.

4. Wolf, N. (2012, 29 December). Revealed: how the FBI coordinated the crackdown on Occupy. *Guardian*.

5. Morrison, A. (2015, 17 September). Occupy Wall Street anniversary: police crackdown on movement cost New York $1.5 million over 4 years. *International Business Times*.

6. Friedersdorf, C. (2015, 25 July). 14 specific allegations of NYPD brutality during Occupy Wall Street. *The Atlantic*.

7. Parveen, N. (2021, 12 February). Priti Patel describes Black Lives Matter protests as 'dreadful'. *Guardian*.

8. Merrick, R. (2021, 9 March). New crackdown on Extinction Rebellion and Black Lives Matter needed due to 'huge inconvenience', minister says. *Independent*.

9. Dodd, V. (2020, 17 January). Greenpeace included with neo-Nazis on UK counter-terror list. *Guardian*.

10. Rielly, B. (2021, 21 April). Activist charged with conspiracy to blackmail for threatening hunger strike. *Morning Star*.

11. Mills, G. (2013, 1 April). The successes and failures of policing animal rights extremism in the UK 2004–2010. *International Journal of Police Science & Management*.

12. Evans, R. (2017, 16 January). Probe into claim that police spy set fire to Debenhams could end by July. *Guardian*.

13. Lewis, P. (2013, 21 June). McLibel leaflet was co-written by undercover police officer Bob Lambert. *Guardian*.

14. Evans, R. (2018, 23 February). Ex-police spy berates Met for revealing her role in mink release. *Guardian*.

15. Lambert, B. (2021, 13 May). Discussion Paper on SDS Targeting Strategy and Deployment in Relation to the Animal Liberation Front. *Metropolitan Police Service*.

16. Calvert, J. (2021, 6 November). New Tory sleaze row as donors who pay £3m get seats in House of Lords. *The Times*.

17. Sabbagh, D. (2022, 20 April). Evgeny Lebedev's nomination for peerage 'paused' after MI5 advice. *Guardian*.

18. Richards, X. (2022, 28 January). Met refuse to say why they won't probe Tory 'cash for honours' culture. *The National*.

19. http://web.archive.org/web/20210221110055/https://unoffensiveanimal.is/2021/01/30/pet-and-laboratory-breeder-raided-80-fire-salamanders-liberated.

20. http://web.archive.org/web/20210718073645/https://unoffensiveanimal.is/2021/07/18/400-guinea-pigs-liberated-in-solidarity-with-the-mbr-beagles/.

21. Farhoud, N. (2021, 22 June). Whimpering dogs forced into cages on UK 'factory farm' ahead of lab experiments. *Daily Mirror*.

22. Leishman, F. (2021, 9 July). Protesters set up camp outside Cambs animal testing breeding facility. *Cambridge News*.

23. Collett, A. (2021, 22 July). Day of action at Camp Beagle as protesters demand release of puppies. *Hunts Post*.

24. Horton, H. (2021, 24 July). Animal testing could end as Priti Patel launches review. *Telegraph*.

25. Barbour, M. (2022, 28 January). Cramped pens & 'bled like vampires to death' for cash: inside harrowing UK beagle farms which breed dogs for lab testing. *Daily Sun*.

26. Collett, A. (2021, 5 October). 'We are here to stay!' High Court allows Camp Beagle to remain. *Hunts Post*.

27. Kelly, E. (2021, 16 November). Will Young cuffs himself to beagle breeding facility in protest of animal testing: 'People do not know about it in this country'. *Metro*.

28. Dalton, J. (2022, 5 June). Footage of beagles bred for lab tests shows puppies 'stressed and confined in cages'. *Independent*.

29. Bruner, T. (2022, 13 June). Envigo tells judge it intends to close dog-breeding facility but wants to profit off animals first. PETA press release.

30. Wadman, M. (2022, 14 June). Beleaguered beagle facility to close; fate of 3,000 dogs bred for research unclear. *Science*.

31. (2022, 13 June). Inotiv, Inc. announces site closures and consolidation plans. Inotiv Inc. press release.

32. Raiken, A. (2022, 24 August). Harry and Meghan adopt dog saved from horror research lab and tattooed with serial number. *Independent*.

33. Watts, H. (2022, 27 August). Prince Harry and Meghan adopt rescue dog to support ban on beagle testing in the UK. *Daily Mirror*.

34. Jones, H. (2022, 19 June). Animal rights protesters occupy dog breeding facility. *Metro*.

35. Davies, D. (2022, 20 June). Beagle puppies freed at MBR Acres after second day of action. *Hunts Post*.

36. Elworthy, J. (2022, 22 June). Police check home of 101-year-old animal rights patron for stolen beagles. *Ely Standard*.

37. (2022, 21 June). Animal Freedom Movement press release.

38. Almond, L. (2022, 23 December). Will Young offers home for beagles held by police. *LBC News*.

Index

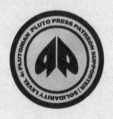

Thanks to our Patreon subscriber:

Ciaran Kane

Who has shown generosity and comradeship in support of our publishing.